SOCIAL SCIENCE AND HEALTHCARE

Nursing Applications in Clinical Practice

Gaëtan Béphage

Lecturer in Social Science and Nursing Studies
School of Health, Hull University ,Hull.

Mosby

Publisher	**Nicola Horton**
Developmental Editor	**Georgina Massy**
Project Manager	**Leslie Sinoway**
Design	**David Hunter**
Cover Illustration	**Andrew Harris**
Production	**Hamish Adamson**

Published by Mosby, an imprint of Mosby International (a division of Times Mirror International Publishers Ltd.), Lynton House, 7–12 Tavistock Square, London WC1H 9LB, England.

Copyright © Mosby, an imprint of Mosby International (a division of Times Mirror International Publishers Ltd.) 1997.

ISBN 0 7234 2324 5.

Originated in the UK by Graphic Ideas, London.
Printed in England by JW Arrowsmith Ltd.

A CIP catalogue record for this book is available from the British Library.

Contents

Preface

My aim in writing this book is to demonstrate the importance and relevance of the social sciences in nursing clinical practice. My students in sociology and nursing often tell me, 'Sociology is about what we already know'. I would like to extend this notion by saying that the social sciences are about what we already think we know about social life, but as health care professionals, fail somehow to apply in our practice. Like many others this book has its limitations. It does, however, give the foundations on which future health care practices may be developed.

The topics I have chosen in this volume (sociology; social anthropology; social economics; social policy and health policy) do not necessarily imply that they are more important than other social sciences such as political science, social philosophy and social history. To attempt to include all the other sciences in such a small volume would have detracted from the essence of the message.

Each chapter follows a standard format: a set of aims and objectives to help the reader focus on the main issues discussed; pure and basic social science theories followed by summaries, and application to practice. A further reading list accompanies each chapter with review questions at the end for consideration.

My rationale in utilising this broad framework is to highlight the links between these important concepts . The chapters should be seen as interrelated and complementary to each other.

Another point to bear in mind is that social life is in a state of perpetual change. By the time this textbook reaches your shelf, more distant cultures will have been explored and new Bills will have passed through Parliament. Health care professionals should therefore be adaptive to change and use their knowledge of the social sciences in addition to their other repertoires.

Change is even more evident in our health care educational system. In care delivery, students are expected to use a holistic perspective based on research findings. This approach is a clear departure from the medical and disease-oriented model of the past. We now emphasise how important it is to assess and identify the patients', social, psychological, biological and spiritual needs.

Health care professionals should therefore look beyond the traditional routine and investigate the broad sociocultural context of their patients. It can in fact be argued that a 'holistic social perspective' be used to ascertain all social needs are met. This is one of the ultimate goals in nursing practice.

A multidisciplinary team approach has now become the basic nursing and medical philosophy. Should social scientists also be consulted within the health care framework? Should care plans adopt a more elaborate, purposeful and meaningful sociocultural perspective? These are some of the questions we need to ask ourselves.

My deepest and sincerest thanks go to : Griselda Campbell who supported my ideas for this book, and patiently waited for the manuscript; my publisher, Nicola Horton who worked very hard in the background and gave useful suggestions; Hannah Tudge, for her understanding and continued support, and who efficiently reminded me of the deadlines!; Georgina Massy who kept me regularly informed of the developments; Leslie Sinoway who had her own deadlines to meet; Imrana Ghumra, Jamie Semple for the library facilities, and finally but not least, Jean Goodwin at Butterwick House, Scunthorpe.

Gaëtan Béphage

The Publishers wish to acknowledge the assistance of Barbara Richell, Senior Lecturer in Nursing Studies, School of Health and Communication Studies, University of Derby who contributed invaluable advice for the chapters on Social Policy and Health Policy.

This book is dedicated to:
Mame et Pape who always paved the way for us; Sophie et Eppie,
my daughters, with love, Papa.

1 The Nature of Sociology and Society

▼ Sociology: A Definition

Sociology may be defined as the study of the social framework developed by groups of individuals over time. Such a study also examines the functioning of the structures that make up society, for example the legal system.

A study of the structure of the legal system examines the social and educational backgrounds of the groups who make up the system, identifies any problems that exist within the framework, and assesses the effectiveness of legal action and how social problems are being handled. Thus, socio-logy is seen as a discipline that examines social life, interprets social action, and develops sociological theories about groups of people and how they organise their lives. In fact, it is a study of human conditions and all activities that ensure survival of the species. Sociology provides us with an insight into the workings of society, these being the interrelationships between individuals, groups of individuals, and the social structures.

To use an analogy, the workings of the human body comprise the coordination of all the various cells and systems, and the physiological relationships and interdependence of each system, to ensure the maintenance of homeostasis. Sociology not only informs us about the

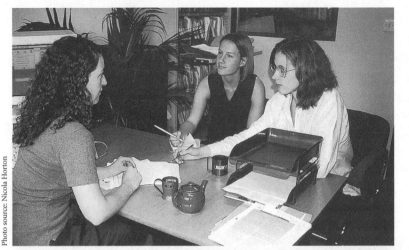

Photo source: Nicola Horton

◄ *Figure 1.1 a and b*
*Social interactions may
vary according to the
setting: groups of
people behave
differently at work and
at home*

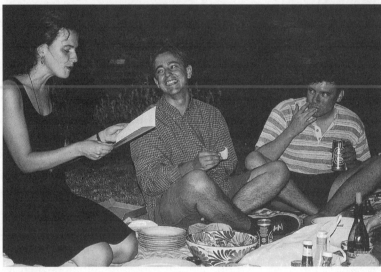

Photo source: Nicola Horton

workings of society and its various components or structures, but also raises our awareness of how 'social life involves patterned regularities' (Bilton *et al.*, 1987). Patterned regularities consist of the social behaviour of people from the cradle to the grave. From birth a baby is socialised into a set way of behaving; a teenager is expected to attend school and not to play truant; on reaching adulthood, an individual is expected to seek employment; in later years, a person is encouraged to retire at a certain age. These are just some examples of social patterns that can be observed

and that possess an element of predictability.

Sociology helps us to identify social problems, to understand the processes that predispose us to them, and to anticipate future social changes. For example, a study of interactions in the classroom helps the sociologist to assess the attitudes of teachers and pupils during the educative process. By examining the subjects taught and the methods by which this is accomplished, one can gain valuable information about the content of the curriculum and how pupils achieve their learning outcomes.

Some pupils display antisocial and rebellious behaviour towards teachers and fellow pupils. A sociological explanation may be that the rebellious pupils have been inadequately socialised at the primary stage within the family setting or that the approach used by teachers towards certain pupils is not educationally sound. Consequently, some pupils may start to play truant and rebel against the institution by disobeying the set rules and regulations. There are many real examples of antisocial behaviour exhibited by pupils and college students. Such behaviour reflects the socio-pathogenic (**an agent causing social disorder**) processes at play in the social framework. They show to both the sociologist and the community that some underlying social influences are undermining the values and beliefs laid down in society's constitutional framework. The following is an account of criminal behaviour manifested by pupils in one school, in Brooklyn, New York (Hall, 1992):

> This is the school where two children were blasted to death last week by a fellow pupil, where metal detectors scour students for pistols and where spot checks revealed 121 weapons tucked away in desks and exercise books.
> Staff too are victims of this reign of terror. Headmistress Carol Beck suffered a heart attack last month, bravely returning only to see two more of her young charges die in the latest shooting.

Such social action illustrates the extent of social problems in the world and offers the sociologist an extensive field for investigation. This then supplies a source of information about certain groups of people, the measures they take to tackle social problems, and the implications of these problems, together with their effects on other institutions such as the police, the legal system, and the policy-making machinery in government.

The family, social class, education, sexual orientation and gender, ethnicity, and race are just some of the topics considered within sociology. For example, sociologists may examine the roles of women in society, their relationships with men and children, their social interactions in a variety of settings—at work and at home—and how they use the services provided.

Sociology should not be seen as another 'ology', as referred to in the British Telecom advertisement in the 1980s, for purely academic interest. It is a discipline that helps to explain the social world, highlights social phenomena, and assists other social scientists in their work.

▼ Distinction between Sociology, Psychology, and Social Psychology

When students first study sociology, they can often experience difficulties in making a clear distinction between this concept and other sciences such as psychology and social psychology. The following statements further highlight the meaning of sociology and provide clarification.

Persell (1990) describes sociology as the analysis of patterned social relationships in modern societies and says:

> It also explores how we take parts of society into ourselves—how we may come to believe, feel, think and act in ways society promotes. Sociology can help us to understand ourselves better, since it examines how the social world influences the way we think, feel and act.

Giddens (1989), on the other hand, refers to sociology in the following way:

Sociology offers a distinct and highly illuminating perspective on human behaviour. Sociology looks at the social influences which shape our lives. Sociology helps to develop a sensitivity towards the wider universe of social activity in which we are all involved. It is the study of human social life, groups and societies. The scope of sociology is extremely wide, ranging from the analysis of passing encounters between individuals in the street up to the investigation of global social processes.

Bilton *et al.* (1987) describe sociology as:

> Not so much **'what'** is studied but **'how'** it is studied, i.e. it is important to indicate what is the particular 'perspective' of sociology, its 'distinct way of looking' at the individual and society.

Moore (1987) states that:

> [Sociology] studies the way that society shapes our lives, by refusing to take for granted the most obvious day to day experiences of people. With a fresh mind and an outlook unclouded by bias, it pulls apart all those excuses and myths about the world that flow around us ...

Townroe and Yates (1987) made the following comments about sociology:

> The word sociology was first used in English in 1843, and it means the study of human societies. Sociologists are interested in how groups in society are changing. They look at the relationships between the different aspects of social life. For example, how religion influences voting, how work influences leisure, etc.

Although both sociology and psychology involve the study of human behaviour, sociology is primarily concerned with how humans behave in social groups (Townroe and Yates, 1987). Psychologists, on the other hand, try to look at human behaviour from a range of different angles, so that they can obtain as complete a picture as possible. A large part of psychology is concerned with what makes people different from one another, the study of personality types (Hayes, 1994).

Social psychology is a study of how people interact with one another and how they make sense of what is going on in their social worlds. A large part of social psychology is concerned with the study of social behaviour, particularly in terms of conformity to social norms, obedience to authority, and how people behave in large groups (Hayes, 1994).

The psychologists McConnell and Philipchalk (1992) defined psychology as the scientific study of human thought and behaviour. In comparison, they see social psychology as a study that focuses on different social factors that lead people to respond in similar ways—for example, how people attract one another, play certain roles, or conform to group pressures.

▼ Sociology as a Social Science

Science is defined as 'a branch of knowledge conducted on objective principles involving the systematised observation of and experiment with phenomena, especially concerned with the material and functions of the physical universe' (*Oxford English Dictionary*, 1991).

The word science conjures up images of people in white coats, working away in laboratories, experimenting and observing changes in matter using 'objective principles'. Sociology, as well as the other social sciences, has constantly been criticised for lacking 'objective principles'. Most sociology textbooks mention concern about whether sociology and the other social sciences should be regarded as scientific in nature. It has been argued that sociology is a scientific discipline in that it involves systematic methods of investigation, the analysis of data, and the assessment of theories in the light of evidence and logical argument (Giddens, 1989).

The following discussions outline the basic grounds for and against sociology being considered a science. The arguments always concentrate on the comparison between the methods used in the natural sciences and the approaches used by sociologists in their study of social phenomena.

■ THE CASE FOR SOCIOLOGY AS A SCIENCE

(a) Although human action can be complex, **observing** and **describing** exactly what is happening is possible. For example, the social life of a group of miners can be observed from the time they finish work. Their social relationships, the numbers of hours worked, what use they make of leisure time, and the types of hobbies they pursue can all be described and recorded. Observation is a method used in the natural sciences. A chemist observes the chemical reaction that takes place when concentrated sulphuric acid is added to copper sulphate, and describes the duration of the reaction, the types of fumes produced, and the gases released.

(b) Collection of data is done by both sociologists and natural scientists. Emile Durkheim, a sociologist, gathered precise statistics from his observation of suicide rates among certain groups of the population. Likewise, a biologist may record the number of red blood cells in a given sample of blood.

(c) Reference is often made to the 'Laws of Nature' and how the physical universe responds to certain rules: clouds bring rain; oxygen supports combustion; an excessive level of carbon dioxide in the blood causes death. Social life has its own laws too: deviant behaviour, such as mugging, rape, and murder, should be punished; the State should provide a system of defence for its people; education should be available to everyone; seatbelts should be worn to promote safety and prevent unnecessary injuries. Social scientists investigate these laws and their impact on the social structure. They make accurate recordings of behaviour patterns as they occur and note any regularities. Sociologists are interested in assessing the social effects of these customs on the social structure and in any patterns that keep recurring. For example, observation of the reduction in severe injuries and in the length of hospital stay associated with the use of seatbelts will show the effectiveness of this practice.

(d) Other arguments that support sociology as a science relate to the similarities in the investigative methods employed by both social and natural sciences. According to Court (1987):

> If a very narrow view is taken in defining science, then sociology and the other sciences can never be truly 'scientific'. If, however, it is accepted that they are each studying completely different worlds, both natural and social science can be considered to be 'scientific' in that they follow the same mode of study or 'scientific approach'.

This scientific approach follows a similar pattern in both sciences in the sense that it can be seen to include:
● Identification of the subject matter to be investigated. For example, the natural scientist may identify the effects of solar radiation on the skin as an area to study, whereas the sociologist may identify the extent of racism in modern society.

- Formulation of the appropriate research questions.
- Identification of the method to be used.
- Collection of the data.
- Analysis of the data.
- An attempt to show that the findings match the hypothesis by interpretation of the findings.
- The making of the results available to the public and other scientists for scrutiny (Court, 1987).
- Repeatability of research process.

Cuff et al. (1990) asserted that the characteristics of scientific approaches include the following components:
- Statements, descriptions, and explanations can be verified or checked in the real world.
- Deliberate use of clear procedures.
- Standards to demonstrate the 'empirical warrant'. (An empirical warrant is a guarantee that the enquiry is factual.)

Using the criteria stated by Cuff et al., one is liable to conclude that a similar process takes place in the research carried out by sociologists, therefore asserting that sociology is a scientific endeavour.

There are, however, counterarguments to suggest that the study of human social behaviour cannot be compared with the study of the natural world.

■ THE CASE AGAINST SOCIOLOGY AS A SCIENCE

a) Human beings are more complex to study than plants and chemical substances.

b) Humans have ideas, thoughts, and emotions, and their perceptions of these are likely to change according to their experiences and the situations they are in. For example, how can a sociologist control the feelings and personal experiences of a group of industrial workers in a factory while studying their attitude towards the routinisation of the tasks they are engaged in? Some of these workers may be experiencing feelings of depression due to a breakdown in familial relationships or fatigue from lack of sleep. These variables are not under the control of the observer. As Giddens (1989) points out, 'We cannot even describe social life accurately unless we first of all grasp the meanings which people apply to their behaviour.'

In laboratory settings, the natural scientist can control the environment: the temperature, the noise level, the amount of fluid to be added to a chemical solution, the intensity of light allowed to penetrate the test tube.

c) Value judgements interfere with the objectivity required in studying phenomena, be they natural or social. According to Nagel (1981), 'The things a social scientist selects for study are determined by his conception of what are the socially important values.' Selection of the material for study thus involves a degree of personal interest. One could argue that an astronomer may possess a particular interest in the position of the stars in the firmament and how their light intensity alters according to climatic changes. In this context, however, the situation is different. Stars do not have feelings; human beings do. When human beings start to observe themselves, they experience a variety of feelings and emotions. There is a social interaction taking place. The researcher is likely to share in the expression of such feelings and to respond to the influences in the environment. This interferes with his/her sense of objectiveness.

d) The education of the researcher will influence his/her perceptual skills. Perception is thus linked with the concept of value judgement. What is perceived is influenced by one's experiences. This is likely to modify the judgement or observational capability of the researcher. For example, a sociologist who played truant at school may identify with the pupils he is investigating, so altering his perception of the situation. Biased interpretation may infiltrate the results of his findings.

The main arguments against sociology, or any of the subjects in the social sciences, being considered as scientific seem to rest on the fluidity of human behaviour. The continuing psychosomatic (mind and body) changes that affect one's perception of both the social world and one's own inner world make it difficult to measure what one is supposed to be measuring. The distinction between external reality and internal reality becomes blurred. Facts and value judgements cannot be dissociated. Facts are related to empirical evidence as it occurs. Value judgements originate from thoughts and ideas, as well as from the emotions of the observer.

▼ The Concept of Society

Society is defined as the 'sum of human conditions and activity regarded as a whole functioning interdependently' (*Oxford English Dictionary*, 1991). It is a concept that is used everyday by individuals all over the world. Its interpretation, however, varies slightly according to individual beliefs, understanding, and personal perception.

Many people use the word to convey the meaning associated with 'community'—a social community made up of groups of people maintaining a particular mode of social life. Within this context one is able to identify 'human conditions'. These are all the social activities that exist among social groups and include such familiar examples as the caring behaviour of parents towards children or the living conditions of homeless people. The human conditions required to survive within the social framework encompass working to earn a wage and the rearing of children in a way that teaches them the values and beliefs of their social environment.

Other examples of human conditions include the requirement to develop social relationships by communicating and expressing one's needs, the demand for love and affection, and the need to succeed and to achieve one's ambitions. Human conditions also embrace such actions as the impulse to avoid pain and to participate in activities that promote health. It must be remembered, however, that there are societies with groups of individuals whose social practices may not be perceived by us as particularly demonstrating pain avoidance or achieving health. For example, the anthropologist Evans-Pritchard, in his study of the Nuer of southern Sudan described how these people collect cow dung, which they then roast and use the ashes to clean their teeth. On the island of Mauritius in the Indian Ocean, it is well known that some religious groups self-inflict pain by walking on burning coal during certain religious ceremonies.

Human conditions also encompass the negative aspects of living: grief following bereavement due to natural causes, such as old age, and the pathological processes associated with the loss; death through the actions of others, as in serial killing, terrorism, riots, and mass violence.

Human conditions and social actions do not occur in isolation, however, because there are social influences at play that contribute in guiding behaviour. Human activity is thus functioning at an interdependent level. The following example illustrates this concept. A student nurse attends college because she wants to develop the skills required to become a qualified practitioner. The activity of learning and developing her professional skills involves the social process of conforming and complying to the rules and regulations of the college. Thus, the student is dependent upon the college. However, the college is also dependent upon the student for survival. To survive and progress, the college has to provide a very high standard of academic learning opportunities that will meet the needs of its students. To achieve this objective, the college must create the right environment by employing teaching staff who are both experienced and qualified to carry out such duties. Accordingly, an element of interdependence can be seen to exist.

▼ Analogy with Biology and Functioning Systems

Society presents itself as a rather complex concept. For this reason, some sociologists attempt to explain its nature by using biology as an analogy.

In biology, the terms structure and function are used when referring to the different systems of the body. Each system originates as a unit, a cell which gradually multiplies and becomes differentiated into organs, which subsequently develop into systems. For example, the cardiovascular system originates from the multiplication of one cell, to produce a multitude of cells, which develop to become the organs (the heart and blood vessels), which then become known as the system.

A similar approach is used by some sociologists to explain the origin, nature, and developing aspects of society. This is an attempt to show the living nature of the social system; its fluidity and movement, the result of all the social processes taking place.

The family is seen as the social unit of the social system. One of its main functions is to reproduce. Without reproduction, the human species and society will not survive. As time goes on, people die and, consequently, groups cease to exist. Similarly, in biology, without cell reproduction the various organs and systems will degenerate and die. Each system of the human body is dependent on each other. Without the cardiovascular system, the respiratory system will malfunction, and vice versa. In society, without the reproductive and socialising functions of the family, other systems will cease to exist. To extrapolate, without the reproductive functions of humans, there would be no children to go to school, therefore no educational system would be needed. No children would also mean no adults in the future, and therefore no workforce and no economic functions, and so on. Accordingly, there is a rippling effect with consequences for the whole of society.

Using biology as an analogy gives us a clearer understanding of the structure and function of the various systems in society and their interdependence.

▼ A Brief Description of Systems and Subsystems within the Societal Framework

The social, or societal, framework is also referred to as the **social structure**. The social structure consists of the distinct arrangement of institutions by which human beings in a society interact and live together.

The State is regarded as a set of institutions comprising the legislature, executive, central and local administration, judiciary, police and armed forces. Its crucial characteristics are that it acts through the institutional system of political domination and has a monopoly of the legitimate use of violence (Abercrombie *et al.*, 1984).

The State thus represents the ultimate superstructure of society. It, like any other structure, is dependent on other systems to survive. The economic system, for example, is an essential component of the framework. Economic activities comprise the production of finance through the buying and selling of resources such as land, iron ore, sand, and buildings. Money generated is then invested to increase profit. To achieve such objectives, the State is dependent on the skills and activities of groups of individuals, both within the economic organisation and within the other systems. Skills and knowledge are gained through the educational system. Furthermore, society is dependent on the socialisation process of the educational system to develop values, beliefs and specific types of attitudes. The rationale is to prepare individuals for employment in the other institutions of society, for example in factories, insurance companies, shops, and the civil service. Without the political and economic intervention from the State, the educational system would not exist. Can the State exist without the educational system? The answer is no. Provision needs to be made to educate and train groups of individuals to acquire the appropriate skills that will be needed by the State and other institutions.

The State needs lawyers and judges for the judiciary and its legislative functions. Similarly, the institutions of the community—the family, kinship, religious structures, voluntary groups, and the many organisations such as the health-care systems, private sectors and local govern-ment—are interdependent and interrelated. Together they form the **whole** of the social structure and decide the activities of its members.

▼ Summary

Several points must be outlined with respect to the nature of sociology. It is in many ways distinct from the sciences of psychology and social psychology. Sociology is concerned with the social framework or structures within which groups of individuals undertake broad social activities. Sociology is about social life. What people do in order to survive. It is a study of human conditions and all the activities that ensure survival of the human species. There are patterned regularities, with many aspects of interdependence between the systems in the societal framework. The study of society informs us about a variety of social functioning as well as social problems.

Psychology is a different discipline. It is a study of mental life. Psychologists are interested in aspects of personality and what makes people different from one another.

Social psychology is concerned with how people interact with one another and their perception of their social worlds, as well as looking at conformity to social norms and obedience to authority.

Sociology is one of the social sciences. Academics have long debated whether sociology is a science or not, compared with the natural sciences. Natural sciences are seen to be more objective, whereas social sciences, which involve the study of human social behaviour, include elements of subjectivity. Human beings have thoughts and feeling, natural matter does not.

Sociology is concerned with social structures, so an awareness of systems and subsystems within the societal framework is essential.

▼ Application to Clinical Practice

An understanding of the nature of sociology can only enhance professionals' insights into the social background of the patients they are in charge of.

Patients in hospital or community settings are the products of their social backgrounds. They represent specific groups in society, they form part of the systems and subsystems of society, and they are influenced by their cultures, the people in their immediate environment, and significant others.

According to Morgan (1991), patients have lay views derived from prior contact with medical professionals, as well as from popular literature, the media, and the advice and experience of family and friends. An assessment of an individual's interpretation of ill health or sickness should be undertaken using a sociological perspective. In other words, during interactions with the patient, sensitivity to their social experiences, which may be influencing their behaviour, should be adopted.

One should also remember that a hospital-ward environment, which represents the micro view of a much wider social structure, can be very daunting to patients. In this context, approaches that help to reduce fears of the unknown will also help to reduce other anxieties, promote comfort, and make patients feel more at ease to express their needs.

As professionals go about their daily clinical activities, they may forget that the wards, hospitals, or community settings are microcosms of a wider society. Healthcare surroundings can have constraining effects on patients and relatives. The clinical environment may not be only anxiety provoking, but also potentially fraught with stressors: pain and suffering, dying patients, embarrassing procedures, invasive treatment, and lack of privacy. Healthcare managers should, therefore, aim at creating environments conducive to patients' comfort. The privacy of side rooms, should the patient so want, ought to be considered. Inviting both patients and relatives to communicate their impressions, anxieties and inclinations for support should be encouraged. Their views are important; so is their participation in care.

Admission to hospital, or being bedridden at home, has social implications for the individual. There is the inherent danger of loss of contact with the outside world and the social structures that the person is accustomed to: contact with family and relatives, social-club members, friends, neighbours, work colleagues, and so on. One must aim to provide facilities that enable continuity with relevant groups in the social framework of the patient. Adopting a sociological approach in viewing the patient as a social individual—regardful of their physical, psychological and spiritual dimensions—is a necessity.

▼ Review Questions

1   Briefly compare and contrast the features of sociology with those of psychology and social psychology.

2   Discuss how sociologists interpret the concept of sociology as a social science.

3   Explain, giving examples, how biology is used to explain the functioning of society.

▼References

Abercrombie N, Hill S.Turner B. *Dictionary of sociology.* London: Penguin; 1984.

Bilton T, *et al. Introductory sociology, 2nd ed.* London: Macmillan; 1987.

Court C. *Basic concepts in sociology.* Wirral: Check Mate/ Arnold; 1987.

Concise Oxford Dictionary, *8th ed.* London: BCA;1991

Cuff E, Sharroc k W, Francis D. *Perspectives in Sociology.* London: Unwin Hyman; 1990.

Giddens A. *Sociology.* London: Polity Press; 1989.

Hall M. *Exclusive: Today goes inside the world's most violent school.* March 4, 1992.

Hayes N. *Foundations of psychology: an introductory text.* London: Routledge; 1994.

McConnell J, Philipchalk R. *Understanding human behaviour.* London: Harcourt Brace; 1992.

Moore S. *Sociology alive!* Cheltenham: Stanley Thornes; 1987.

Morgan M. The doctor–patient relationship. In: Scambler G, ed. *Sociology as applied to medicine.* London: Bailliere Tindall; 1991: 47–64.

Nagel E. The value orientated bias of social enquiry. In: Potter D, Anderson J, Clarke J *et al.*, eds. *Society and the social sciences.* Oxford: Oxford University Press; 1981:406–417.

Persell H. *Understanding society.* New York: Harper & Row; 1990.

Townroe C, Yates G. *Sociology for GCSE, 2nd ed.* Harlow: Longman; 1987.

▼ Further Reading

Haralambos M. Culture and socialisation. In: *Sociology: a new approach, 2nd ed.* Ormskirk: Causeway Press; 1986:1–17.

O'Donnell G. What is sociology? In: *Mastering sociology, 2nd ed.* London: Macmillan; 1988:3–11.

O'Donnell G ibid. 12–26.

Ryan A. Is the study of society a science? In: Potter D, Anderson J, Clarke J, *et al* eds. *Society and the social sciences.* Oxford: Oxford University Press; 1981:8–17.

2

Basic Perspectives in Sociology

▼ Introduction

Sociologists use different sets of perspectives, or viewpoints, to help them understand and interpret social phenomena. This also happens in other disciplines. For example, a student nurse may have one viewpoint of how to study biology or sociology, whereas a fellow student may have a completely different viewpoint.

Linked with the concept of perspective is the term 'theory'. A theory is a set of ideas that claims to explain how something works. There are many sociological theories in use. The most common ones are listed below.

STRUCTURALISM:

● Functionalism (consensus).
● Marxism (conflict).

SOCIAL ACTION AND MEANING:

● Symbolic interaction.
● Ethnomethodology.

The aims of this section are to outline the meanings attached to these different perspectives and to explain how their use contributes to making sense of the social world.

Structuralism is a sociological concept that encompasses the two main perspectives in sociology: functionalism and Marxism. These perspectives are considered to reflect the broad structures of society. Thus, structuralism relates to social structures within the societal framework or the social system. A social structure may be defined as 'a distinctive arrangement of institutions whereby human beings in society interact and are able to live with each other' (New Encyclopaedia Britannica, 1992). When sociologists refer to social structure, they very often associate it with changes in society and the different social forces that influence such changes.

Social scientists started using the word 'structure' in the nineteenth century. Before then , it was applied to other fields such as biology. Biologists study the structure and function of living organisms. Both of these terms have since become popular in sociology. Structures are the components or framework of society and, when viewed as a whole, conjure up the image or representation of a system. It is therefore not surprising that the term 'social system' is used synonymously.

▼ Functionalism

The word 'function' is used in everyday language: for example, the function of a car is to carry passengers from one destination to another; the function of a bridge is to allow travellers easy communication across the river, road, etc., that it spans.

When sociologists refer to function, they are using the term in the same way as natural scientists do. Human biologists study the functions of the individual organs and systems within the human body, and their relationships to each other, to gain an understanding of the organism as a whole. Sociologists who emphasise the different functions of the various parts of society in their interpretations of the social world are known as functionalists.

Emile Durkheim (1858–1917) and Talcott Parsons (1902–1979) are two well-known functionalists.

■ DURKHEIM'S THEORY OF SOCIETY

This centres on Durkheim's belief that there are **social facts**. Many aspects of social life form the concept of social facts; for example, work, mental illhealth, suicide, death, religious beliefs, and marital discord. Durkheim argued that individuals in any society are influenced by the need to live in harmony with each other because they are bound by their own morality. Individuals have a need to show good behaviour because this is what is expected of them. Good behaviour originates from the moral values laid down by society. Thus, morality is in itself a social fact.

Durkheim assumed that for any group of people to live together in harmony they must have some basic agreements on what their priorities are as a group and on how they ought to behave to each other and arrange their relationships (Cuff et al., 1990). He described the basic agreements that individuals in society share as 'collective consciousness'. For example, the collective consciousness of all staff within a healthcare organisation include the belief that each worker will show basic hygiene practices. According to Durkheim, this 'consciousness' provides the foundation for the maintenance of 'group solidarity'. Thus, solidarity refers to some form of unity or agreement of feeling or action. It is this cohesiveness that develops the integration of groups and all the various structures of society.

The idea of integration is better explained by considering the functions of religion. Religious practices bind people together. All members of a religious community share the same beliefs and practices, and a social relationship develops. This process reaffirms their unity and common agreements, therefore stabilising the solidarity and integration of the group.

Durkheim's theory of society rests on his belief that morality, as well as other shared values, helps to maintain solidarity and integration. Social facts form the very fabric of sociological knowledge and social structures. Durkheim is therefore seen as a 'structural' functionalist. This means that he viewed the structures of society as performing set functions and influencing the behaviour of groups in the process.

∎ TALCOTT PARSONS' THEORY OF SOCIETY

This theory is formulated from the amalgamation of the following fundamental concepts:

- The person.
- Culture.
- The social system.
- Values, norms, beliefs.
- Adaptation.
- Goal attainment.
- Pattern maintenance and tension management.
- Integration.

1 **The person.** It is the person or individual who creates society. Individuals have personalities that are the sum of all their characteristics. They need social action to survive. People are driven to enter social relationships. These relationships involve the sharing of emotions, feelings, and ideas. This need for sharing and discussion forms the basis of social life for the social group concerned.

2 **Culture.** Persons and personalities are also linked to culture. Culture is the accumulation of ideas, knowledge, and ways of behaving (social habits) that are transmitted from one generation to another in any particular society. Culture is generated by people; there is thus an interrelationship between the two. A common culture binds people together, stimulating a consensus or collective agreement about what will benefit the members of that society. For example, there is a consensus on the clothing one should wear to a religious ceremony or the diet one should eat if one belongs, say, to the Islamic religion.

3 **The social system.** Person and culture provide the two dimensions of Parsons' theory, but also interrelate with the social system. According to Parsons, the social system consists of all the structures within society, at both the micro- and macro-level. At the micro-level there are the smaller units of the social system, such as the family, the church, the bank, and schools. At the macro-level, there is the state, the legal system, the political system, etc. These structures all interrelate and are highly interdependent. At the micro-level, the family depends on the educational and legal systems, as well as on the economic system, for survival. The state and the government rely on the family to socialise the young and to provide future generations for the workforce and so on.

4 **Values, norms, beliefs.** The elements referred to above can only take shape and develop into differentiated structures consequent to agreed values, norms, and beliefs. Health, for example, is one concept highly valued in society. Individuals develop systems of healthcare organisation to promote and maintain health. To be able to maintain such functions, however, it is essential that people follow the norms. According to Bilton et al. (1987), norms and values are ideas about what persons should do, about what behaviour is 'proper' or 'fitting'. Exercising specific types of behaviour in

particular social contexts, nevertheless, requires a set of beliefs. Believing that health is important simultaneously expresses an attitude and a value.

5 Adaptation. For a social system to survive, there must be some control over the environment; for example, there is a need to extract resources such as food and shelter to meet the physical requirements of the group members. Society creates institutions to ease the adaptation process; for example, the teaching of science and technology helps individuals to gain insight into the natural world and to develop strategies to deal with the forces of nature.

6 Goal attainment. All societies need to set goals towards which social activity is directed. Once goals have been established and prioritised, resources must be allocated to enable them to be achieved.

7 Pattern maintenance and tension management. It is essential that the basic pattern of values is maintained. Institutions such as the family, the educational system, and religion can help to achieve this. However, the social system is not free from tension. Tension and stress can disturb what Parsons called 'the social equilibrium'. The people must take measures to counteract such tendencies and to maintain stability. Social provision of facilities for leisure, recreation and holidays can provide the necessary relief from the environment of work. When tension causes mental illhealth, there should be appropriate institutions to deal with such problems. The aim of these activities is to ensure that the regulated pattern of the social system is not disturbed, therefore maintaining equilibrium and stability.

8 Integration. Ensuring the integration of groups within the social system is a task performed by institutions such as the church and the educational system. The church teaches codes of moral conduct to individuals. Schools and colleges socialise children and adults according to the values and beliefs of the social system, and prepare them for the outside world.

Parsons' theory of the social system highlights some fundamental values that are the foundation upon which the framework of society rests.

Using a similar approach, Cuff *et al.* (1990) proposed that the basis of the functionalist perspective rests on the following concepts:

- Consensus.
- Equilibrium.
- Systems.
- Functions.
- Functional prerequisites.
- Interdependence.
- Solidarity and integration.

■ CRITICISMS OF FUNCTIONALISM

(a) Functionalists reify society; that is, they perceive society as a material thing by endowing it with the ability to think and act intentionally in a way that only humans can (Jones, 1993). The social system is seen as controlling and constraining the action of individuals. Individuals thus appear not to be able to cause social change, but to be under the influence of the social structures they live in.

There is also the emphasis on social order and integration. In fact, disorder and disintegration are common features of society. One may therefore argue that there is also a degree of dysfunction in society, as pointed out by Merton (1957).

(b) According to Giddens (1989), the approach of the functionalists is unrealistic because it views society as possessing human qualities with 'needs' and 'purposes'. As he points out, societies are not endowed with will-power or purposes; only human individuals have these.

(c) Cuff *et al.* (1990) support Merton's criticism of functionalism by expressing his view that it contains some 'contestable assumptions'. These workers question the idea of 'functional unity' by arguing that any particular element of society cannot be functional for the maintenance of the whole of society, particularly in modern complex social systems. However, they concede that this approach may have been valid for small-scale societies.

(d) Court (1987) does not believe that functionalism adequately accounts for social change. Individuals in society are seen as passive, working towards the maintenance of group cohesion and stability, not displaying any purposive action

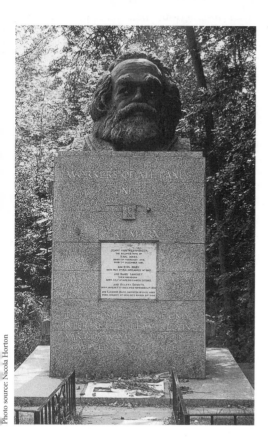

Photo source: Nicola Horton

▲ *Figure 2.1. Marx's memorial in Highgate cemetery, London.*

to create social change. This view is reflected in the comment made by Jones (1993): 'Functionalism seems to promote a static and conservative picture of society.'

▼ Marxism

Karl Marx (1818–1883) was born in Germany. Most, if not all, sociologists feel the need to refer to his extensive writings, because his perspective provides a sharp and illuminating contrast to the other viewpoints.

Marxist theory is based on some core concepts. According to Marx, society consists of a base and a superstructure. The base consists of the 'proletariat' (the working class). The proletariat are involved in the 'mode of production', the means by which a society produces material goods, including not just the technology but also the social relations of the producers (Giddens, 1989). The superstructure consists of the other elements in the system; namely the beliefs, values, and ideas transmitted by the 'bourgeoisie' (the people who own the technology and have the power to recruit members to undertake the work required). The bourgeoisie is often called the capitalist class: the landowner, for example, who has the capital (the wealth) to invest to produce more wealth. The production of more wealth cannot take place without the proletariat; they form the workforce. The superstructure also consists of the collection of institutions and activities carried out by the legal and administrative components of the state, which is an institution itself (Weeks, 1982).

In Marx's view, two types of relationships can be identified in this framework: the exploiter and the exploited. The relations that exist between the owners of production and the workers. Marxist theory says that there is conflict between the working class and the capitalists. The capitalist is seen to exploit the proletariat by controlling wages and maximising profit for the benefit of other capitalists. While managing the workers, the capitalists create a 'false consciousness' among them. False consciousness refers to the impressions the workers have of the world or society they live in that do not reflect the reality of their conditions, in particular the exploitation they are under. This false consciousness is produced through the 'ideology' generated by the capitalists at the level of the superstructure. Ideology can be seen as a set of beliefs and values that express the interests of a particular social group. In Marxist interpretation, capitalist ideology is a viewpoint that distorts reality and justifies and legitimates the position of that group.

Jones (1993) emphasised that capitalism stands as an ideological force because it contains a doctrine of social justice that justifies inequalities of income and wealth.

It is the conflict created by such inequalities that, according to Marx, will lead to social change. The working class will eventually realise their false consciousness and overthrow the capitalist system.

Marxist theory of society provides a different perspective to the functionalist approach. It stresses the economic influences of the mode of production and the conflict in society generated by the relations of production: the relations between the dominant class and the working class. The dominant class aim to increase profit and exploit the workers. The working class offer their labour and rely on the dominant class to supply them a wage.

■ CRITICISMS OF MARXISM

(a) Marx is often accused of being an economic determinist, emphasising that social change can only occur through changes in the economic base of society (Court, 1987).

(b) Marx's vision of the future, that the working class will overthrow the capitalist system, has not realised itself. This is evident in many societies where there is still a high level of inequality.

(c) Giddens (1989) pointed out that political and military power is often a 'means' of accumulating wealth, rather than the result of it.

▼ Symbolic Interactionism

Symbolic interactionism, in contrast to the perspectives outlined above, considers the detailed social interactions that take place between individuals. Therefore, this perspective is considered to focus mainly on the micro-social aspect of human life.

Symbolic interactionism was developed by Herbert Mead (1863–1931), a philosopher at the University of Chicago, and Charles Cooley (1864–1929), from the University of Michigan. According to Mead and Cooley, society is in a state of constant change, with groups of individuals in a continuous process of interactions. During this interacting process, people use 'symbols'. A symbol may be defined as the representation of an idea, a sign, or a figure; for example, white represents purity, whereas black is associated with darkness, dirt, or impurity. When individuals are communicating and interacting, they use words to convey impressions and meanings, and these words are subsequently interpreted. Thus, symbolic interactionism is sometimes called interpretive sociology.

As Haralambos (1988) pointed out: 'Symbols provide the means whereby man can interact meaningfully with his natural and social environment. They are man made and refer not to the intrinsic nature of objects and events but to the ways in which men perceive them.' Accordingly, the process of interacting with the environment and the people around also involves a psychological element. Mead felt that the act of perceiving the action of others belonged to the whole concept of interactionism. As humans interact, they require feedback from the persons they are interacting with to confirm that their behaviour is compatible with the norms of that social situation. To ensure such compatibility, it is essential for the individuals concerned to reflect upon their behaviour and to be able to interpret the signals and symbols that become apparent while interacting. According to Mead, it is during the process of social interactions that the 'self-concept' develops. The self-concept is the awareness or image of oneself as an individual in relation to others.

The concept of 'self' is a perspective developed by Goffman (1981), a Canadian sociologist, in his interpretation of symbolic interactionism. Briefly, Goffman's theory consists of the following ideas:

● Humans interact and communicate with each other. This process involves a 'display of self'. We project our 'selves' by creating impressions that will act to our advantage and favourably influence others.
● Humans define the situations they find themselves in. They perceive the situation, interpret it, then define it. For example, we see a large crowd of people shouting and raising banners on the street. We may decide that there is a strike on. The observation that these people are angry and the words written on the banners confirm our suspicion.
● Individuals display social relationships and membership.
● We all have a 'front stage' and a 'back stage'. Here, Goffman is using dramaturgy as an analogy to explain the different roles we play when in public and when in the privacy of our homes. For example, a judge is expected to act in a certain way when in court; when he or she is off-duty, we expect a more relaxed and unofficial behaviour.

■ CRITICISMS OF SYMBOLIC INTERACTIONISM

(a)   Too much emphasis is placed on face-to-face social interactions at the expense of the influences of the social structures on human social behaviour.

(b) Symbolic interactionists omit the fact that social action is constrained. There is a tendency to think that all human social interactions are free of constraints and that individuals have complete freedom.

(c) The historical and social settings within which the interactions take place and their influences are not, as such, considered .

(d) The origins of the meanings of the interactions are not discussed (Haralambos, 1988).

▼ Ethnomethodology

This perspective, which was developed by the American sociologist Harold Garfinkel (1967), is an extension of symbolic interactionism. The difference, however, lies in the detailed study of the **methods** and approaches used by individuals to make sense of their social world.

Ethnomethodologists are thus concerned with the content of conversation and communication. They aim to analyse how individuals see, describe, and explain social order. To explain their social world, humans give meanings to events occurring around them. They do this through interpreting and communicating their perception with others. The focus is on 'the meaning of the interaction through words, but can only be explained through knowledge of the context in which it occurs' (Persell, 1990). The context in which the interaction occurs is referred as 'indexicality'.

Fundamentally, ethnomethodology identifies the accounts and interpretations of the members of society; it assesses their views of what makes their social world a reality.

■ CRITICISMS OF ETHNOMETHODOLOGY

(a) Ethnomethodologists do not seem to consider the importance of motivation in the social behaviour of people they study (Haralambos, 1988).

(b) The effects of class and power inequality, and how members of society can be affected by them, are not discussed.

(c) When sociologists use the ethnomethodological approach to study group behaviour, they are themselves attempting to make sense of the world they are studying by using 'methods' that are similar to those used by their subjects. The question is, how accurate is their interpretation of reality?

▼ Summary

Sociologists examine their subject matter by utilising a combination of theories or perspectives. Functionalism/consensus and Marxism/ conflict are classified as macro-sociological theories because they consider the broad structures of society. Symbolic interactionism and ethnomethodoloy are classified as micro-sociological theories because they focus on the detailed aspects of human behaviour: the meanings of interactions and the sense people make of their world.

Functionalism refers to the functions of the social system. Marxism focuses primarily on the economic aspects of society and the degree of social conflict between capitalist and working classes. Symbolic interactionism is concerned with social interactions between people and the symbols or signs they use during the process of interacting. Ethnomethodology relates to the meanings people give to their social world—and their interpretations of these meanings—to make sense of what is happening around them.

Although these theories are of relevance in giving us an insight into the nature of society, they do have limitations.

▼ Application to Clinical Practice

■ THE SOCIOLOGY OF THE WARD ENVIRONMENT

When healthcare students begin their clinical experience, they often wonder how to relate sociological perspectives to nursing practice. One aspect worth identifying is the ward environment, which is a micro-structure within the macro-structure of the hospital organisation. As with other systems in the social framework, it carries out specific functions; for example, it provides a place of safety and security for the patients. Safety and security can only be ascertained by the groups of professionals (nursing, medical, paramedical staff, and others), whose main aim is to deliver care to meet the needs of patients.

At this micro-level of the social system, one finds different groups of individuals with their own sets of roles and functions. The medical staff diagnose and provide the medical framework within which the nurses operate. The nurses function by making nursing diagnoses, delivering care at the bedside, and ensuring patients' comfort. To achieve such aims, healthcare professionals must be able to:

(a) Adapt to the changing environment. Sullivan and Decker (1988) acknowledge that environmental factors in the healthcare field are in a state of rapid and constant change. The changes that occur within the ward climate are numerous. Basic examples include:

- Emergency situations and crises: cardiac arrests, respiratory arrests, patients falling out of bed.
- Doctors rounds, staff sickness.
- Emergency admissions, list-case admissions, deployment of staff, meal times, drug administration rounds, patients going for radiographs and so on.

Nurses must possess the skills and knowledge to cope with such changes. Adaptation of the healthcare team is essential to ensure that the working environment is stabilised and that care delivery is kept at the optimal level. The aim is to guarantee that patients' needs are met. The functions of the ward manager are to plan, to organise the workload, and to anticipate further changes in the working environment, thus ensuring that eventualities are dealt with efficiently and the equilibrium of the ward is maintained.

(b)   Maintain a standardised pattern of nursing intervention and manage tension. A systematic approach to nursing care is important to achieve a comprehensive and competent assessment that will meet the needs of patients. A standardised intervention provides healthcare professionals with a framework for nursing action. The nursing process involves assessing, setting objectives, and implementing and evaluating care.

The ward is an ideal environment for the development of tension since there are so many different groups of professionals involved in care delivery. Other factors such as the nature of the work itself (procedures, emergencies, dying patients), also contribute towards the tension. Nursing staff use a variety of coping strategies to manage such tension; for example, they make use of counselling sessions and frequently attend meetings to discuss their problems.

(c) Integrate. Integration is essential for the efficient coordination of human resources to make sure that patients' needs are met. The ward manager must create steps to unite the staff under his or her control and management. According to Sullivan and Decker (1988), integration may be achieved by the parties jointly identifying the problems and their needs. They explore a number of alternative solutions and come to a consensus on a solution.

By using the basic theory of functionalism at this micro-level of the social system, one can identify how nurses, in conjunction with other healthcare professionals, are able to maintain the equilibrium in clinical practice.

■ INTERACTIONS BETWEEN PATIENTS AND HEALTHCARE PROFESSIONALS IN NURSING PRACTICE

Nursing practice is associated with an endless number of social interactions: interactions between patients and nurses, nurses and nurses, medical staff and nurses, patients and medical staff, and so on. During the course of such interactions, numerous 'symbols' are used. Many of these symbols are expressed nonverbally. For example, the type of uniform worn informs the onlooker about the position occupied by the wearer in the hierarchical structure of nursing or medicine.

Symbols are also expressed verbally, by the choice of specific words. These words are the technical terms commonly used by healthcare professionals in their daily interactions. Patients find it extremely difficult to make sense of symbolic terms. The difficulty is compounded by the fact that patients may feel anxious and threatened by the unfamiliar environment. The variety of uniforms worn by the staff adds to the perplexity of the situation. It is, however, the language used by care professionals that interferes with how patients comprehend their social world.

Ley (1988) researched patients' understanding of what they are told and came to the following conclusions:

> It is likely that patients will not understand and will misinterpret much of what they are told. There are two main reasons for these failures in comprehension. The first is that clinicians often present information to patients in too difficult a form. The second is that patients often have their own theories about illnesses and naturally enough interpret new information within the framework of their existing ideas.

Ley argued that technical terms such—as 'peristalsis', 'lumbar puncture', 'sphincter', and 'labia'—will baffle the patient. Unless the meanings of such terms are adequately explained, patients are unable to make sense of the treatment they are receiving and the social reality they are in.

It is also important for care professionals to assess any existing ideas patients may have about their illnesses. This background knowledge will help the clinician to identify any psychological or social problems the patient may be experiencing.

By examining the clinical environment from an interactional or ethnomethodological perspective, healthcare profesionals can work towards making the social interactions more purposeful and meaningful, and can hence improve the quality of care that they are providing.

▼ Review Questions

1   Define the following sociological concepts:
(a) Functionalism.
(b) Marxism.
(c) Symbolic interactionism.
(d) Ethnomethodology.

2   Compare and contrast the features of functionalism, Marxism, symbolic interactionism, and ethnomethodology.

3   Discuss how healthcare professionals may apply sociological theories in healthcare settings.

▼ References

Bilton T, Bonnett K, Jones P, *et al* . *Introductory sociology, 2nd ed.* London: Macmillan; 1987.

Court C. *Basic concepts in sociology.* Wirral: CheckMate/Arnold; 1987.

Cuff E, Sharrock W, Francis D. *Perspectives in Sociology.* London: Unwin Hyman; 1990.

Garfinkel H. *Studies in ethnomethodolgy.* Englewood Cliffs: Prentice Hall; 1967.

Giddens A. *Sociology.* London: Polity Press; 1989.

Goffman E. The presentation of self. In: Potter D, *et al.*, eds. *Society and the social sciences.* Oxford : Oxford University Press; 1981:373–384.

Haralambos M. *Sociology: themes and perspectives.* London: Unwin Hyman; 1988.

Jones P. *Studying society: sociological theories & research practices.* London: Collins; 1993.

Ley P. *Communicating with patients.* London: Chapman & Hall; 1988.

Merton R. *Social theory & social structure.* New York: Free Press; 1957.

New Encyclopaedia Britannica, 15th ed Vol. 27 Social Sciences 380–414: Social Structure and Change Chicago University Press: Chicago;1992:414–420.

Persell H. *Understanding society.* New York: Harper & Row; 1990.

Sullivan E, Decker J. *Effective management in nursing, 2nd ed.* Harlow: Addison-Wesley; 1988.

Weeks D. *Social sciences. A second level course. An introduction to sociology.* Oxford: Oxford University Press; 1982.

▼ Further Reading

Armstrong D. An outline of sociology as applied to medicine. Bristol: Wright & Sons; 1980.

Bottomore T, Rubel M. *Karl Marx: selected writings in sociology & social philosophy.* Harmondsworth: Penguin; 1963.

Goffman E. *Stigma.* Notes on the management of spoiled identity Harmondsworth:Penguin; 1970.

Goffman E. *Presentation of self in everyday life.* Harmondsworth:Penguin; 1971.

Locker D. Social causes of disease. In: Scambler G, ed. *Sociology as applied to medicine, 3rd ed.* London: Bailliere Tindall; 1991:18–30.

Morgan M. The doctor–patient relationship. Parsons' model of the doctor–patient relationships. In: Scambler G, ed. *Sociology as applied to medicine, 3rd ed.* London: Bailliere Tindall; 1991:47–64.

Parsons T. *The social system.* New York: Free Press; 1951.

Origins of Social Processes

The Family (Primary Socialisation)

▼ The Concept of the Family

The concept of the family as an important unit within the social structure cannot be underestimated. Its importance and influences are so great that sociologists and anthropologists never fail to highlight its facets and to discuss its nature. The family may be regarded as the milieu from which values, beliefs, and attitudes, and the various social processes originate and develop through social interactions. The family is where primary socialisation takes place, where children learn the culture, values, and beliefs of society. The facilitation of primary learning is the responsibility of the parents.

Interpreting the characteristics that make up the family is a major task. The complexity is compounded by the fact that the individual perception of its nature is varied. As Harris (1969) pointed out, the term 'family' is much used by the inhabitants of the technologically advanced societies with which sociologists are concerned. It is possible, therefore, that confusions could arise due to differences between popular and academic uses of the term.

In his assessment of the various interpretations given by the lay individual, Harris formulated the following 'complications':

● There are instances when one family may be simultaneously two families—the husband's family and the wife's family. The 'in-laws', in combination, make one family.

- There is an inclination for people to refer to their relatives as 'the family'.
- The term 'whole family' may be used when referring to both parents and their offspring.
- People may refer to parents and children in connection with the household as well; for example, individuals comment that the family has 'broken up' due to the children leaving home to live elsewhere.

According to Mitchell (1979), the family is: 'A group of persons united by the ties of marriage, blood, or adoption; constituting a single household, interacting and intercommunicating with each other in their respective social role of husband and wife, mother and father, brother and sister; creating a common culture.'

A slightly different perspective is adopted by Hill and Mattesich (1979), quoted by Clarke- Stewart *et al.* (1988): '[The family] can be viewed as a social system, established when two adults marry, added to by the births of children, subtracted from by the departure of various family members, dissolved when marriage partners divorce or die.' These authors also emphasised that within this system, a change in any one part—such as the birth of a child—affects all other parts.

The basic features of the family may be outlined as follows:

- It consists of a group of individuals: a husband, a wife, and their offspring.
- There is an element of legal binding through the marriage process by which marital status is obtained.
- There is also the characteristic of 'ties by blood', which means that the offspring are blood-related. This consequently strengthens the family bond and its structure.

- The adoption of children, who may or may not be blood-related, still constitutes the family concept.
- These individuals (husband, wife, and children) together create a single household.
- There is a strong element of social processes social interactions, intercommunication, and the development of a common culture. Within this social framework, or particular household, values, beliefs, and knowledge are transmitted.
- The family is perceived as a social system in its own right. In this instance, one can argue that it is a micro-social system in comparison with the wider social framework.
- Separation caused by divorce or the death of a partner leads to family disintegration and its nonexistence.
- Social relationships between partners and offspring are in a state of constant change. As children are born, family members must adapt to new social relationships.

There are additional facets that need to be considered to clarify the concept further. Gittins (1993), for example, argued that the family is a highly controversial concept, full of ambiguities and contradictions. Childbearing, childrearing, the construction of gender, allocation of resources, mating and marriage, sexuality, and ageing all loosely fit into our idea of 'family'. The concept therefore encompasses many dimensions.

One dimension frequently linked to the concept of family is that of 'household'. Gittins (1993), quoting Murdock (1949), stated that household is a defining characteristic of the family and vice versa: 'A household therefore will comprise a married couple, or parent and child(ren). In a household the family is perceived as carrying out specific social activities—such as the nurturing— of the young, developing relationships, food preparation, entertaining relatives and friends, and so on.' Thus, 'household' may be applied to social instances where the family lives under one roof; the two concepts are interlinked.

However, 'household' may also be used when one or more family members live away from the home. Examples of this include families where the husband is in the armed services, is a travelling salesman, or travels abroad frequently. Similarly, families where partners have jobs some distance away from one another may maintain a second household where one of them lives during the week (Gittins, 1993).

It is important to emphasise that the term 'household' is not synonymous with the term 'family'. Rather, it is a concept related to the idea of shared social activities undertaken by groups. As Gittins (1993) pointed out, 'household' does not necessarily conjure up images of mothers and fathers undertaking specific social activities. There are households where similar social activities take place but the members are not blood-related, for example a group of students living together. In this context, although they may sleep under the same roof, they do not consider themselves a family.

There is another perspective that is frequently used by sociologists and anthropologists when attempting to clarify the family terminology. This is the concept of 'kinship'. Gittins (1993) argued that kinship is a social construction and does not necessarily imply a straightforward biological relationship. Edholm (1982), on the other hand, defined kinship as:

...the ties which exist between individuals who are seen as related both through birth (descent) and through mating (marriage). It is thus primarily concerned with the ways in which mating is socially organised and regulated, the ways in which parentage is

assigned, attributed and recognised, descent is traced, relatives are classified, rights are transferred across generations and groups are formed.

'Ties' provide another social perspective. Sometimes they relate to the perception of the individual and his or her definition of the social relationships that exist. 'Ties' also mean the bond, the closeness that creates attachment, social or biological, between individuals. For example, in some cultures the ties between friends are so intense that they refer to one another as brothers and sisters.

▼ Family Types

Gittins (1993) suggested that the plural term 'families' may be more appropriate, as it encompasses the various permutations that exist in society. To say 'the family' may imply that only one type exists. It is worth outlining the various types of families that have existed throughout history to illustrate some of the stages concerned with their development. Giddens (1989), for example, identified six developmental phases outlined below:

■ THE OPEN LINEAGE FAMILY

This comprises a small family unit living in a small household. The concept is similar to that of the 'nuclear family': husband, wife, and offspring. This was, apparently, a dominant family form in the 1500s to 1800s. The distinctive feature of this family type was evident in their involvement with community relations and other kin. It was a transient institution. The death of a partner or the very early departure from the home of children caused its dissolution.

■ THE RESTRICTED PATRIARCHAL FAMILY

This family type was characterised by its authoritarian attribute and the strong emphasis that was placed on 'marital and parental love'. In comparison with the open lineage family, this institution gradually severed its connection with the wider kin and community, thus becoming a more separate entity (Giddens, 1989).

■ THE CLOSED DOMESTICATED NUCLEAR FAMILY

This institution is the one we are all familiar with today. It is a family type characterised by close emotional bonds, a high degree of domestic privacy, and a preoccupation with the rearing of children. The nuclear family consists of two adults living together in a household with their own or adopted children (Giddens, 1989).

Haralambos et al. (1986) pointed out that the typical family unit (the nuclear family) was the norm in pre-industrial England: between 1564 and 1821, only about 10% of households contained relatives beyond the nuclear family.

Young and Wilmott (1973) coined the term 'symmetrical family' to describe the typical nuclear family. In this context, 'symmetrical' means the proportionate or well-ordered nature of family roles, in particular the conjugal roles (matrimonial expectations, that is the functions of partners concerning their responsibilities).

■ THE EXTENDED FAMILY

This family form may be defined as a group of three or more generations living either within the same dwelling or very close to each other. It may include grandparents, brothers and their wives, sisters and their husbands, aunts, uncles, nieces or nephews (Giddens, 1989).

It is often assumed that the extended family unit was the norm in the pre-industrial era. However, the social historian Christopher Hibbert (1987) argued that, contrary to popular belief, families were not large during this period, even though many women spent most of their adult lives pregnant. From the late sixteenth century until the early twentieth century, the average household in England contained fewer than five people. Couples had parents or parents-in-law living with them less often than they do now, partly because the parents did not live as long as their modern counterparts and partly because housing was both easier to come by and cheaper. In a similar vein, Worsley (1978) argued that the extended family has seldom been found in any society, pre-industrial or industrial. Historical evidence supports the view that the nuclear family was the prevailing residential unit long before the industrial revolution.

■ STEP FAMILIES

A step family contains one biological parent—the natural mother or father—and a social parent, known as the step-parent. For example, a woman living with her children and a man other than her husband forms the step family, the man living-in being called the stepfather.

■ ONE-PARENT FAMILIES

One-parent families result from the death of a parent, unmarried parenthood, or divorce, and are not new. Widowed one-parent families were a relatively common phenomenon in the pre-industrial and early industrial period (Elliot, 1986).

The stereotype of the modern family is of a married couple with dependent children. However, the social reality portrays evidence of increasing numbers of single-parent families and cohabiting couples. Based on data from the statistical office, Worsley *et al* (1987) stated that 5% of households in 1985 comprised lone parents with dependent children, a low figure compared with the 30% of households having married couples with dependent children. However, in a 1991 publication, Blackburn argued that the proportion of single-parent families was growing rapidly—the number had doubled since 1961—because of an increasing number of births to single mothers and a rise in the divorce rate.

Population trends in the 1990s reinforce these findings. According to Reeves et al. (1994), the number of lone-parent families is increasing, and many of these live in situations of socio-economic disadvantage. These authors asserted that in 1991 there were estimated to be 1.3 million one-parent families in Great Britain, the majority headed by a lone mother. According to the statistical office, in 1992 one in five women with dependent children was a lone mother. The proportion of lone fathers has changed very little (under 2% of all families with dependent children) (Social Trends, 1995).

▼ The Functions of the Family

The family has many functions in society. Whether the society is pre-industrial or industrial, westernised or nonwesternised, family systems have recognised basic functions. These functions are outlined below using three sociological perspectives of the family.

■ THE FUNCTIONALIST PERSPECTIVE

This perspective explains family functions as follows:
- It is the function of the family to procreate and to control sexual activity.
- One important aspect is for parents to participate in childrearing.
- Families function by socialising children to conform to the values and beliefs of the society they live in, a process known as **primary socialisation**.
- Families provide sociopsychological support for its members. This is an important function, because the release of tension, conflict, and stress helps the individual to cope with life.
- Families have economic functions. They participate in the economy of their society by acting as consumers of production. In other words, they consume the produce manufactured by the different organisations in their society.

■ THE MARXIST PERSPECTIVE

According to Gomm (1990), Marxists consider that the functions of the family are:
- To control sexuality.
- To reproduce to provide the labour power for work in capitalist industry.
- To reinforce the ideologies that prop up capitalism.
- To act as a safety valve and shock absorber to handle the tensions and frustrations generated in the work place.
- To allow men to exploit women.
- To provide 'free' services necessary to maintain the workforce.
- To motivate people to consume the products of capitalist society.

■ THE FEMINIST PERSPECTIVE

This perspective considers that the main functions of the family result in the following:

- Exploitation of women at home and perpetuation of patriarchy.
- Reproduction of the labour power for work in the capitalistic industry (Gomm, 1990).
- Oppression in the family functions: the regulation of women's labour through the housewife role; the control it gives men over women's sexuality and fertility; its structuring of gender identities (Elliot, 1986). Oakley (1974) pointed to the 'alienating nature of women's work in the home'.
- Fletcher (1966) emphasised that, although the smallest of the formal associations in society, the family is one of the most influential and important. In response to the concern that the family is declining in importance, he argued that it is no less stable than hitherto; that the standards of parenthood and parental responsibility have not deteriorated. He summed up the functions of the family by stating the following:

The modern family fulfills more functions, and in a far more detailed and sophisticated manner, than did the family before or during the development of industrialisation in the 19th century.

Although its productive functions are not as evident as in the cottage-industry periods, its economic functions are still a reality.

The family remains an important economic unit of consumption.

Much more money is being spent on household goods (the consumer function), an expenditure also known as the 'consumer outlay'.

The family is an educative unit. It socialises its members, thus ensuring that the culture of society is transmitted from one generation to the next.

Parents in the modern family are expected to have an informed awareness of educational provisions provided by the state.

Parents are responsible for ensuring that healthy practices are maintained within the home for the 'secure and healthy development of the child's whole personality'.

▼ Cultural Comparisons

Sociologists often question whether the family is a universal institution. In other words, is what we know about the family—its composition, its functions and its organisation—similar to that in other societies?

Barbara Littlewood (1978) provided an interesting insight into the family network of couples living in Quercio, a town of about 11000 inhabitants in the province of Bari in Apulia, the 'heel' of Italy. The box below summarises of some of her findings, obtained after 14 months' fieldwork

---

1 When couples marry, their choice of home tends to be based on the proximity of the wife's mother. As Littlewood pointed out, many daughters never live (in Quercio) 'more than 10 minutes walk away'. Similarly, Young and Wilmott (1957), in their study of kinship in East London, reported: 'Mr Gould, when he married, moved away from his parents and went about 10 minutes walk away to live near his wife's parents elsewhere in the borough, in this case in Bow.'

2   In Quercio, the mother cares for and has responsibility for all small children. After puberty, however, the father and brothers become publicly responsible for a girl's sexual activities, although the mother is still held ultimately responsible for character defects.

3   After marriage, the tie or bond between a mother and son is likely to be broken. In contrast, the bond between mother and daughter remains strong.

4   There is a degree of rivalry between the mother and daughter-in-law with respect to gaining the son's affection.

5   Although most married couples have a separate home, it is common for young couples to eat at the homes of one set of parents, usually the wife's parents.

6   The family is a more important social unit than the couple in terms of the orientation of the individuals. The couple's behaviour is controlled by others. Their relationship cannot be understood in isolation from this.

7   During illhealth, a wife will be helped by her daughters in the cleaning and cooking, not by her husband. A sister or a neighbour may help if the children are too young.

8   The home lives of some men (local government officials, members of trade unions) are subject to scrutiny by the local community.

In contrast, Helmut Morsbach (1978), in his study of family relationships among married couples in traditional Japanese societies, found the relationships summarised in the box below:

1   The strong relationship between mother and son remains unbroken after marriage.

2   The bride occupies the lowest social position inside the household.

3   The mother-in-law is influential in socialising the wife into the 'ways of the family'. A degree of jealousy and conflict exists between the two, because the mother is reluctant to lose the affection of her son, who now has a wife upon whom he can devote his emotional needs.

4   Although the husband has autonomy and sexual rights, the wife is still influential and manages the household, a task shared with the mother-in-law. Financial or economic management of the home can still be seen to be the wife's responsibility.

5   Many changes have taken place in the lives of Japanese families since the Second World War. Women are now more ambitious and western-oriented. They are more motivated to occupy a respected position in society; it is perceived as desirable both financially and sociopsychologically. Morsbach attributed this new philosophy to 'improved post war education of women generally'.

▼ Summary

The family is an important institution in the social structure. Other concepts are often used to clarify the definition of 'family':

- **Household**—a term normally used to refer to co-residence (Gittins, 1993).
- **Kinship**—this may include a nonbiological connection and is 'socially constructed'.

'Family' is defined as a group of persons united by the ties of marriage, blood, or adoption; forming a single household; interacting and intercommunicating with each other in their respective social roles. The main basic features of a family can be summarised as follows:

- It is a group of individuals—husband and wife and their offspring.
- There is an element of legal binding through marriage.
- There is the characteristic of 'ties' by blood, which means that the offspring are blood-related.
- These persons, in combination, create a single household.
- Social interactions and intercommunication take place within the family household. Values, beliefs, and knowledge are transmitted through the process of socialisation.

Gittins (1993) suggests that it is more appropriate to refer to the plural 'families', because there are so many types, rather than to use the singular term, which connotes only one variety. Family types include:

- The nuclear family (wife, husband, and their child or children).
- The extended family (several generations living either under one roof or in the vicinity).
- The one-parent family (the husband or wife is either dead or separated, which leaves the other partner to rear the children).
- The step family (the presence of one biological parent and/or a social parent or 2 social parents, known as the step-parent).

The family has important functions in society: namely, reproduction, production (allocation of resources, economic partnership), and the construction of gender. Different perspectives are used when considering the functions of the family. Functionalists view the family as functioning to meet the needs of the social system in order to maintain social equilibrium. Feminists view the family as perpetuating patriarchy and the exploitation of women. The plight of women at home has been highlighted by authors such as Ann Oakley (1974). Marxists, on the other hand, see the family as functioning to create a workforce for a capitalist society. The family reproduces the ideologies that maintain capitalism.

Cultural comparison shows that some aspects of family life are similar in different societies: women stay at home to look after the children; after marriage most couples tend to reside near their parents. However, there are many differences in cultural beliefs and practices among families throughout the world.

Ronald Fletcher (1966) has discussed how the family has gained in importance, rather than declined, by emphasising the many functions it now performs.

▼ Application to Clinical Practice

▪ ASSESSING THE NEEDS OF FAMILIES IN COMMUNITY SETTINGS

The needs of families in the community are met by healthcare professionals such as health visitors, district nurses, and community midwives. As Turton and Orr (1985) pointed out, the main roles of the health visitor are those of prevention, health promotion, and monitoring the health needs of all the family members in the community.

The functions of the family are very important to society. Families maintain cohesion by socialising their members. To perpetuate these essential activities, families need to be in a state of good social health. The health visitor or community nurse should utilise the following criteria to assess the health status of families (Turton & Orr, 1985):

- Family and individual perceptions of their health state.
- Family and individual medical histories.
- Sociological factors.
- Physiological factors.
- Environmental factors.
- Social policy factors.

In this way, the health visitor can identify the needs of the family and any potential problems. It is important to take a broad approach to include external influences from other family members, such as the extended family of grandparents and so on. A comprehensive assessment of sociological factors that may impinge on the health status of the family must be taken. It is essential to bear in mind the sociocultural background of the family, so that any specific needs are assessed appropriately. For example, as Turton and Orr (1985) argued, it would be important to know the dietary beliefs of an Asian family before discussing nutrition. Turton and Orr (1985) also emphasised how the social background of families has implications for their health status:

> There is a notable difference between the life style of a hospital consultant and a hospital porter, and this is reflected nationally in the different levels of mortality and morbidity, with those in the professional and managerial professions having fewer illnesses and a longer life expectancy (Turton and Orr, 1985).

Turner and Chavigny (1988) discussed the need for community nurses to be aware of the many factors that might be mobilised to help the family meet its physical and emotional healthcare needs. They recommended that the assessment should include the financial status of the family and any 'substantial health and life insurance coverage'. Acknowledging that finances and insurance are sensitive issues, Turner and Chavigny (1988) advise the community professionals to obtain this sort of information using skilful interview techniques after some degree of therapeutic relationship has been established.

According to Turner and Chavigny (1988), the aim of the assessment is to detect any anomalies that may affect the entire family unit. The psychological and emotional health needs are identified. The health practices of the family are also assessed, such as the use they make of recreational activities and their leisure time (walking, cycling, gardening, etc.). The type of diet consumed by the family, including the use of mineral supplements and vitamins, should also be noted.

HEALTH NEEDS OF THE ELDERLY IN THE FAMILY

Healthcare professionals have to assess the holistic needs of the elderly by considering their broad social network. Elderly members of the family appear likely to suffer the consequences of health malpractices: lack of exercise; nutritionally inadequate diet; and psychological problems related to being isolated, which are compounded by a lack of understanding about health-education measures. It is thus imperative that the whole family is educated to raise awareness of health-education issues, which can then be transmitted and reinforced to the elderly members in the home.

Barnes (1987), referring to the 1957 study by Young and Wilmott on family and kinship in East London, discussed the intricate network of care and mutual support that existed within families and the community at that time. The extended family network has not totally disappeared, as the 1982 Study Commission on the Family confirmed. It is essential to identify during assessment whether the elderly individual possesses any such links with other family members. The aim is to encourage and maintain any therapeutic relationships that are available. As Barnes (1987) states: 'When the time comes that they do need caring for, it is usually the family who offer most support.' Williams (1989) reinforces the point by arguing: 'The most important members of the caring team are the informal or prime carers. Usually, although not always, these carers are members of the family. Family members can include spouses, children, siblings or grandchildren.'

Although there are problems associated with ageing, professionals must not underestimate the positive roles of elders in the family unit. They can help to stabilise family unity, by sharing experiences and participating in childrearing.

Although the prime carers have an important role in care-giving, their own psychosocial needs must be met. Caring for an elderly relative is a stressful task, and can cause conflict and tension in the family circle that will undermine any health practices being implemented. This has implications for family health. As Williams (1989) argued: 'Families are caring for dependants at great cost to themselves . . . disturbed nights and dangerous behaviour, particularly falling, were aspects of caring that caused most distress to carers'. Assessment, therefore, must encompass the whole family network, bearing in mind the intricacies of human needs in their social environment.

ASIAN FAMILIES AND THEIR NEEDS

Britain is a multicultural society. The results of the 1991 Census show that slightly over three million people, 5.5% of the population, described themselves as belonging to an ethnic minority group. The largest individual ethnic minority group was Indian, constituting 1.5% of the population or 28% of the ethnic minority population as a whole (Social Trends 24:25, 1994).

Asian families form part of the social system. They participate in a variety of ways in the socio-economic functioning of society. Healthcare professionals have the responsibility to show cultural sensitivity towards these families. According to Leininger (1991) cultural sensitivity refers to the imperative need for 'professional nurses to respect common human needs and humanistic aspects of people care worldwide. Leininger (1995) reiterated this philosophy by explaining: 'nurses are not only expected to be culturally competent to work effectively with individuals, but to work with families, cultural groups and in communities.' Openmindedness and sensitivity to moral and ethical decisions are necessary'.

It is the client's cultural background that influences his or her present social behaviour. The family exerts considerable influence on the behaviour of its members. Barnes (1987) commented how adolescents in Asian families can experience problems if the family is very restrictive and fails to recognise their need to share a social life with friends. Social isolation, which can lead to depression and nervous breakdown, may be the consequence of familial restrictive behaviour. As Barnes pointed out, Asian girls are expected to be chaste, and so their relationships and movements are normally severely restricted. This approach may cause conflict and tension in the family. Barnes argued that anxiety and uncertainty can be found among immigrant girls from Pakistani families. The community nurse should exercise a tactful approach while assessing and identifying the psychosocial needs of such clients.

As well as identifying tension within the family network and attempting to alleviate it, the community nurse should work towards breaking the barriers to communication. This may be achieved by employing an interpreter, who will both advise the nurse and undertake the task of translating the information.

Williams (1989) advised that it is wise to ask clients how they wish to be addressed, because different epithets are considered insulting in different cultures. Sensitive communication skills are therefore essential.

If intervention procedures are to be effective, the community nurse must have a thorough understanding of the sociocultural background of the individual. To meet comprehensively the needs of Asian families, the nurse must be familiar with the features outlined below:

- Asian families may have differing attitudes to roles, responsibilities, and authority.

'British health professionals must avoid imposing ethnocentric views of normal family life on their Asian patients. Topics requiring particular sensitivity and understanding include moral responsibility and obligations, arranged marriages and family honour' (McAvoy & Donaldson, 1990).

- The burden of caring for the sick, handicapped, or elderly individuals tends to fall disproportionately on women (McAvoy & Donaldson, 1990).
- Asian families make little use of services available in the community. Badger *et al.* (1989), for example, found that community nursing services are inadequately used among this ethnic group.
- Some Asians have to fast at set times in the year; for example, Muslims fast between dawn and dusk during the month of Ramadhan. This may result in an Asian client with diabetes becoming hypoglycaemic.
- They may avoid certain types of food: pork and its products.
- It could be offensive to some Asians, such as Sikhs, to be asked if they smoke, because smoking is forbidden to them.

FAMILIES WITH MENTAL HEALTH PROBLEMS

Lyttle (1986) commented: 'Families are the building bricks of which society is constructed and each family unit tends to develop rhythms, practices and norms which maintain the stability of that unit. This stability may be greatly threatened by mental disorder in any one member of the family unit, not just the patient.'

It is the responsibility of all healthcare professionals in the community to identify the psychological needs of families in distress. It is, however, the role of the community psychiatric nurse to provide specialised mental health nursing intervention for these families.

Mental disorder encompasses a variety of psychological problems such as depression, schizophrenia, anorexia nervosa, drug dependence, obsessive–compulsive neurosis, anxiety, and mania. These disorders very often interfere with the coping mechanisms of the family, rendering them ineffective. Beck *et al.* (1988) defined this situation as 'A state of coping wherein the family typically manifests a pattern of destructive behaviour in response to the inability to manage internal or external stressors as a result of inadequate resources (physical, psychological, cognitive, and/or behavioral).'

Beck *et al.*(1988) provided a framework to be used in assessing the needs of individuals in the family. This is summarised as follows:

- **Physical**: are the physical needs of all the family members being met?
- **Emotional**: are the emotional needs of members being met?
- **Intellectual**: are problems being solved effectively?
- **Social dimension**: does the family seek or accept help appropriately? Are they failing to adapt to crisis? Is there ineffective communication between family members?
- **Spiritual**: is the family able to meet the spiritual needs of its members? Are members preoccupied with religious thoughts?

These dimensions focus on the mechanism that may interfere with family health. Intervention should therefore be aimed towards reducing and eradicating the stressors that cause the problems.

■ AN OUTLINE OF THE EFFECTS OF HOSPITALISATION ON THE PATIENT'S FAMILY AND THE ROLE OF THE NURSE

Hospitalisation causes stress—not only to the patient, but also to the relatives or family. Lobiondo-Wood *et al.* (1992) examined the impact of a child's liver transplant on the family. In a review of literature, they identified the following:

- A chronically ill child in the family is a major life stressor, continuously affecting the functioning of the family.

- Families have a strong need to develop coping strategies because of the stresses that a chronic illness causes in families, along with role strain, social isolation and a variety of unique family factors
- The family and child have to adapt to many long-term healthcare needs and related stressors.

The role of the nurse is to:
- Assess the adaptation needs of the family and develop their confidence in coping with the changes in their life patterns. The nurse must remember that the resources needed to move towards adaptation are not necessarily the same for all families (Lobiondo-Wood *et al.*, 1992).
- Provide adequate and correct information to the family in order to promote understanding. A lack of information and understanding will impair family functions (Luckmann & Sorensen, 1987).
- Support the client and relatives in the management of emotional conflicts and personal sufferings.
- Create a framework or environment in which the family may adapt and cope with the disorganisation and role changes.

As Hinchcliff *et al.* (1989) pointed out: 'The nurse must be aware of her feelings and beliefs about these various family forms and how they might influence her nursing practice.'

Caring for not only the client but also the relatives and family places a heavy demand on the skills and resourcefulness of healthcare professionals. The family is in need of support in a variety of clinical settings, as well as for a variety of reasons. To achieve this goal, care professionals must endeavour to anticipate these needs and to mobilise all the possible resources available.

▼ Review Questions

1   Define the term 'family'.

2   Discuss the role and functions of the family in society.

3   Outline and describe the types of family.

4   Compare and contrast the views of the functionalist, Marxist, and feminist sociologists with reference to the family.

5   Compare and contrast family features in some societies.

▼ References

Badger F, Atkin A, Griffiths R. Why don't general practitioners refer their disabled Asian patients to district nurses? *Health Trends* 1989, **21**:31–32.

Barnes A. *Personal & community health*. Family and social life. London: Bailliere; 1987:127–129.

Beck C, *et al. Mental health— psychiatric nursing—a holistic life cycle approach, 2nd ed.* St Louis: Mosby; 1988.

Blackburn C. *Poverty & health: working with families*. Buckingham: Oxford University Press; 1991.

Clarke-Stewart A, Perlmutter M, Friedmann S. *Lifelong human development*. New York: Wiley and Sons; 1988:497–500.

Edholm F. The unnatural family. In: Whitelegg E, Arnot M, *et al.*, eds. *Changing experience of women*. Oxford: Martin Robertson; 1982:116.

Elliot F. *The family: change or continuity*. Basingstoke: Macmillan; 1986.

Fletcher R. *The family and marriage in Britain. An analysis and moral assessment*. Harmondsworth: Penguin; 1966.

Giddens A. *Sociology*. London: Polity Press; 1989:389.

Gittins D. *The family in question. Changing households and family ideologies*. Basingstoke: Macmillan; 1993.

Gomm R. *'A' level sociology course. National extension.* Cambridge: National Extension College; 1990.

Haralambos M, Smith F *et al. Sociology: a new approach.* Ormskin: Causeway Press; 1986:183–217.

Hibbert C. *The English—A social history 1066–1945.* London: BCA; 1987: 386-387.

Hill R, Mattesich P. *Family development theory and life span development*. In: Baltes P, Brim O, eds. *Life Span development and behaviour*. Vol. 2 New York: Academic Press; 1979:161–204.

Hinchcliff S, Norman S, Schrober J. *Nursing Practice and Healthcare*. London: Edward Arnold; 1989.

Leininger M. Transcultural Care Principles, Human Rights, and Ethical Considerations. *Journal of Transcultural Nursing* **3**:(1) 1991, 21–23.

Leininger M. Editorial: Teaching Transcultural Nursing to Transform nursing for the 21st Century. *Journal of*

Transcultural Nursing **6**: 2 1995, 2–3.

Littlewood B. South Italian couples. In: Corbin M, ed. *The couple.* Harmondsworth: Penguin; 1978:30–50.

Lobiondo-Wood G, Bernier-Henn M, Williams L. Impact of the Child's Liver Transplant on the Family : Maternal Perspective, Paediatric Nursing **18:** (5) 461–466 1992.

Luckmann J, Sorensen K. *Medical-Surgical Nursing: A Physiologic Approach, 3 ed.* Philadelphia: WB Saunders; 1987.

Lyttle J. *Mental Disorder: its care and treatment.* London: Bailliere; 1986.

McAvoy B, Donaldson L. *Health Care for Asians.* Oxford: Oxford University Press; 1990.

Mitchell D. *A new dictionary of sociology.* London: Routledge & Kegan Paul; 1979:80–81.

Morsbach H. Aspects of Japanese marriage. In: Corbin M, ed. *The couple.* Harmondsworth: Penguin; 1978:84–99.

Murdock G, *Social Structure.* New York: MacMillan; 1949.

Oakley A. *The sociology of housework.* London: Martin Robertson; 1974.

Reeves J, Kendrick D, Denman S. Lone Mothers, their health and lifestyle. Health Education Jrnl (1994) 53: 3 291–299.

Study Commission on the family. Values and the changing family London: Study commission on Family; 1982.

Turner J, Chavigny K. *Community Health Nursing:* an epidemiologic perspective through the Nursing Process Philadelphia: Lippincott Co; 1988.

Turton P, Orr J. *Learning to Care in the Community, 2ed:* London: Hodder and Stoughton; 1985: 44–46.

Williams I.*Caring for elderly people in the community, 2ed,* London: Chapman and Hall; 1989.

Worsley P, ed., *Modern Sociology Introductory Readings, 2nd ed.* London: Penguin; 1978:159–166.

Worsley P, *The New Introducing Sociology.* London: Penguin; 1987: 125–162.

Young M, Wilmott P. *Family and kinship in East London.* London: Routledge & Kegan Paul; 1957:111.

Young M, Wilmott P. *The symmetrical family.* London: Routledge & Kegan Paul; 1973.

▼ Further Reading

Carson C, Manchersaw A. Mental illness: support for relatives. *Nursing Standard* 1994, **6:**28–31.

Harris C. *The family: an introduction.* London: Allen & Unwin; 1969:62–63.

Kane C. Family social support: toward a conceptual model. *Adv Nurs Sci* 1988, **10:**18–25.

McGee P. Culturally sensitive and culturally comprehensive care. *Br J Nurs* 1994, **3:**789–792.

Miles A. Caring for the family left behind. *Am J Nurs* 1993, **93** (12):34–36.

Murphy K, McCleod-Clark J. Nurses' experiences of caring for ethnic minority clients. *J Adv Nurs* 1993, **18:**442–450.

Thorne S, Robinson C. Guarded alliance health care relationships in chronic illness. *J Nurs Schol* 1989, **21:**153–157.

Webb L, Morries N. Wilson's model of family care giving. *Nursing Standard* 1994 **8:**(16) 27–30.

4

Origins of Social Processes

Education (Secondary Socialisation)

▼ CHAPTER AIMS

To explain the relevance of education in society.
To present the sociology of education and its functions in secondary socialisation processes.

▼ CHAPTER OUTLINE

Education: a definition
Theories of achievement and underachievement in education
Functions of education
Summary
Application to clinical practice

▼ LEARNING OBJECTIVES

The reader will be able to:
- Provide a clear definition of education as a concept.
- Discuss the issues pertinent to level of attainment in schools.
- Identify the functions of the educational system and education.
- Compare and contrast achievement among middle-class pupils with those of working-class and ethnic minority pupils.
- Provide a written account of the perspectives used in the sociology of education.

▼ Education: A Definition

As Byrne and Padfield (1990) pointed out, there is no general agreement about the meaning of the term 'education'. Is it restricted to the acquisition of theoretical knowledge in an institutional setting, or should it include what one learns 'from ordinary conversation, the television or general experience of life'? Byrne and Padfield (1990) put forward two definitions: 'A formal process of training the intellect' or, more broadly, 'The development of the all-round person, including intellectual, spiritual, moral, creative, emotional and even physical facets.'

Gould and Kolb (1964) interpreted the sociology of education to mean any form of instruction or training of an individual 'whether or not it is concentrated in the early years of life, undertaken through the agency of specialised institutions, directed generally to the promotion of consensus and integration, through the inculcation of attitudes and values to the formation of personality, or specifically to vocational training'. They concluded by saying that its subject matter is the 'assimilation of individuals into a cultural tradition'.

Whether education is a formal process or not, it is a concept that has been studied by sociologists for many years. The educational system forms one of the most important social institutions of the societal framework. Sociologists are interested in finding out how individuals in the wider society are influenced and socialised into behaving in ways that will conform to the social rules built into the social structure. It is the educational system that reinforces the values, beliefs, and attitudes learned from one's parents during the early years ('primary socialisation'). Education gained outside the family milieu is described as 'secondary socialisation'. In secondary socialisation, the knowledge is acquired about the world outside the home through contact with other personalities—teachers, priests, peers, etc.—and by becoming members of groups. There is a strong element of interaction with other people, which involves a degree of 'internalisation'. Persell (1990) described internalisation as 'taking social norms, roles and values into one's mind'. Education, therefore, incorporates some essential features: an interactive process with people in the learning environment—the formation of socialised behaviour and the internalisation of the learned behaviour.

The sociology of education is concerned with the functional relationships between education and the other great institutional orders of society: the economy, the polity, and kinship (Mitchell, 1979). The educational system, with its production of education, is perceived by sociologists as a unit amid the wider context of society.

Education and the educational process mould the individual into the cultural values of the social system. From a sociological viewpoint, the process of education is to prepare people to meet the socio-economic demands of society. This can only be achieved by socialisation. Socialising involves 'the transmission of basic moral education, literacy and numeracy for specialised training', so that individuals can become skilful workers (Mitchell, 1979).

Several writers have made reference to important issues related to education in society.

These issues comprise some of the major components of the sociology of education and are outlined below.

a) Educational achievement is based on one's social status:

> The overwhelming weight of evidence confirms that social class origins are strongly and clearly implicated in educational success or failure (Bilton et al., 1987).

> When groups are compared, socially disadvantaged children tend to get lower test scores and poorer grades and to drop out sooner (Persell, 1990).

> Inequalities imposed on children by their home, neighbourhood, and peer environment are carried along to become the inequalities with which they confront adult life at the end of school (Giddens, 1989).

> Children from less well-off families are both less likely to have graduated from high school and more likely to attend inexpensive, two year community colleges rather than a four year BA program if they do make it to college (Worsley, 1978).

b) The influence of gender differences has implications for educational achievement:

> Girls fare better than boys in primary school and the early stages of secondary education. Girls thereafter tend to fall behind, and are disproportionately represented in some subject areas rather than others (Giddens, 1989).

> Generally girls begin school intellectually ahead of boys [but] somewhere in high school their performances begin to sag (Persell, 1990).

> When inequality of the sexes was discussed in education in the 1970s, the focus was on girls and the curriculum. A government enquiry was instituted in 1974 with the federal Minister for education Mr Kim

Beazley announcing that For too long girls have been underachieving in school and ending their formal education early. This has restricted the career and life chances open to them (Malloch, 1989).

c) There is inequality of educational opportunity for the ethnic minority. The concept of desegregation is mentioned by Persell (1990), concerning educational practices in the United States. Desegregation is the abolition of racial isolation as far as ethnic minorities are concerned. In Persell's study, desegregation refers to the integration of ethnic groups with the majority groups so that they can participate on an equal basis in the educational process. Giddens (1989) reported that almost 80% of American schools attended by white students contained 10% or less black students. These findings suggest that educational opportunity is not as easily available to minority groups.

> The goals of desegregation include equal educational opportunity, equal achievement, reduced prejudice between members of different races, equal self-esteem, and increased respect among members of different races (Persell, 1990).

> In capitalist societies, equality of opportunity is the organising principle of state education. Despite the introduction of comprehensive schooling and related initiatives, there remains a significant difference in the academic achievement levels of pupils from working class and middle class backgrounds (Cashmore, 1988).

▼ Theories of Achievement and Underachievement in Education

It is argued that the cultural environment of the school may predispose certain pupils to poor scholastic achievement; the culture generated by the presence of middle-class influences in the educational system. Dearlove and Saunders (1991) put it in this way: 'Some researchers claim that middle class influences are the fault of the schools themselves, that an implicit and sometimes explicit white middle-class culture pervades the educational system, and that this clearly favours white middle class pupils while alienating others.'

Other arguments are based on the belief that practices within the homes of middle-class parents are conducive to learning: the availability of textbooks, study rooms, and other related learning resources. These features reflect the attitudes of middle-class parents. Worsley (1977) commented on the other factors likely to influence the educational careers of pupils: 'The parent's interest in education, their own educational histories, their occupational aspirations for their children, the degree of insecurity in the family (whether deriving from poverty, illness or absence of a parent), size of family, and the child's position in the birth order'. One should also consider the attitude of middle-class parents regarding their careful selection of schools. Worsley commented on how middle-class parents often choose the neighbourhood in which they wish to live by first finding out where the 'good' schools are. Quoting Jackson and Marsden's study of education (1962), Worsley used this excerpt: 'They [the middle-class parents] chose one which not only promised well for a grammar school place, but pointed firmly in the direction of college or university.'

Another aspect frequently used in the debate of educational success is the concept of language. It is asserted that middle-class parents and teachers use an 'elaborated code' in their communication. This theory was developed by Bernstein in the early 1960s. In the elaborated code, communication is seen to be more explicit, 'and the speaker leaves his meaning less open to interpretation and dependent on shared assumptions, thus filling in the detail of his behaviour, providing explanations for that behaviour and so on' (Worsley, 1977). In contrast, working-class children and their parents use a 'restricted code', which tends to be implicit in character. According to some analysts, for example Worsley (1977) and Bilton *et al.* (1987), language intervenes in the educational process, rendering working-class children at a disadvantage in the schooling system.

■ PEER GROUP AND TEACHER INTERACTIONS

Peer group influences are other factors considered in the causation of success or failure. According to Dearlove and Saunders, (1991): 'The explanation [is] in the peer group and its support for antisocial values (especially marked it seems among certain groups of adolescent working class boys for whom manual labour has a strong symbolic value as against the non virility of brainwork).'

Dearlove and Saunders also point out that 'Teachers and pupils alike tend to internalise the labels which come to be applied as a result of academic selection.' Consequently, as Cashmore (1988) put it: 'Teachers perpetuate these differential patterns of achievement through their expectations and treatment of working class pupils. These pupils are stereotyped as low achievers and are offered educational opportunities in accordance with these assessments.'

■ ACHIEVERS AMONG THE ETHNIC MINORITIES

Although the achievement of ethnic minority black pupils, who, as Cashmore (1988) indicates, come from working-class families, has been moderate, a government document from the HMSO (1991) highlighted the progressive achievement of the ethnic minorities in society, as the following excerpts show:

- The House of Commons now has five ethnic minority members.
- In the professions, a growing number of black and Asian people are achieving distinction. In Law for example, two Circuit Judges and a number of Recorders of the Crown Court are of ethnic minority origin, as are an estimated 6% of practising barristers.
- In the media, Trinidad-born Trevor McDonald, appointed in 1973 as the first black newsreader, is currently with Independent Television News (ITN). Moira Stuart, London-born of Bermudan and Barbadian parents, has been a newsreader with the BBC since 1981.

▼ The Functions of Education in Society

a) Education is seen as a framework through which individuals are carefully selected so that they attain a social position that reflects their skills or abilities. For example, not everyone can become prime ministers, hospital consultants, or brain surgeons. These individuals went through a process of education to gain relevant skills that eventually led them to reach certain goals.

b) Society needs people with specific qualities, aptitudes, skills, and so on, to ensure that the economic structure remains stable and functions effectively. Therefore, one may deduce, education has economic functions. For example, the production of food requires individuals with technological skills and managerial skills. It is the role of education to ensure that the relevant knowledge is transmitted. Bilton et al. (1987) see the educational system as 'a vehicle for developing the human resources of an industrial nation'.

c) As mentioned earlier, education functions by transmitting knowledge about the particular culture of society. Culture contains values and beliefs, 'the attitudes which people must share if there is to be social stability' (Gomm, 1990). 'From a functionalist perspective, schooling contributes to the cohesion of society by transmitting to new generations the central or "core" values of that society' (Bilton *et al.*, 1987).

The functionalist perspective, however, does not explain the incongruity that is evident in relation to schooling and the level of productivity in the outside world. In other words, theory taught in school does not match the practical and technical skills that are needed in industries. Bilton *et al.*(1987) argued that the cognitive skills taught in schools and the technical requirements of efficient production are far from clear. Lawton (1980), too, acknowledged the discrepancy by commenting that people engaged in industry 'are often critical of the schools on the ground that basic skills have been neglected and that insufficient pupils pursue studies in science and mathematics'.

Other criticisms put forward accentuate the lack of correspondence between higher achievement and high productivity in the workplace (Worsley, 1978). There is also the argument that only selected aspects of knowledge are transmitted, when in society there are other types of values (Bilton *et al.*, 1987).

Bowles and Gintis (1976), cited by O'Donnell (1993), gave a critical analysis of the functions of education within the American state system. Their theory reflects a Marxist perspective of the role of education. The foundation of their theory rests on the close links they identify between education, inequality, and the economy. In their

view, the educational system reproduces inequality by teaching 'people to be properly subordinate and render them sufficiently fragmented in consciousness to preclude their getting together to shape their own material existence'. They identify a hierarchical structure in the social system, which perpetuates the division of labour. Division of labour is seen by sociologists to be the cause of 'unequal positions in society and legitimizing that allocation on the basis of test scores or grades that may not be a valid indication of merit' (Persell, 1990).

The debate on the sociology of education will continue for many years. The importance of education as one of the units of the social structure cannot be underestimated; it is the machinery concerned with the process of socialisation.

▼ Summary

The main aim of the educational system is to transmit knowledge. The knowledge is related to cultural tradition. It is within tradition that the values and beliefs of a particular society are contained. Values are learned during the early years of primary socialisation and are subsequently reinforced by the educational system. Education is thus seen as part of the process of socialisation. Sociologists refer to it as secondary socialisation. There is a relationship between education and the other systems of society: the polity, religion, economy, and kinship.

Education has important functions in society: it prepares individuals to reach a certain social position by ensuring that the relevant skills are acquired; and it helps to maintain social order and stability. Functionalists view education as contributing to the cohesion of society by transmitting to new generations the central or 'core' values of that society. Marxists, however, see education as perpetuating inequality by teaching people to be subordinate. They argue that education represents the hierarchical structure in society; for example, the hierarchy between teachers and pupils, and between administrators and teachers.

The main issues regarding the sociology of education are concerned with whether the school curriculum adequately prepares people to meet the technical requirements for efficient production in industries. Arguments are also centred around the debate of educational attainment. The question often asked is: 'Why do working-class pupils underachieve?' The answer seems to lie in the social background of working-class pupils—the attitudes of their parents with regards to their values and beliefs about education. Middle-class pupils do better because they are brought up in an environment conducive to learning. Some authors find a similar trend among the ethnic minorities, who, they say, come from working-class families. West Indian pupils, in particular, tend to underachieve compared with their white and south-Asian peers. To contrast with the evidence showing underachievement among the ethnic minorities, a government document (HMSO, 1991) has highlighted the progressive achievement of distinction among some ethnic groups.)

▼ Application to Clinical Practice

■ THE SOCIALISATION OF STUDENT NURSES

Before working in healthcare settings, student nurses go through a progressive process of socialisation. This process moulds the attitudes, values, and beliefs of the individual to match the philosophy of the institution. The philosophy of the institution is reflected in the nursing curriculum; this sets out the learning outcomes to be achieved, the process to be implemented to reach these goals, and the framework within which the student has to operate.

Aswegen and Niekerk (1994) see professional or occupational socialisation as a very important part of adult socialisation. They note that when adults enter a profession or a type of training, they bring with them personal experiences that reflect their values and beliefs. These authors argue: 'The socialisation process often involves changes in knowledge, attitudes and values.' They perceive nursing to be a professional culture; a culture, they feel, which needs to be transmitted for the profession to survive. The concept of nursing contains some key values—it is a practical profession encompassing norms, values, beliefs, and attitudes. These core elements are fundamentals. It is imperative for the institution to impart knowledge that will exemplify these characteristics. The students will, over time, internalise these beliefs. Aswegen and Niekerk (1994) assert that the educational institutions (colleges and universities) are not competently socialising the students into the professional roles that are expected of them. In other words, the professional culture is not being transmitted effectively to the students; consequently, students are not internalising the core values and attitudes of the profession. The following extract (Seed, 1994) illustrates how the socialisation of the student from a theoretical perspective is fragmented and does not match the reality of clinical practice:

> While the students recognised that topics for conversation such as the weather might be inappropriate, they lacked the knowledge and skills to answer patients' questions or to deal with highly emotive situations such as those described by Pat. Although the

students had strategies for dealing with situations which might involve demonstrating concern through the use of touch, they nevertheless felt they lost credibility. Pat points out that she was not prepared in school for the interpersonal aspects of nursing. Such views reflect the findings of Gott (1984) who suggests that student nurses require more practice in communication skills.

Bradby (1990) identified the various stages involved in the socialisation process and detailed how some practices may interfere with the acquisition of relevant professional skills. The first stage identified is described as a 'status passage'. Bradby defined this as the process of change from one social status to another. Other features of the 'passage' include the 'anticipation and anxieties experienced prior to the event'. There is also the motivation to anticipate future events and an attempt to reduce the anxieties likely to be associated with such events. For example, a student who is to enter nurse training will anticipate the stress of the unknown, the fear of meeting unexpected situations, and may attempt to deal with such forthcoming events by personal preparations. This may involve seeking information and reassurance from, for example, friends who are qualified nurses. The student may, on the other hand, actually attempt to experience this fear to some extent or gain work experience in a similar work setting (Bradby, 1990). The other characteristic of status passage is how the individual feels the need to relinquish 'some aspects of a previous status'.

Bradby (1990) identified several stages of the status passage. These stages, also discussed by Aswegen and Niekerk (1990), are related to the realities of the clinical areas the student has to face: the feelings of incompetence, the lack of skills to cope with demanding and unknown situations; 'being overwhelmed, of feeling lost,

bewildered, strange and useless, regardless of the practice undertaken during the induction course' (Bradby, 1994). The student assimilates these experiences (elements of surprise and reality shock on entering the wards). These experiences represent some aspects of the socialisation process, which is divided into **serial passage**, **disjunctive passage** and **divestiture and personal identity**.

SERIAL PASSAGE

This stage of socialisation is defined as the transmission of knowledge and skills to new recruits following a traditional pattern. Sometimes this is described as 'the way we do it here'. This approach is criticised because it socialises new recruits into a pattern of thinking that may discourage innovative ideas and can result in outmoded, incorrect, or poor practice (Bradby 1990). As Bradby asserted, it encourages conformity to the accepted norms at the expense of developing ideas.

DISJUNCTIVE PASSAGE

This stage is described as the exposure of the student to clinical situations that he or she has no expertise in dealing with. In such circumstances, some students manage to cope 'without help or guidance'. As Bradby (1990) pointed out: 'Much of the essential care for patients was undertaken in this manner. Students were left alone to attend to patients' hygiene needs feeling anxious and embarrassed.'

The implication here, as far as the socialisation of the student is concerned, is the internalisation of poor practical skills and knowledge that may endanger the patient. The lack of knowledge may also be reflected in the transmission of wrong information and the teaching of inappropriate skills to other junior peers. The disjunctive passage contains the tendency for a lack of supervision and a failure of the mentoring system, which result in poor practice.

DIVESTITURE AND PERSONAL IDENTITY

This stage comprises the remoulding of the person by imposing the values of the institution. 'Divestiture' can be defined as 'the attempt of an organisation to deprive an individual of his identity so that conformity with the institution's needs will occur' (Leathart, 1994). Bradby (1990) gave examples of a similar process occurring in other institutions, such as the armed forces and the church. Both Bradby and Aswegen and Niekerk (1994) commented that the whole process, although degrading, contributes to reshaping the social and psychological identity of the person. This degradation process, they asserted, is not obvious to the student or the institution. The student, however, feels overwhelmed and has to cope with the 'sensory overload'. The stimuli from the educational institution and the healthcare setting bombard the student's senses, causing alarm and anxiety. The clinical staff, however, perceive the student as lacking in purpose and confidence and 'not pulling their weight'.

Bassett (1993) commented on the dichotomy between the theoretical knowledge taught in colleges of health and the clinical practice. She pointed out: 'There is constant tension between schools of nursing and the wards or department. How does the student nurse adapt and survive the two different environments?' It is this dichotomy that forms one of the components that causes personal anxiety in the student. This anxiety is compounded by the need for the student 'to establish a personal identity which has been lost during this rapid transition from a previous social status' (Bradby, 1990).

The healthcare setting, for example the ward environment, is the arena where the student learns the rules of conformity; what to do to feel accepted by the other healthcare professionals. According to a Bradby (1990): 'Feeling part of the ward team was far more important than the quality of care which had to be delivered to patients.' There was, however, another dimension to the socialisation process. The students learned that some patients would provide them with reassurance; the patients would respond to them in a 'friendly' or 'parental' way, thus boosting their self-esteem and reinforcing their self-realisation of a personal identity.

Personal identity is retrieved after six to ten months of socialisation. The attitudes of the learner change from being overwhelmed, unsure, and unassertive, to a more positive acceptance of the new role, that of the nurse. Bradby outlined the change in the following way:

> By six months the students felt more comfortable with the clinical areas and had grasped the theoretical concepts. They often stated that they felt more adult and had become more independent, showing that this occupational socialisation had also hastened their status passage into the adult role.

The role of socialisation, therefore, is to expose the student to a learning environment. The climate of the educational setting (including both the institution where theory is taught and the clinical environment) represents the reality of the nursing profession. The student progresses through definite stages of change. These stages are the conceptual framework of the 'status passage', and are described by Davis (1975) as:

- Initial innocence: the new recruit comes into college filled with the popular view of nursing.
- Labelled recognition of incongruity: the student realises that his or her view of nursing is not accurate.
- Psyching out: the student nurse begins to accept the new and serious reality.
- Role simulation: the nurse tries out the new reality.
- Provisional internalisation.
- Stable internalisation.

The last two stages demonstrate the change that has occurred from lay person to socialised nurse, and acceptance of this. The stage of stable internalisation is when the student integrates all the learning that has taken place into his or her value system, and feels more assured in the role of the nurse and of the expectations of others about this role.

Seed (1994) conducted a longitudinal study of student socialisation and reported the following findings:

- The practice of nursing occurs in a constrained environment where there is a lack of information.
- Trained staff keep information to themselves.
- Early in their training, students see themselves as mostly workers and hardly students.
- Students realise that they have been 'depersonalised'.
- Students experience feelings of 'exploitation' in the clinical areas and report that most of the tutorial staff do not treat them as 'people'.

These are some of the beliefs likely to be internalised by the students from the impact of socialisation.

Socialisation is, however, an ongoing experience that affects qualified nurses too. Leathart (1994) applied Bradby's (1990) theory of status passage in her exploratory study of nurse–patient communication in an intensive therapy unit (ITU). Leathart theorised that qualified nurses go through a similar process of socialisation. She pointed out that the mentoring system, where knowledge and skills are passed on from one nurse to another, is characteristic of serial passage.

Compared with a student nurse, a qualified nurse new to the ITU may not be mentored because of a shortage of staff. Consequently, the nurse has to face the stressors associated with intensive-care nursing of a critically ill patient. Leathart (1990) argued: 'Because most tuition is given at the bedside on a one to one basis, as "the way we do it here", there is little scope for the nurse to become aware of alternative practices, or what are outdated or incorrect practices.' This creates alarm and anxiety in the nurse, who may feel inadequate under such circumstances. Because intensive care is highly technological, the new nurse 'will be expected to be able to provide everything from the most basic nursing needs to the most complex technical tasks'. The tendency to attempt to 'cope without help or guidance', as discussed above, is again seen in the behaviour of qualified nurses. Leathart (1990) pointed out the 'disjunctive passage' stage of socialisation in this instance.

Conformity resulting from 'divestiture' takes place because the organisation has a specific perception of the trained nurse in an ITU; he or she is expected to be confident, to have technical knowledge, to be competent in the delivery of care, and thus to be 'a valuable member of the team'. To deviate from these expectations is likely to cause stress to the nurse, by not being accepted in the team. Leathart (1994) pointed out: 'Two nurses identified strategies that they felt promoted their acceptance into ITU: conforming to what others are doing, and demonstrating a willingness to progress.' To express feelings of apprehension or to show hopelessness in clinical practice is seen to be acceptable in new nurses, who must quickly conform to the ideals of the ITU: staff or succumb to the stress such persistent feelings produce and leave the unit (Leathart, 1994). Recovery of identity occurs when the nurse is accepted as a member of the team.

To conclude, the socialisation of the nurse takes place in a climate full of stressors. The practitioner has to use many strategies to cope. The strategies selected are likely to create a favourable impression on others, who will consequently accept the new recruit as a member of the team.

Values and beliefs concerning the working environment are internalised, as are experiences gained. Conforming to the needs of the organisation is a common feature. The 'socialised' nurse finally becomes accepted and regains her personal identity after going through the stages discussed above.

▼ Review Questions

1 Explain the meanings given to the sociology of education.

2 Describe the social functions of education.

3 Compare and contrast perspectives used by sociologists with reference to the concept of education.

4 Discuss the theories related to the debate on achievement and underachievement in schools and society in general.

5 Describe the concept of secondary socialisation.

6 Goopal Singh is a 20-year-old student in nursing. He left his homeland in India two months ago. He lives with a cousin in rented accommodation five miles from the city of London.
(i) Discuss how Goopal Singh's cultural background may influence the process of socialisation.
(ii) Identify the factors that may be considered in assessing his educational needs.
(iii) Explain the features of the educational system that may hinder his achievement.

7 Tom Evans is a new recruit in the steel industry. He is 30 years old. His father is a coalminer. His mother is a part-time secretary at a local council.
(i) Give an account of the issues that need to be considered to explain his present social position.
(ii) Discuss the possible effects of socialisation on him.

▼ References

Aswegen E, Niekerk K. *Socialising future professionals.* Nursing RSA Verpleging 1994, **9**:23–27.

Bassett C. Socialisation of student nurses into the qualified nurse role. *Br J Nurs* 1993, **2**:179–182.

Bilton T, *et al. Introductory sociology 2nd ed.* London: Macmillan; 1987:308–313.

Bowles S, Gintis H. Schooling in capitalist America 1976. In: O'Donnell M, ed. *New introductory reader in sociology.* Walton-on-Thames: Nelsons & Sons; 1993:204–205.

Bradby M. Status passage into nursing: another view of the process of socialisation into nursing. *J Adv Nurs* 1990, **15**:1220–1225.

Byrne T, Padfield C. *Social services—education.* St Yves: Clays; 1990:212.

Cashmore E. *Dictionary of race and ethnic relations, 2nd ed.* London: Routledge & Kegan Paul; 1988:304–306.

Davis F. Professional socialisation as subjective experience: the process of doctrinal conversion among student nurses. In: Gould J, Kolb WL, eds. *A sociology of medical practice.* London: Collier McMillan; 1975:116–131.

Dearlove J, Saunders P. *Introduction to British politics, 2nd ed.* London: Polity Press; 1991:431–434.

Giddens A. *Sociology.* London: Polity Press; 1989:416–449.

Gomm R. *Sociology 'A' level.* Cambridge: National Extension College; 1990.

Gott M. *Learning nursing.* London: RCN; 1984.

Gould J, Kolb W. *A dictionary of social sciences:* education. London: Tavistock; 1964:228–229.

HMSO. *Aspects of Britain: ethnic minorities.* London: HMSO; 1991.

Lawton D. *The politics of the school curriculum.* London: Routledge & Kegan Paul; 1980:41.

Leathart A. Communication and socialisation (1): an exploratory study and explanation for nurse patient communication in an ITU. Communication and socialisation (2): perceptions of neophytes in ITU

nurses. *Int Crit Care Nurs* 1994, **10**:93–104, 142–154.

Malloch M. Women in the state of Victoria. In: Walker S, Barton L,(eds). *Politcs and the Process of Schooling.* Milton Keynes: Open University Press; 1989:166–190.

Mitchell D. *A new dictionary of sociology.* London: Routledge & Kegan Paul; 1979:210–212.

Persell C. *Understanding society. An introduction to sociology, 3rd ed.* London: Harper & Row; 1990.

Seed A. Patients to people. *J Adv Nurs* 1994, **19**:738–748.

Worsley P. *Introducing Sociology, 2nd ed.* Milton Keynes: Open University; 1977:217–223.

Worsley P. *Modern Sociology: introductory readings, 2nd ed.* Harmondsworth: Penguin; 1978.

▼ Further Reading

Berger P, Luckmann T. Secondary socialisation in: *The social construction of reality: a treatise in the sociology of knowledge.* . Harmondsworth: Penguin; 1966:157–166.

Cave W, Chesler M. Socialisation: educational emphasis in primitive perspective. The socialisation community in: *Sociology of education: an anthology of issues and problems* New York: Macmillan; 1974:3–6, 18–27, 338–361.

Sills D ed. Socialisation: anthropological aspects II. Adult Socialisation IV. In: Sills D ed: *International encyclopaedia of the social sciences, Volumes 13 & 14.* New York: Macmillan; 1972:545–549, 555–562.

5

Belief Systems: *Religion*

▼ LEARNING OBJECTIVES

The reader will be able to:
● Formulate a definition of religion.
● Explain its functions in the modern world.
● Compare and contrast religious beliefs
  and practices in different social contexts.
● List the perspectives used in the sociology
  of religion.
● Discuss comparatively the role of the nurse
  in meeting the spiritual needs of patients
  from various cultural and religious
  backgrounds.
● Outline some effects of religion on health.

▼ The Nature of Religion

Religion is a mystifying concept that has been
pervading human existence for centuries. To
explain the meanings attached to it is not easy.
Sociologists, anthropologists, philosophers, and
other social scientists have all experienced difficulties in elucidating its nature. Most people tend
to associate the word 'religion' with a certain
belief system. This belief system, when examined
closely, unwraps a multitude of related attributes,
which require scrutiny so that the true nature of
religion can be explained.

North (1973) proposed that, from a sociological viewpoint, religion has two dimensions: the
social aspect and the cultural aspect. The social
aspect includes activities such as being a member
of the church, participating in the activities
organised by the church, and attending mass on
set days. The cultural feature is demonstrated in
the individual interpretation of what one believes
in and commitment to those beliefs. However, as
North argued, the social dimension and the cultural dimension do not necessarily integrate into
each other: church attendance, which is a social
activity, does not necessarily convey a belief in
God; similarly, nonattendance of church does not
imply disbelief in God.

Belief or disbelief in God is a very common
theme when discussing the concept of religion.

Associated with the word 'religion', therefore, are other terminologies used to describe man's relation to divine or superhuman powers, as well as the various organised systems of beliefs and worship in which these relations have been expressed (Chambers Encyclopaedia, 1973).

To belong to a particular system of belief or religion reflects a general human conviction—common to all people and to all stages of culture—of the relations that exist with divine powers. The evidence that people in most societies (from the preliterate to western culture) have maintained a relation with the divine or supernatural is available from anthropologists who have charted the progress of ethnological (the comparative scientific study of human people) knowledge. For example, a form of religion can be identified among the people of Sumatra, the Andaman islanders, and the natives of Tierra del Fuego (Chambers Encyclopaedia, 1973).

As one investigates the nature of religion, the concept becomes even more complex. 'Religious' beliefs and practices are different in various parts of the world. Haynes (1993) pointed out: 'Whereas ethnicity may be defined as the shared characteristics of a racial or cultural group, this tells us little about religion per se. It is clear that no consensus exists as to what religion is.'

The complexity is further increased when one assembles the multitude of definitions provided by social scientists. Anthropologists perceive that religion makes up one component of the 'cultural' aspects of social life, whereas sociologists seek its 'social' rather than its political significance. Theologians, however, promote religion by exposing the doctrine in its 'purest' form and by teaching about the charismatic founder of the religion, be it Moses in Judaism, Jesus in Christianity, or Muhammad in Islam (Haynes, 1993).

However, an awareness of the approaches used by these various groups does not clarify the concept of religion. The search to find an essential ingredient in all religions (e.g. the numinous, or spiritual, experience; the contrast between the sacred and the profane; beliefs in one God or in many gods), so that 'an essence' of religion can be described, is the goal of many students of religion, as well as social theorists.

The sociology of religion is based on the social interpretation of its nature. Emile Durkheim's theory of functionalism, as applied to religion, highlights its social functions: that it is a system of beliefs and rituals concerning the sacred that binds people together into social groups (Abercrombie et al., 1984). In contrast, the sociologist Weber and the theologian Tillich argue that religion is a set of coherent answers to human existential dilemmas—birth, sickness, and death—which make the world meaningful (Abercrombie et al., 1984). However, this latter definition is rather inadequate; it assumes that all people are religious because we all have to face 'existential' problems and are trying to make sense of our worlds.

In attempting to make sense of world phenomena, cultures throughout the world have recourse to religion. Belonging to a particular religion is an attitude that is expressed in the act of worship. In some cultures, for example in the Trobriands, religious rites may become detached from the attitude of worship and these then become 'magical techniques'. Magical techniques or rites are ceremonies performed in some cultures to ward off 'spirits' and 'to supply man with the power and the means to defend himself and, if properly applied, to frustrate all the nefarious attempts of the "mulukwaausi" (the flying witches)' (Malinowski, 1922). In some social contexts, therefore, assessing the true nature of religion can present problems because magic and worship may intermingle.

Other writers, for example Calvert and Calvert (1992), consider that the definition of religion comprises those aspects of life that are beyond proof and hence entail commitment of faith that a certain view of things is true; for example, faith in superdominant beings who possess the power to control and hurt the 'nonsubmissive'. These superdominant beings communicate their power through agents called 'holy men' or priests. Morris (1978) outlined the influence of religions and religious beliefs by describing how 'intelligent' men have succumbed to the pressures and fears generated by images of punishment in the afterworlds; images created by 'holy men' endowed with special powers from the gods.

Although the essence of religion is the concern with submissiveness, faith, love, kindness, and fraternity, there is also a dimension that depicts the breeding of conflicts and violence. Morris (1978) illustrated this viewpoint by asserting that religion breeds sects and sectarian violence, such as that seen in Northern Ireland: 'Despite preaching love and kindness, many religious organisations have a long history of holy wars, repression and intolerance.'

To understand the meaning of religion, therefore, involves the assimilation of the various attributes that encompass its nature. In practice, a religion is a particular system or a set of systems in which doctrines, myths, rituals, sentiments, institutions, and other similar elements are interconnected (New Encyclopaedia Britannica 1992).

▼ Types of Religion

■ ISLAM

The religion of Islam belongs to the Semitic (relating to the languages of Hebrew and Arabic) family, and is known the world over. The doctrines of Islam were disseminated by the Prophet Muhammad in Arabia in the seventh century ad. Islam means 'surrender'. This illuminates the whole concept of Islam and its fundamental principles. Followers of Allah (arabic for God) surrender themselves completely to Him. Allah, in Islamic religion, is the Almighty. He is the sole God—creator, sustainer, and restorer of the world. His will and commandments are written in the Qu'ran (Koran). In Islam, Muhammad is considered to be the last of a series of prophets (including Adam, Noah, Jesus, and others), and his message simultaneously consummates and abrogates the 'revelations' attributed to earlier prophets.

SOME SOCIO-ETHICAL PRINCIPLES BASED ON ISLAMIC BELIEFS

Islam promotes the institution of marriage. The family therefore forms the core structure; '[it] is central to Muslim life and Muslim society' (Henley, 1982). The foundation of this centrality is found in the scriptures of the Qu'ran. These recommend the practice of accepting the value of the family, its role as 'a source of support, love and security'. The Qu'ran specifies the type of behaviour expected of a Muslim; his or her role, obligations, and rights. Muslims believes that they are controlled by the power of Allah and that all men and women are His servants. Celibacy is discouraged as much as possible by the Qu'ran, except in exceptional circumstances —'resorted to only under economic stringency' (New Encyclopaedia Britannica, 1992).

There are some religious duties that Muslims are expected to perform in accordance with the Islamic scriptures: they have to believe in Allah, participate in daily prayer, fast during Ramzan (Ramadan—the ninth month of the Muslim year throughout which a strict fast is observed during the hours of daylight), give alms, and go on a pilgrimage to Mecca (the believed birthplace of the Prophet Muhammad and the holiest city of the Muslim world).

Henley (1982) described some other fundamental principles that guide the behaviour of the Muslim by referring to the Sharia—the Islamic legal system evolved by scholars and based entirely on the Qu'ran and on the recorded sayings and actions of the Prophet Muhammad. To the Muslim, therefore, adhering to the Holy Scriptures of the Qu'ran is the ultimate acceptable form of religious behaviour.

CHRISTIANITY

Whereas the Prophet Muhammad spread the content of the Holy Scriptures from the Qu'ran to the Muslims, in Christian religion it was Jesus of Nazareth—the Christ or Anointed One of God—who preached the Holy Scriptures of the Bible to the people. Christianity is believed to have been founded by Jesus in the first century AD, and it is considered to be the world's largest religion.

The focus of Christianity is founded on the faith in the Lord Jesus. Jesus is seen as God's messenger; hence, He is God's follower and has the power and charisma expected of a religious leader. Christians sometimes refer to Jesus as the Messiah ('deliverer'). To practise the Christian religion, therefore, is to worship Jesus. He is the agent of redemption (the saving or delivering of oneself from sin or damnation). Redemption is achieved by religious practices: attending church, praying, fasting, reading the Bible, and following the Ten Commandments, and by demonstrating in various ways that one is a good Christian by acknowledging the presence of God in the Lord Jesus.

There is also the understanding that God has created Man in His own image. 'This idea views God and humans joined with one another through a mysterious connection. God is thought of as incomprehensible and beyond substance; yet God desired to reflect the divine image in one set of creatures and chose humans for this' (New Encyclopaedia Britannica,1992).

In Christianity, the agent responsible for spreading the gospel is the church, with all its groups of believers who support its functions, beliefs, doctrines, and culture.

BUDDHISM

Buddhism originated from India and is one of the well known world religions. It is categorised into the School Of Elders in southern Asia and the later Mahayana in northern Asia.

The essence of Buddhism is based on enlightment; Buddha is the Enlightened One. The teachings of Buddha are founded on the search for the four Truths: the fact of pain or ill; that pain has a cause; that pain can be ended; and the Noble Eightfold Way leading to a state of peace, 'Nirvana', which is the attainment of perfect serenity through the control and abolition of desires.

The fundamental doctrines of Buddhism are beliefs in:

- *Karma*: the belief that any actions or deeds on this earth are met with future rewards or punishment.
- *Rebirth*: one is reborn to experience the fruits of past deeds in either a happy or painful new existence.

In Buddhism there is no belief in the permanent self. The aim of the Noble Eightfold Way is to break the chain of karma, binding the individual to rebirth by attaining Nirvana, when the body is finally dissociated (*Hutchinson 20th Century Encyclopaedia, 7th ed.*, 1987).

■ HINDUISM

Hinduism refers to the religion practised by the Hindus (originally, the inhabitants of the land of the Indus River). Hinduism encompasses the worship of many gods and local deities. However, the core of the religion does not depend on the existence or nonexistence of God, or whether there is one God or many. It is an amalgamation of religions. In contrast with Islam (founded by the Prophet Muhammad) and Christianity (founded by Jesus of Nazareth), Hinduism has no founder; it has no church, no central decision-making organisation to prescribe religious dogmas or uniform rules for all its followers; it has no authoritative body to reject certain beliefs or practices as heretical and non-Hindu (Henley, 1983).

The Veda is the ancient body of religious literature for the Hindus; it contains the essence of Hinduism. However, although some Hindus— especially those who are traditionally oriented— may refer to the Veda, it appears that the majority rarely quote the book: 'It is seldom drawn upon for literal information or advice; but is venerated from a distance' (*Encyclopaedia Britannica*, 1992). The content of the Veda is, nevertheless, still influential in socialising the Hindus into the spirit of Hinduism.

The Brahmans constitute another component of Hinduism. Brahmans are priests who promote the scriptures of the Veda. Their aim is to preserve the purity of Hinduism and to encourage Hindus to follow the message of the Veda. Hindus have the highest respect for the Brahmans; they believe that Brahmans have Holy Powers and represent the best role models of social status and religious purity.

SOME BELIEFS AND PRACTICES IN HINDUISM

According to Henley (1983), Hindus believe in one Ultimate Reality, one Supreme Spirit. This spirit is the life force that resides in every human being. To the Hindus, the Brahmans may represent the Supreme Spirit. However, this Supreme Spirit has no gender and cannot be described in any way because it has no particular features. Its presence pervades throughout human life and the world.

There are three main gods in Hinduism— Brahma, Vishnuo and Shiva—which together constitute the Trimurti (Hindu Trinity). These gods symbolise the cyles of life in general: Brahma symbolises Creation; Vishnu, Preservation; and Shiva, Destruction. Hence, in life there is growth, preservation, decay, and death.

Other beliefs include:

- *Karma*:   how one's deeds or actions in one's present life will be evaluated on rebirth; if one's actions are praiseworthy, appropriate rewards will be obtained in the afterlife.

- *Ahimsa*:   fundamental in Hinduism is the concept of 'noninjury' or the avoidance of killing; it is sacrilege to kill a cow in India; to kill a cow to eat its flesh goes against the belief of ahimsa; to some extent ahimsa is related to vegetarianism; to avoid eating meat is to practise one's belief in ahimsa.

- *Dharma*:   proper behaviour according to one's status is important; a Hindu is expected to pray daily and to worship and respect the gods; respect is also expected to be shown towards the elders, priests, and teachers, as well as to parents; this duty is known as dharma.

The maintenance of self-purity by avoiding certain agents and contact with certain people is another aim of the practising Hindu. Fluids or substances excreted from the body are considered impure. Water and fire are considered to be purification agents and are utilised accordingly in some religious ceremonies. It is common practice for Hindus to wash themselves prior to praying.

The fundamentals of Hinduism are intricate in nature. To understand Hinduism is also to gain insight into the culture and social framework of a complex society.

▼ Perspectives on Religion

■ THE FUNCTIONALIST PERSPECTIVE

A leading figure in the study of religion, and quoted by many writers, is Emile Durkheim. Durkheim (1961) *Elementary forms of religious life,* argued that religious beliefs are classified into two groups: the 'sacred' and the 'profane', or the 'religious' and the 'secular'. The sacred, in Durkheim's view, is concerned with any concepts an individual in a particular culture perceives to be the representation of something. Hence, this category not only includes symbolic concepts—for example, deities to be venerated—but also objects such as a tree, a mountain, an ornament, or an animal.

Durkheim illustrated his argument by drawing upon his knowledge of Australian Aborigines. He pointed out how a 'totem' (a natural object, especially an animal, adopted by North American Indians as an emblem of a clan or an individual) becomes a sacred symbol for the Aborigines; it becomes the outward and visible form of the totemic principle or God (Haralambos, 1985). God is an invisible personality, incomprehensible and powerful; the totemic symbol provides a more visible, realistic, and tangible form that can be worshipped through a ritualistic process. The totem is also a representation of the beliefs of the clan. The rit-

uals that accompany the worship of the totem make it sacred. 'Durkheim treated the totem as symbolic of the God; he inferred that the God is a personification of the clan' (Encyclopaedia Britannica, 1992). Since God is a personification of the clan made visible by the totem, it is argued that the Aborigines are indirectly worshipping society (the society of the Aboriginal clan). In Kpelle in west Africa, group totems are used in the form of animals. These animals are said to be the residence of the ancestors; accordingly, they are well respected and are given offerings.

Although the theory put forward by Durkheim enlightens the reader about the possible sources and explanation of religion from a sociological and theoretical perspective, a counter argument is provided by Tyler (1970) *Religion in Primitive culture.* He was opposed to the idea that totems are the basis of religion and saw totemism as people's attempt to classify the world and its phenomena.

FUNCTIONALIST INTERPRETATION OF THE FUNCTIONS OF RELIGION

Functionalists argue that religion functions by causing group cohesion and integration. According to Durkheim, people in society exhibit a degree of cohesiveness and integration among themselves because they share the same beliefs, have the same values, and express similar attitudes in their understanding of environmental phenomena. The rituals, ceremonies, and sociocultural practices that form part of the particular belief system are social expressions of a 'collective consciousness'; for example, the church congregation on a Sunday morning is a display of group solidarity, shared values, and consensus about one belief system in the institution of religion. Functionalists such as Durkheim interpret this solidarity as the factor that empowers the people to maintain social integration, thus ensuring group cohesion. The anthropologist Malinowski (1954) made a similar argument to support his theory of the social solidarity created by religion. However, it is argued (Haralambos, 1985) that the approach used by Durkheim in showing the positiveness of religion can only be applied to small-scale societies; in a large multicultural society, social solidarity is not easily achieved because there may be a variety of belief systems.

Other functions of religion from a functionalist perspective may be summarised as follows:

- It is a sociocultural concept that contains knowledge and principles regarding form of conduct.
- It provides the means by which human action can be evaluated in terms of what is right or wrong; it acts as a guiding principle.
- Some values and beliefs contained in religion support the beliefs found in the legal system. As Haralambos (1985) commented, 'Thou shall not kill' is a commandment that influences the integration of beliefs into the value system: 'The norms that direct these areas of behaviour prohibit manslaughter, murder and euthanasia.'
- Religion provides the framework of consensus that helps to maintain order and stability in society.
- It is a tonic to self-confidence, by allowing tension and frustration to be moderated through rituals and religious ceremonies (Haralambos, 1985).
- Religion, according to Talcott Parsons, provides meaning to problems (e.g. suffering, exploitation, and oppression).

The major argument against the functionalist view of religion is the obvious display of social disorder that occurs in the world because of religious organisations in conflict, for example the Catholics and Protestants in Northern Ireland: 'On every side it would seem that religion threatens social integration as readily as it contributes it.

The history of Christianity, with its many schisms, manifests the great power of religion not merely to bind but to divide' (Haralambos, 1985).

■ THE MARXIST PERSPECTIVE

Marx's view of religion in society is concerned with the 'illusory' element of its nature; an illusion experienced by the masses, in particular the oppressed and the exploited. In religion, Marx argued, the proletariat find the rationale for their present depressed social situation. To become religious or to become a member of a religious organisation is an 'expression of a real distress and the protest against the real distress'. According to Marx, the real distress is found in the exploitative nature of capitalist society. Religion 'clouds the consciousness of the people'; it is an ideology that reflects the value system and beliefs of the upper class. To criticise religion, therefore, is to criticise the present state of affairs and expose the truth of human conditions.

The Marxist approach emphasises that social change can only be carried out through political struggles, rather than by relying on religion to deal with one's oppressed state.

MARXIST INTERPRETATION OF THE FUNCTIONS OF RELIGION

- Religion functions by dulling the pain of oppression.
- It provides a justification for social order, by stating and explaining why society is the way it is.
- It is one of the tools used by capitalist society to maintain the ideology (the collective beliefs that help to legitimise or delegitimise social order).
- It is an instrument of oppression.
- It helps to maintain a false class-consciousness.
- It has a gentling and controlling influence.

WEBERIAN INTERPRETATION OF THE FUNCTIONS OF RELIGION

- Religion functions by exposing a particular aspect of the world.
- The principles and guidelines obtained from religion motivate people to evaluate their social environment and to assess its meanings. Because religion represents principles and guidelines about human conduct, an understanding of their meanings direct people's action into appropriate channels.
- Religion and beliefs are linked with the spirit of capitalism and profit-making; religion provides the driving force behind business enterprise.
- Religion influences capitalism; for example, it highlights the 'Protestant ethics', which glorify the benefit of hard work for the 'glory of God'.

▼ Secularisation

Secularisation may be defined as nonreligious beliefs and practices, shown in a lack of church attendance and a lack of belief in one God or many gods. Calvert and Calvert (1992) made reference to how it involves a loss of religion's social significance. Abercrombie and Warde (1988) noted a decline in individual adherence to Christian religious belief evident by the number of people regularly attending church. They quoted statistics that showed that the Christian churches had lost 1.3 million members between 1970 and 1985. The reasons for this decline, they argue, are related to disempowerment of the church—caused by the state being more in control—and a lack of political involvement by the clergy. This does not mean, however, that the church has lost power altogether; there are still many religious-oriented groups, rituals, and ceremonies that reflect obedience to principles of religious beliefs and practices.

Another factor that may have contributed to the decline in adherence to religious institutions is the behaviour exhibited by some members of the clergy. The media fairly frequently broadcast various 'misdemeanours' committed by vicars and priests: 'Bishop forced to speak out by gay group' (The Independent, March 1995); 'Bishop says he is willing to ordain homosexuals' (The Independent, March 1995). Allegations of child abuse and other sex and financial scandals may also contribute to the situation.

Smith (1992), in a survey report of the aftereffects of the US Televangelists Scandals of 1987–1988, concluded that 'a series of sex and financial scandals and several lesser controversies' had rocked public opinion of televangelism and American Protestantism. One member was caught in sex and money improprieties and was later convicted; another member was exposed hiring prostitutes for pornographic purposes. Smith's survey (1992) revealed a decline in the rating of televangelists as 'trustworthy' from 41% in 1980, to 23% in 1987 after the first scandal broke, to 16% in 1989 near the end of the disclosures. Other after-effects were noticeable in standard religious activity: church membership dropped from 69% in 1986 and 1987, to 65% in 1988; and the per cent who prayed daily fell from 58% in 1985, to 53% in 1989. Smith's findings are disturbing; it is possible that similar nonreligious, scandalous activities are covertly taking place but go undiscovered, only occasionally reaching public notice.

There are other possible factors that may lead to secularisation. Abercrombie and Warde (1988), for example, explained that the family may have become the milieu in which the individual expresses his or her beliefs at a very personal level, although church attendance is nonexistent or minimal. Bilton et al. (1987), on the other hand, argued that scientific advances may have been a precipitating factor in the advent of secularisation: people's reliance is now on modern technology that can solve problems more speedily, with greater ease, control, and efficiency, and to an increasingly higher standard.

Whatever the reasons for secularisation may be, there is evidence that, in some parts of the world today, religiosity is declining in intensity. Gellner (1992), however, argued that there is an exception to this rule—Islam: 'To say that secularisation prevails in Islam is not contentious. It is simply false. Islam is as strong now as it was a century ago. In some ways it is probably stronger.' Secularisation, therefore, can only be observed among some groups in the modern world. To what extent secular practices will continue to erode the foundations of traditional religious institutions is difficult to predict.

▼ Sects and Cults

Sects are small groupings, detached initially from the main church organisations: for example, the Sufis and Shiites are sectarian organisations separate from Islam in eastern countries; Calvinists and Methodists are sects in western culture. Sects have their own religious beliefs, but can show opposition to established groups and demand higher standards of their members (Calvert & Calvert, 1992). Sects are normally classified as 'new religious movements' or 'alternative religions'.

Whenever the word 'cult' is used, it conjures up images of mystical groups that exert control and use coercive behaviour to manipulate people. According to Richardson (1993), it was Troeltsch (1931) who developed the term as 'something of a residual category in his theoretical scheme of religious forms in western cul-

ture'. Richardson (1978) defined the term 'cult' as follows:

> A cult is usually defined as a small informal group lacking a definite authority structure, somewhat spontaneous in its development (although often possessing a somewhat charismatic leader or group of leaders), transitory, somewhat mystical and individualistically oriented, and deriving its inspiration and ideology from outside the predominant religious culture.

Examples of such informal groups include the People's Temple, the Unification Church (Moonies), the Church of Scientology, and the Hare Krishnas. As mentioned above, the image of these organisations perceived by most people is one of coercion and even of fear:

> Devious and coercive practices are identified popularly as the means by which these groups maintain members' allegiance to such deviant standards. Concerned parents, official religious leaders, and others in mainstream culture continue to be troubled by the perceived threat of these groups (Cartwright & Kent, 1992).

The anxieties generated by cult groups are so great that 'countercult' groups are sometimes formed. The aims of these anticult groups are to kidnap members (sometimes of their families) who have joined the cult movement, to deprogramme them, and to use 'intense confrontation' in their attempts to deconvert them.

The research carried out by Barker (1993) into the Moonies, however, presents a different perspective on this organisation:

> There is no evidence that any kind of coercion is used by the Moonies, or that the diet or workshop activities seriously impair the biological functionings of the guests to the extent that they would be judged incapable of behaving 'normally' were they in another social environment at the time.

▼ Summary

The concept of religion is a mystifying one. It consists of many features that depend on the sociocultural context being considered. Christianity, Islam, and Hinduism are some religions in the world today. Each is structured differently and contains a variety of sectarian movements. Beliefs are often based on religious scriptures, which often contain the moral and legal guidelines that the believer should follow. Hinduism is based on the worship of many deities. Christians believe in God who made Man according to His image. Jesus of Nazareth (the 'Messiah') is the Son of God, who, according to legend, came to preach the gospel. Islamic religion is founded on the belief that there is only one God (Allah) and one prophet (Muhammad) (see p.53). The scriptures of Islam are embodied in the Qu'ran (Koran).

Sociologists have attempted to explain religion from different perspectives: functionalism and ideology (conflict theory—i.e. Marxism and the Weberian theory). Religion has many functions in society. According to functionalists, it stimulates group cohesiveness and social integration. On the other hand, it can be seen as an ideology that 'clouds the consciousness' of the people: Marx referred to it as 'the opium of the people'. Another interpretation is that it is people's way of explaining an aspect of their social world.

It is believed that religion is losing its force in the world. The term used is 'secularisation'. The theories of secularisation are based on: religion's loss of social significance, as evidenced by a reduction in church attendance; a loss of influence by the church; the arrival of scientific advances that explain natural phenomena and ease the manner in which problems are dealt with; the negative image of the clergy resulting from scandals about sex, pornography, and child abuse.

Sects and cults are terms used when referring to new religious movements. Sects and cults are small groups that are separate from the main organised groups of churches. Cults are perceived by many as mystical, coercive organisations that exercise social control over their groups and that are the source of fears and anxieties for families whose members have been recruited. Compared with cults, sects have a more positive image.

▼ Application to Clinical Practice

■ PRINCIPLES OF CARE

Caring for patients, either in hospital or in their own homes, involves a thorough understanding of their basic religious or spiritual needs. Each individual possesses a set of values, which may include belief systems very different to our own. Attempting to gain knowledge of these beliefs and empathising with the patients will facilitate therapeutic interactions. Religious beliefs influence and control the behaviour of the devout believer. Sometimes patients may appear to be uncooperative, such as refusing to take medication when it is evident to the nurse that they are in pain. As McGee (1992) asserted, communicating effectively with the patient will ensure that potential misunderstandings do not occur. Sometimes communication may be impossible because the patient has no knowledge of the English language and the nurse is unable to communicate in the patient's language. In these circumstances, one should resort to an appropriate interpreter.

MUSLIMS IN HEALTHCARE SETTINGS

Admission to hospital is a frightening experience for any individual, from whatever sociocultural background. However, for practising Muslims, the healthcare environment may have constraining effects on their religious practice and interfere with their beliefs. There are several aspects that the nurse must consider to ensure that the patient's requirements are met:

● The need to pray.
● The need to fast.
● The need to maintain family contact.
● Dietary needs.
● The need to maintain dignity and privacy.

1 The need to pray. The Holy Qu'ran specifies five daily prayers: after dawn, around noon, in the mid-afternoon, early evening (after sunset), and at night (Henley, 1982). It is important for Muslims to wash before praying, thus ensuring physical cleanliness. The nurse should discuss with patients the times of day they are planning to pray and their need to wash, so that appropriate provisions may be made. The need to wash before prayer often requires special facilities in British institutions (Henley, 1982). Anticipating the patient's need, by providing a bowl of water at set times if the patient is bedridden or ensuring that the bathroom is available after toiletting, will help prevent any psychological distress. Muslim men and women will be reluctant to pray if they feel unclean. This is likely to happen if the patient has used a commode or bedpan after defecation and is not provided with any washing facilities. It may also happen following certain procedures when items of clothing are soiled with blood or other body fluids. If the patient is ambulant, a shower is recommended.

Certain patients may be exempt from daily prayers: those who are seriously ill (Henley, 1982), those with mental illhealth, and women for 40 days postnatally.

2 The need to fast. Muslims need to fast during Ramzan (Ramadan), the ninth month of the Muslim year. Fasting is a way of their spiritual life. Muslims are socialised into the practice of fasting at a very early age. It is one way of showing their commitment to the Holy Qu'ran; it also demonstrates self-discipline and helps them 'to share and understand the suffering of the poor and hungry' (Henley, 1982). During the 29–30 days of Ramzan, Muslims abstain from food, including liquid, between dawn and sunset. They do, however, eat before starting the fast and at the end, after sunset.

Patients whose health status is in jeopardy need to be reassured that they are exempt from fasting because it is stated in the Qu'ran. Certain patients, for example those with diabetes, require close observation by the nurse, as they may become hypoglycaemic. Patients who are severely dehydrated will require intravenous infusion to stabilise their fluid and electrolyte balance. It is the role of the nurse to explain the rationale for the nursing intervention and to reassure the patient that fasting may be undertaken once health is regained.

If fasting is allowed, it is important to discuss with the patient how essential it is for them to report any adverse effects of this practice, so that nursing staff can act appropriately. Involving the patient's relatives in the care will encourage communication and improve interactions with healthcare professionals.

3 The need to maintain family contact. The family has an essential role to play in maintaining social support, love, and security: 'The family is central to Muslim life and to Muslim society' (Henley, 1982). To ensure that family ties are not severed, a system of open visiting may be set up after having negotiated with the patient's relatives regarding their specific needs. Encouraging visiting by the family will help the patient to keep in touch with the out-side world.

4 Dietary needs. There are some dietary observations that have implications in healthcare settings. A Muslim will not eat meat that has not been prepared in 'a ritual humane way' (McAvoy & Donaldson, 1990). Halal meat comes from animals killed with a quick cutting of the throat while invoking the name of Allah and draining all the blood away before cooking (McAvoy & Donaldson, 1990). Patients are likely to refuse food provided by the kitchen staff of a hospital or by the meals-on-wheels service in the com-munity. Patients deal with this problem by using food provided by relatives. Again, it is the nurse's role to discuss with the patient and relatives the types of food that may be brought in.

Certain dietary products are completely for-bidden: pork and its products, fish without fins or scales, alcohol, and blood (McAvoy & Donaldson, 1990). Some types of insulin are manufactured from pork products; also, many medications contain alcohol. Finding alternative medications should be considered. In situations where this is not possible, McAvoy and Donaldson (1990) suggested involving the 'Immam' or priest, who will reassure the patient to take the medications.

5 Dignity and privacy. Muslim women do not usually fully undress for physical examination, but uncover only parts of themselves at a time (Henley, 1982). It is preferable for the examining profes-sional to be female, as this will help the patient to feel more at ease and she will be more likely to communicate readily. Some women may wear jew-ellery that has a deep religious significance, for example an amulet or a medallion containing words from the Qu'ran. Physical contact between men and women who are not husband and wife is forbidden. However, contact between members of the same sex shows friendship, support, and understanding (Henley, 1982).

Ensuring privacy for personal washing rituals is important. During menstruation, women con-sider themselves 'unclean' and do not pray. However, their preoccupation with keeping themselves clean may cause anxiety if washing facilities are not available. Privacy and dignity should also be maintained by ensuring that patients are not given clothing with an open back (e.g. a theatre gown).

It is important to be aware of the procedure to follow in situations of dying and death. The dying patient needs the presence and comfort of relatives, who will recite verses from the Qu'ran. The patient, if possible, should be positioned so that his or her face is turned towards Mecca. Seeking the advice of the family or a religious leader from the Mosque may be necessary. On death, the body should not be touched by non-Muslims; wearing gloves to carry out any proce-dures (e.g. removing an intravenous cannula or a nasogastric tube) is advisable. The family should be consulted if other nursing interventions are required (Henley, 1982).

HINDUS IN HEALTHCARE SETTINGS

The requirements of the Hindu while in hospital or in community care are, in some aspects, quite similar to those of the Muslim. The holistic needs of the individual must be considered. The needs for cleanliness and the sustainment of purity must be observed. A shower is preferred to a bath; lying in a bath is seen as impure because it means soaking oneself with water that contains dirt from the body. Washing and clean-ing before praying are rituals of the devout Hindu. The use of toilet paper after defecation is not a favoured practice; Hindus would prefer to use water to wash themselves. Offering the patient a jug of water or any other alternative that satisfies his or her needs is recommended.

The bedridden patient will require much reassurance and support. The nurse should empathise and allow the patient to express any particular needs related to religious practices.

Food provided in hospital may not be readily accepted by the patient as the content is unknown. Most Hindus do not eat meat or fish or anything made from these products (Henley, 1982). Hindus will not eat food served with utensils that have been used for dishing out other food such as gravy and meat stews. Many hospitalised Hindu patients will have their meals prepared by their relatives.

CHRISTIANS IN HEALTHCARE SETTINGS

To ensure that the spiritual needs of Christian patients are met, on admission the nurse should ask about any particular religious practices. If, for example, the patient expresses a need to attend mass, this may be arranged with the hospital chaplain. Most hospitals have a small chapel where patients who are not seriously ill or bedridden can go for prayers and to receive Holy Communion (the Eucharist: the Christian sacrament commemorating the Last Supper in which bread and wine are consecrated and consumed). For the seriously ill or bedbound, the nurse should discuss with the patient and relatives the possibility of arranging for the chaplain to carry out a small ceremony on the ward, in the privacy of a sideroom.

Most hospital wards will have a small Bible in the locker. However, some patients may find the particular edition not suitable for their needs; therefore it is courteous of the nurse to ask the patients if they would prefer to bring their own Bible.

The devout Christian wears a crucifix around the neck. If it is necessary to remove it (i.e., preoperatively), one should explain to the patient the rationale behind this request and ask his or her permission or, if communication is impaired due to illness, ask the permission of the family.

Christians have other beliefs and practices regarding dying and death, and some dietary restrictions. The nurse should discuss the various needs patients may have with the hospital chaplain.

■ THE IMPACT OF RELIGION ON HEALTH

In 1910, Professor Osler made a tentative reference to faith and its effect on health in the *British Medical Journal:* 'The most characteristic development of Christian faith healing has been in connection with certain saints and shrines'. He elaborated on the concept with evidence from the cures witnessed by many people after visiting the most popular faith resort in Lourdes: 'More people, it is said, frequent Lourdes than all the hospitals of France, and the same is true in Canada of the most popular shrine of the New World—St Anne de Beaupré.'

Can religion affect health? Troyer (1988) studied the life styles of four religious groups (Seventh Day Adventists, Mormons, Hutterites, and the Amish) and related them to their incidence of cancer. His findings can be summarised as follows:

● Breast cancer was significantly reduced among Mormons.
● All four religious groups studied had greatly reduced rates for lung cancer.
● There was a deficit of bladder cancer among Seventh Day Adventists.
● Rates for ovarian cancer were lower than expected in all four groups.

The health perspective is connected to dietary and personal habits. As Troyer stated (1988), the Seventh Day Adventists have a well-defined dietary code that is strongly advocated by the church and widely followed by its constituency. For example, they do not eat meat, poultry, or fish, and they especially avoid pork and other biblically 'unclean' meats; the consumption of coffee, tea, and alcohol is prohibited; smoking is discouraged. Their dietary habits consist of the consumption of health-promoting food: fresh fruit, vegetables, nuts, and whole grain. These dietary practices may well contribute towards their state of health.

Although dietary practices vary across the groups studied (for example, the Amish and Hutterites have no dietary restrictions), Troyer, having assessed the other possible variables such as socio-economic and demographic considerations, concluded that their dietary habits resulted in 'reduced overall rates of cancer, suggesting that the lifestyles of all four groups have merit in terms of reducing the overall risk of cancer'.

The dietary needs of individuals are important aspects of care. As described above, there are many factors—beliefs, values, rituals—that become part of certain groups' religious practices. Regardful of their own beliefs and practices, healthcare professionals have the responsibility to implement care that will objectively match individual needs. A holistic approach embodies all the dimensions that impinge on the person's sociopsychological, physical, and spiritual life.

▼ Review Questions

1 Examine the concept of religion and discuss the perspectives used by sociologists to explain its nature.

2 Describe how religious groups require specific care interventions in clinical practice.

▼ References

Abercrombie N, Hill S, Turner B. *A dictionary of sociology*. London: Penguin; 1984:207.

Abercrombie N, Warde A. *Contemporary British society*. Cambridge: Polity Press; 1988.

Barker E. The making of a Moonie: choice or brainwashing? (1984) In: O'Donnell M, ed. *New introductory reader in sociology*. Walton-on-Thames: Nelsons; 1993:449–457.

Bilton T, *et al. Introductory sociology: 2nd ed*. London: Macmillan; 1987.

Calvert S, Calvert P. *Sociology today*. Education and belief systems. Hemel Hempstead: Harvester Wheatsheaf; 1992:215–222.

Cartwright R, Kent S. Social control in alternative religions: a familial perspective. *Sociological Analysis* 1992, **53**(4):345–361.

Chambers Encyclopaedia. Vol. **11** 'Religion'. London: ILSC; 1973, 586–587.

Durkheim E. *Elementary forms of the religious life*. London: Collier Books; 1961.

Gellner E. Post modernism: reasons and religion. (1992) In: O'Donnell M, ed. *New introductory reader in sociology*. Walton-on-Thames: Nelson and Sons; 1992:443–448.

Haralambos M. *Sociology: themes and perspectives*. London: Unwin Hyman; 1985.

Haynes J. *Religion in Third World politics.* Milton Keynes: Open University Press; 1993.

Henley A. *Asians in Britian: caring for Muslims and their families.* Cambridge: NEC; 1982.

Henley A. *Asians in Britain: caring for Hindus and their families.* Cambridge; NEC; 1983.

Hutchinson 20th Century Encyclopaedia *7th ed 'Buddhism'.* Horsley E. ed. London: Hutchinson; 1987, 205–207.

Malinowski B. *Argonauts of the Western Pacific: an account of native enterprise and adventures in the Archipelagoes.* London: Routledge & Kegan Paul; 1922.

Malinowski B. *Magic, science, religion and other essays.* New York: Anchor Books; 1954.

McAvoy B, Donaldson L. *Health care for Asians.* Oxford: Oxford University Press, (1990).

McGee P. *Teaching transcultural care.* London: Chapman & Hall; 1992.

Morris D. *Man watching*—Religious displays. London: Grafton; 1978.

New Encyclopaedia Britannica (Macropaedia). Christianity. Chicago: University Chicago; 1992, **16**:251–254; ibid **20**:519–525; ibid **22**:1–44; ibid **26**:509–510.

North P. *People in society — An introduction to sociology.* London: Longman; 1973:189–194.

Osler W. The faith that heals. *Br Med J* 1910, **18**:1470–1472.

Parsons T. *The social system.* New York: Free Press; 1951.

Richardson. An oppositional and conceptualisation of cult. *Annual Review of the Social Sciences of Religion* 1978, **2**:29–52.

Richardson J. Definitions of cult, from sociological-technical to popular–negative. *Review of Religious Research* 1993, **34**:348–356.

Smith T. The polls: poll trends. Religious beliefs and behaviours and the Televangelist Scandals of 1987–1988. *Public Opinion Quarterly* 1992, **56**:360–380.

Troeltsch E. *The social teachings of the Christian Chuches.* New York: MacMillan; 1931.

Troyer H. Review of cancer among four religious sects: evidence that life styles are distinctive sets of risk factors. *Soc Sci Med* 1988, **26**:1007–1017.

Tyler E. *Religion in Primitive culture.* Gloucester: Peter Smith; 1970.

▼ Further Reading

Hickling F, Griffith E. Clinical perspectives on the Rastafari movement. *Hosp Community Psychiatry* 1994, **45**:49–53.

Kliger R. Somatization: social control and illness production in a religious cult. *Culture Med Psychiatry* 1994, **18**:215–245.

Koenig H. Research on religion and mental health in later life: a review and commentary. *J Geriatr Psychiatry* 1990, **23**:23–53.

Levin J, Schiller P. Is there a religious factor in health? *J Religion Health* 1987, **26**:9–36.

Vanderpool H, Levin J. Religion and medicine: how are they related? *J Religion Health* 1990, **29**:9–20.

6

Organisations and Work in Society

▼ LEARNING OBJECTIVES

The reader will be able to:
- Distinguish the main features of organisations in society.
- Discuss the concepts of bureaucracy as applied to systems of organisations.
- Compare and contrast perspectives on organisations.
- Define the nature of work.
- Outline work processes in society.
- Describe the meaning and significance of work.

▼ Organisations

■ CHARACTERISTICS OF ORGANISATIONS

In setting a framework for a definition of 'organisation', Silverman (1987) identified two distinguishing features: their 'formal' and 'social' aspects. By 'formal', Silverman meant organisations like the military and the Church, and enterprises such as ICI, the Health Service, MI5, Scotland Yard, etc.; the 'social' (or informal) component of organisations refers to families, friendship groups, communities, and so on. The focus of this chapter is on the formal aspects of organisational structures: their features, and the theories put forward to explain their features and their aims in society.

Organisations in any society have set aims to achieve. One can argue that organisations are born as a direct consequence of a particular need of a society—for example, health. Silverman (1987) proposed that, to achieve the goals stated, formal organisations formulate rules and guidelines 'designed to anticipate and to shape behaviour in the direction of these goals'. He listed three main features of organisations:

- Organisations arise at a particular point in time. They have definite purposes, and their founders define the rules and aims. The process involves the exercise of authority by management and a system of communication.

- The participants in an organisation seek to coordinate and control. Their relationships follow set patterns, according to their roles and fuctions—not to be underestimated.
- The concern of the organisation is to discuss and execute any planned changes in social relations; also, to examine the 'rules of the game'.

Stewart (1991), although agreeing that one central feature of organisations is the 'collective achievement of goals', stressed their complex nature, the result of the multitude of activities and functions they perform. For example, the Health Service comprises many different organisations—such as community health councils, the hospital service, the general practitioners' service—each with its own specialised function. Stewart (1991) explored the other common characteristics of organisations:

- The structure.
- The policies, rules, and procedures, including the decision-making and communication systems.
- The technology.
- The people.
- The environment of the organisation.

The structure refers to the organisation of labour: who does what, where, and when. Structure also encompasses the specialties of various departments and the professionals with the expertise to perform these specialised tasks. For instance, the biochemistry department of a hospital is differentiated from the haematology department; the operating theatre undertakes different functions to a scanner unit or an intensive-care department. These multifaceted functions make the organisational structure more complex. According to Stewart (1991),

structures are easy to alter by managers, who can reallocate jobs, regroup departments, or centralise and decentralise.

All organisations have rules and procedures to guide the workers and, to some extent, to control and coordinate behaviour. For example, the Health Service obtains its directives from the Department of Health in government, which is also an important part of the policy-making machinery.

Technology is another aspect of the complex framework of organisations. Computerisation affects the structure of an organisation. Technology demands technical skills. It is therefore essential that work is allocated according to relevant skills and experience. This may involve the setting up of a Resource Technology Centre within the organisation. According to Stewart (1991), technology 'offers more choice in the form of organisation because it can make either more centralisation or decentralisation possible'.

People are the most important resources in any organisation. They affect the way in which even the most clearly designed organisation will work in practice (Stewart, 1991). The interactions between the people, the technology, and the overall organisations are complex, and must not be underestimated or ignored. Some writers (Silverman, 1980; Stewart, 1991) have made reference to the theory of socio technical systems—the relationships between the worker, the organisation (technology), and the environment—which emphasises the humanistic nature of organisations.

▼ Theoretical Perspectives of Organisations

∎ TALCOTT PARSONS

Talcott Parsons (1960) viewed an organisation as: 'A broad type of collectivity that has assumed a particularly important place in modern industrial societies—the type to which the term "bureaucracy" is most often applied.' To Parsons, an organisation is another system in the social system, with specific goals to attain. He saw this aspect as the defining characteristic of an organisation. He argued that there is a relation between the organisation and other systems in society; for example, an organisation manufacturing intravenous infusion pumps, blood arterial lines, and other technical items, will relate with the Health Service to sell its products, the Health Service being the other organisation or system.

To carry out its functions and attain its goals, an organisation needs to make use of resources. Parsons (1960) identified these as land, labour, and capital. Furthermore, for an organisation to succeed, it requires power. 'The mobilization and utilization of power is the central focus of the operations of organizations' (Parsons, 1960). Power is obtained by consensus as to society's value systems. If, for example, society values health as an essential commodity, and the goal of the organisation is to prevent illhealth and promote health, resources will be mobilised for the benefit of the organisation to enable it to achieve its goal. Power is obtained both outside and within the organisation. As Parsons (1960) put it: 'Every organization, whatever the nature of its functional primacy—for example manufacturing or medical care—is part of the polity and a generator of power, but is also a recipient of the power generated at higher echelons in the polity.'

Parsons (1960) also identified types of organisations according to their particular functions in society. Thus there are organisations whose specific goals are to maintain the integrity of the economic system; for example, manufacturing industries, ICI, gas companies, and so on. Other organisations have set objectives in 'the generation and allocation of power in the society', such as governmental departments. Parsons (1960) also identified organisations with integrative and pattern maintenance functions. The courts and the legal profession fit in the former category; churches and schools are examples of the latter.

Parsons' (1960) interpretation of organisational structures is based on their functions in society, their roles in the attainment of specific goals.

∎ MAX WEBER

Max Weber's perspective of organisations is centred on the concept of their 'bureaucratic' nature. Weber (1946) identified the characteristics of bureaucratic organisations as follows:

- They are governed by principles of administrative rules.
- Official duties are the essence of their activities.
- The officials have the authority to command the implementation of such activities.
- Duties are fulfilled in a methodical way by people who possess relevant qualifications.
- Bureaucracy segregates official activity from the sphere of private life.
- The bureaucratic machine (officials in management, including the 'files' and equipment needed to function) is impersonal.

- The professional bureaucrat is chained to his or her activity by his or her entire material and ideal existence.
- Bureaucratic organisations develop from capitalism.
- There is a system of hierarchy.

■ DAVID BEETHAM

Weber's theory defines in many ways the concept of bureaucracy and the features of organisations. One theorist, Beetham (1987), argued that Weber's perspective is mechanistic in nature and that organisations are not so impersonal. Beetham proposed an alternative interpretation based on the social network of organisations. He focused his argument on the humanistic nature of individuals who work in organisations, pointing out that: 'In practice, however, people's personalities are never so totally subsumed into their roles; they come to the organisation as individuals with personal needs and expectations for which they seek satisfaction', in particular from social interactions with other workers.

Beetham also argued that organisations may be viewed as models of 'information systems'. Communication is important for the transmission of information. This should not be seen as a one-way process: from the top downwards; it also requires effective channels of communication upwards from the 'grass roots' (Beetham, 1987).

The other approach used by Beetham is the consideration given to the expertise possessed by individuals within the organisation, other than the superiors. He pointed out: 'Subordinates possess their own powers, which reside in informal social networks, in the control of information, or in their own expertise.'

▼ Summary

Organisations possess several common characteristics. Using Talcott Parsons' (1960) perspective, organisations have set goals to attain in society. Some organisations function to ensure that the economic needs of society are met; others, such as the courts and the legal profession, have integrative functions; yet others, for example churches and schools, have 'pattern maintenance functions'; whereas political systems of organisations are concerned with the generation and maintenance of power, and the Health Service manages healthcare provision.

Weber's (1946) approach in explaining organisations is very different to Parsons'. He argued that organisations are bureaucratic machines. The main feature is the presence of officials with specialist knowledge, who control the work place and have impersonal relationships with the rest of the workforce. Their (officials) activities are governed by administrative rules. Bureaucracy segregates the individual from the sphere of private life. A hierarchical structure dominates the organisation.

Beetham's theory is based on the human-relations perspective, evident in the relationships between the workers. Organisations are also models of communication systems. To Beetham, every individual in an organisation has some form of expertise that is useful for the running of that organisation.

▼ Application to Clinical Practice

■ BUREAUCRACY IN HEALTHCARE

In a critical evaluation of the changes that have

taken place in the National Health Service (NHS), Macara (1994) asserted that: 'Rather than improving efficiency, the reforms imposed on the NHS have increased bureaucracy, reduced patient choice, limited the range of core services, and led to inequity of treatment.' Macara (1994) argued that the increase in bureaucracy was, for example, preventing patients from receiving treatment locally because of a lack of facilities, thus forcing some to travel out of their locality for treatment.

It appears that with increased bureaucracy there is also an increased level of technology in the shape of computer systems, which, as Macara (1994) noted, have drawn the attention of the media and official investigation in relation to levels of waste. Wasted technology is evident because nursing practitioners are yet unable to internalise the relevance of computer systems. As Wood (1993) pointed out: 'Nursing technology has been described as a maturing market, but there are signs that disillusionment is creeping in. Doubts are growing about whether the first generation systems have met nursing needs or gained "the hearts and minds" of the nurses using them.'

Healthcare organisations operating in this bureaucratic framework are under increased pressure to implement information technology systems in the work place. This is likely to result in fragmentation of care. As Wood argued, improving care planning, for example, is not easily achieved with computerised nursing systems. Care plans produced by such systems are likely to be rigid and standardised, whereas individualised care demands flexibility. 'The kind of sensitive, individualised assessment of patient needs described by Benner and Wrubel are not easily incorporated into previously agreed timed units of care or listed tasks' (Wood, 1993).

In an interpretative study of the process of discharging patients from hospital to care at home, McWilliam and Wong (1994) in Canada argued that healthcare professionals 'worked with several persistent characteristics of a bureaucratic context': centralised control, fragmentation of work, and anonymity among workers.

According to McWilliam and Wong, the charge nurse at ward level is seen to control activities that ensure the provision of good patient care by other professionals, including bedside nurses. It is the charge nurse who is the liaison agent for the social worker; who 'does the actual communication' when discharge is being planned; and who communicates the relevant information to the homecare nurse. This approach, to some extent, reduces the autonomy of other professionals on the ward.

McWilliam and Wong highlighted work fragmentation as another common theme of the bureaucratic context. They saw this to be a result of 'designed work assignments and specialisation of professionals'. Nurses were not always able to maintain continuity of contact with their patients. Consequently they had to compensate for the fragmentation by making a 'comprehensive assessment of patients needs so that [they] could provide appropriate care'. The authors made particular reference to a nurse who had been able to maintain contact with her patient for 24 hours only during a 16-day hospitalisation.

There was also role confusion: who should do what and when. In-hospital nursing practitioners involved in discharge planning assumed the homecare 'case manager' would be educating the patient in readiness for discharge, and vice versa. McWilliam and Wong pointed out: 'In-hospital nurses had limited understanding of the homecare setting, and therefore of how their nursing efforts might contribute to the patient's preparation.' Thus one can identify fragmented knowledge of the community-care setting.

Lack of knowledge about each other's role is another characteristic of employees in large bureaucracies. McWilliam and Wong noted that nurses, eager to make certain that organisational goals were met, simply assumed responsibility for anticipating and initiating discharge planning, without involving collaboration from the other health-team members, including medical staff.

The above research points to an aspect of a bureaucracy that is prevalent in some healthcare organisations. In spite of the bureaucratic system—a feature of modern society—healthcare professionals manage to maintain autonomy in the implementation of care to meet individualised needs. The British system, for example, shows evidence of a central control from the Department of Health. At the level of care delivery, however, healthcare professionals are encouraged to exercise autonomy and individuality. The main emphasis of healthcare training is founded on the principle of exercising self-direction with the client's individual needs in focus. This is achieved by the implementation of primary nursing and by teamwork. The aims of the NHS reforms are to minimise bureaucracy and to ensure cost-effective care delivery.

Work

▼ The Nature of Work

'Work' may be simply defined as: 'The application of mental or physical effort to a purpose; the use of energy. A task to be undertaken; a person's employment or occupation' (*Concise Oxford Dictionary*, 1991). However, defining the

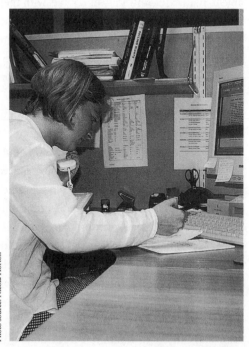 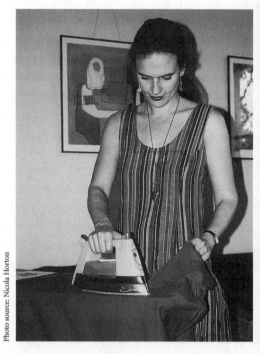

▲ *Both these women are workers: one is part of the formal economy, the other is part of the informal or household economy*

concept of work is not so easy. It is sometimes used synonymously with the term 'employment' or 'occupation'. Deem (1988) suggests that any consideration of the concept of work should be viewed in its historical and social context. She argued: 'Work is something we are obliged to do, like writing an essay, sitting an exam or earning a living, whilst leisure is something that we choose to do and find enjoyable (such as swimming, listening to music, playing football, going out for a meal) when we are not working.' Therefore, comparing work with leisure provides a contrast that, to some extent, helps to clarify its characteristics.

In a formal aspect, work is associated with organisations and bureaucracy, together with all the characteristics of bureaucracy as previously outlined. Work may also be connected with the earning of money in formal settings (e.g. industry, nursing, and education). Deem (1988) points out that there is specialisation of tasks within work, with a marked difference between economic activities and other aspects of society (such as the family and religion). Work is also distinguished from leisure and holidays or time-off, when the worker is free to relax. From a historical and social perspective, having time off work is not a common occurrence, as Creed and Coult (1990) point out in their account of steelworkers in Scunthorpe in the 1890s: 'In later years we got proper holidays but when I started you didn't you worked from year to year like. I mean you could ask for the odd day off, if you could afford it, but you hadn't to be away o'er long, or you'd may be lose your job.'

The informal aspect of work includes tasks done within the home environment by the family, for example washing and cleaning windows. According to Abercrombie and Warde (1992), in the sociology of the 1960s the activities of the family:

had nothing to do with work, other than servicing men so that they could leave the household to return to it; work had nothing to do with women, whose responsibility was (in Parsons' phrase) for the 'expressive' functions of the family, including the socialisation of children and the emotional and sexual refurbishment of men.

Nowadays, however, work is seen to be 'one of the dominant themes and activities of households of all kinds and types' (Abercrombie & Warde, 1992).

▼ The Social Context of Work

Deem (1988) provides three classifications of work:

- Formal economy type of work, e.g. car and steel production.
- Hidden or underground economy type of work, e.g. furniture making in a shed at home for cash.
- Household or communal economy type of work, e.g. sewing, knitting and DIY (do-it-yourself).

The formal economy type of work is characterised by its relationship with the economy. Work is done in order to meet the economic requirements of society. The manufacturing of cars and lorries, for example, is essential for the transportation of workers and the distribution of goods. This relationship, which is an important one, has implications for education, the family, and the community (Deem, 1988). Abercrombie et al. (1988) referred to this interrelationship as the 'labour process'; the relationships established by employers, supervisors, and employees while meeting the requirements of society. They identified the main dimensions of the labour process as follows:

- The range of tasks to be involved.
- The degree of discretion given to the worker to decide how to accomplish those tasks.
- The mode of control used by managers and supervisors to ensure that those tasks are completed satisfactorily.

Using the theory put forward by Braverman, Abercrombie et al. (1974) argue that workmen's skills are fragmented in the labour process, because the tasks they do are fragmented. For example, the fixing of headlights on a car in a factory is a task carried out continuously by a group of assembly-line workers. The organisation of work takes this form because, it is argued, managers want to exercise control over the workers. This hierarchical, scientific approach to management, which is aimed at maximising productivity, is known as 'Taylorism' (O'Donnell, 1993). It is characterised by the fragmentation of tasks that do not require a high level of skills; there are repetitive movements, and there is a rigid division between mental and manual labour. Deem (1988) explained the mental manual divide by arguing that some types of jobs in the work place, for example soldering two metal plates together, do not involve any abstract thinking and therefore do not demand any intellectual agility. It is argued that the shaping of work organisations by the scientific management of Taylorism has 'deskilled' the workers.

■ THE LABOUR MARKET

The labour market refers to the jobs or employment available in society. As Deem (1988) points out, it is connected with the supply of labour (i.e. how many people are looking for jobs) and the demand for labour (i.e. what jobs are available, where, and to whom).

Several factors influence the availability of work to individuals in society. If a job demands a high level of skills and qualifications (such as for judges, lawyers, and doctors), this will affect the number of people who can apply. Job protection is another factor. Some organisations will only recruit staff who they already employ (the 'internal labour market'; Deem, 1988). There is also the concept of 'job sheltering', where the eligibility to join an organisation is decided by a group of workers who specify the skills needed (Deem, 1988). Another term commonly used is the 'reserve army of labour': the groups of people in society (e.g. women and ethnic minorities) who are employed in poorly paid occupations, which are also insecure and temporary. When demands for labour in other occupational spheres arise, these 'reserves' will be encouraged to apply. This process was particularly evident during the First and Second World Wars, when housewives found employment in ammunition factories. Similarly, in the 1950s and 1960s, recruitment from the West Indies and Commonwealth Countries increased due to demands for workers in nursing and the London Underground Railways.

The labour market therefore shows that work in society is a complex social phenomenon, its availability being subjected to a multitude of social influences.

■ THE IMPORTANCE AND SIGNIFICANCE OF WORK

Work is of the utmost importance, both from a global perspective—for the economic functioning of society—and at a personal level—for the economic needs of the individual. The money earned enables the worker to buy goods and resources, thus helping him or her to maintain a certain standard of living (Deem, 1988). Work also gives a structure to the days and weeks. It offers the individual the means to be independent, and helps to maintain self-esteem and one's sense of identity. Being at work is also an opportunity for people to develop social relationships and to be in contact with others who share similar aspirations and beliefs regarding the organisations they work for. However, for some people, work may not be as fulfilling and meaningful. Certain occupations may be stressful and less rewarding, and conflict at work may sometimes be the cause of personal discontent.

Having a job and going to work, therefore, has an impact on the lives of people in society, as well as on the social structure. Unemployment or 'work loss', a common social problem, is dealt with in Chapter 13.

▼ Summary

Work, be it mental or physical, is a social activity. It is sometimes used synonymously with 'employment' or 'occupation'. It may be informal (such as the type done in the home: gardening, sewing, child care, and so on) or formal, often referred to as the formal economy type of work (such as that done in formal organisations, bureaucratic in nature, whose goals are to meet specific economic needs). Individuals in formal work will reap monetary rewards or wages from the organisations.

The relationships between the worker, the economy, and the managers are referred to as the 'labour process'. This concept pinpoints the fragmentation of tasks, as observed on an assembly line in a factory. This form of work process is known as 'Taylorism'—a scientific approach to management that ensures the production of goods at a much faster rate—and has been criticised for 'deskilling' the workforce.

Another concept frequently used in discussions about work is the 'labour market'. This term applies to the availability of job opportunities in society at any particular time. Some social factors may influence the uptake of certain jobs: gender, ethnicity, job sheltering, class, aptitudes, and skills.

Work (or employment) has a high profile in society: it is economically meaningful to the individual; it can boost self-esteem and give a sense of identity. However, other people may perceive and experience work differently, depending on the type of occupations they do and how stressful and worthwhile these are.

▼ Application to Clinical Practice

It is an essential aspect of the nurse's role to encourage patients to discuss their feelings regarding the effects of hospitalisation on their work situation. The admission assessment should include an initial identification of the patient's occupation. Being out of work due to illness or disability is likely to provoke anxiety in patients and their relatives.

Roper *et al.* (1985) identified a set of questions nurses should ask about a patient's 'working and playing' situation to obtain a profile of the patient's needs:

- What kind of working and playing activities does the patient usually engage in?
- How much time does the patient spend working and playing?
- Where does the individual work and play, and with whom?
- What factors influence the individual's working and playing?
- What does the individual know about the relationship between working and playing, and health?
- What are the individual's attitudes to working and playing?
- Has the individual any longstanding

problems with working or playing?

- What problems, if any, does the individual have at present with working or playing, and do any seem likely to develop?

As Roper *et al.* (1985) noted, patients in hospital have a need to escape the monotony and boredom of the confined environment. They argued that work gives the individual a sense of belonging and acceptance. This psychological and social need somehow becomes more intense because of hospitalisation. It is therefore necessary for healthcare professionals to be perceptive to these needs.

It is suggested that an environment more conducive to relaxation should be created in clinical practice. The hobbies and activities of individual patients should be identified. Recreational and diversional therapies should be considered in a variety of clinical settings (such as paediatric wards and wards for the elderly). According to Roper *et al.* (1985), there is no reason why patients should not continue with work activities, if possible, providing these are not detrimental to their health and do not interfere with their treatment. These authors give examples of how students may read and write essays in preparation for exams; children on paediatric wards may benefit from the ward teacher's lessons; business people may make phone calls and prepare plans of action for post-discharge business meetings; or a housewife may write a list of shopping or washing instructions for the family at home.

Some patients, however, may engage themselves in work activities during hospitalisation that cause them more harm than good; for example, patients whose reasons for admission are related to the high stress factor of their occupation such as executives and air traffic controllers with gastro-intestinal ulcers. These patients may need to be convinced that doing work, or even worrying about it, could jeopardise their recovery (Roper *et al.*, 1985).

■ WORK THERAPY FOR PATIENTS WITH MENTAL ILLHEALTH

Patients with mental illnesses, receiving treatment either in an institutional setting or in the community under the management of the community psychiatric nurse, may have a need to learn or relearn work skills. Work provides 'a common status and position in the community, it draws people together' (Bauer & Hill, 1986), it gives structure to the days, and it boosts the self-worth and self-esteem of the individual.

Healthcare professionals in this field should provide opportunities for clients to escape periods of inactivity by engaging them in activities they can easily do. Bauer and Hill (1986) suggested tasks like clearing and washing tables, sweeping and washing floors, and outdoor work such as mowing the lawn and weeding. These activities would be appropriate for clients who exhibit anxious behaviour patterns, demanding of time and attention. The authors argued that the aim of work therapy is to 'gradually reintroduce the client into a vocational setting to reduce the shock of transition from hospital to work'. An assessment of occupations available in the community should be made, with the client being involved in the decision-making process. Employers may be contacted regarding the type of work available, the standards expected, and the hours to be worked.

Encouraging clients to do volunteer work is another avenue to be explored. Although this form of work therapy does not involve monetary rewards, it is meaningful in the sense of preparing the individual for the world of competitive employment.

■ NURSES' WORK

The work of nurses in clinical practice is being increasingly extended. This may be seen in the responsibilities they now have in the treatment and care of patients; for example, the insertion of an intravenous cannula before infusion therapy, the taking of blood samples for analysis, and the suturing of wounds. The United Kingdom Central Council (UKCC) (1992) refers to the 'adjustments to the scope of professional practice', and allows for nurses to 'adjust' their practice, as long as certain principles are met, one of them being that 'each aspect of practice is directed to meeting the needs and serving the interests of the patient or client'.

The interests of the patient or client are best served by the nurse and allied care professionals on the basic principle of the health-promotional nature of their work; the promotion of a safe psychological and physical environment; the treatment of illhealth and its prevention.

▼ Review Questions

1   Discuss the concept of bureaucracy and organisation using relevant sociological perspectives.

2   Explain the importance and nature of work in society.

3   Describe the role of care professionals in clinical practice with reference to the concept of work.

▼ References

Abercrombie N, Soothill K *et al. Comtemporary British society*. Cambridge: Polity Press; 1988.

Abercrombie N, Warde A. *Social change in contemporary Britain*. Cambridge: Polity Press; 1992.

Bauer B, Hill S. *Essentials of mental health care. Planning and interventions*. Philadelphia: WB Saunders; 1986.

Beetham D. Bureaucracy. In: O'Donnell M, ed. *New introductory reader in sociology*. Walton on Thames: Nelsons & Sons; 1993:266–274.

Braverman H, *Labour and monopoly Capital*. New York: Monthly Review Press; 1974, 45–58.

Consise Oxford Dictionary 8th ed., Allen R, ed. London: BCA; 1991.

Creed R, Coult A. Steel town. *Real life drama of the men and women who built an industry*. Beverley: Hutton Press; 1990.

Deem R. *Work, unemployment and leisure*. London: Routledge; 1988.

Macara A. Reforming the NHS reforms. *Br Med J* 1994, **308**:848–849.

McWilliam C, Wong C. Keeping it secret: the costs and benefits of nursing's hidden work in discharging patients. *J Adv Nurs* 1994, **19**:152–163.

O'Donnell M. *New introductory reader in sociology.* Walton on Thames: Nelsons & Sons; 1993.

Parsons T. Social systems. In: Grusky O, Miller G, eds. The sociology of organisations: basic studies. New York: Macmillan; 1970:75-82.

Roper N, Logan W, Tierney A. *The elements of nursing – 'Working and playing'.* Edinburgh: Churchill Livingstone; 1985:274.

Silverman D. Social technical systems. In: Lockett M, Spear R, eds. *Organisations as systems.* Milton Keynes: Open University Press; 1980:66–72.

Silverman D. *The theory of organisations. A sociological framework.* Aldershot: Gower; 1987.

Stewart R. *Managing today and tomorrow.* Basingstoke: Macmillan; 1991:23–29.

UKCC. *The Scope of Professional practice.* London: UKCC, June 1992.

Weber M. Bureaucracy. In: Grusky O, Miller G, eds. *The sociology of organisations: basic studies.* New York: Macmillan; 1970:5–23.

Wood H. New technology—what has it done for nursing? *Surg Nurse* 1993, Vol 3:13–16.

▼ Further Reading

ORGANISATIONS

Blau P. Functional theory. In: Grusky O, Miller G, eds: *The sociology of organisations: basic studies.* New York: Macmillan; 1970.

Crozier M. The French bureaucratic system of organisation. In: Grusky O, Miller G, eds: *The sociology of organisations: basic studies.* New York: Macmillan; 1970:549–556.

Etzoni A. Compliance theory. In: Grusky O, Miller G, eds: *The sociology of organisations: basic studies.* New York: Macmillan; 1970:103–126.

Warwick D. *Social processes: bureaucracy.* London: Longman Group; 1974.

WORK

Deem R. *All work and no play: the sociology of women and leisure.* Milton Keynes: Open University Press; 1986.

Hendry J. *Understanding Japanese society.* London: Routledge; 1987:135.

Orlando I. Nursing in the 21st century: alternate paths. *J Adv Nursing* 1987, **12**:405–412.

Seymour J. *Changing life styles, living as though the world mattered.* London: Victor Gollanz; 1991.

Class Systems in Society

▼ What is Social Class?

In lay terms, class denotes a category, a particular
position one holds in the social structure. People
are often referred to by their occupation, which
also indicates their class; for example, 'He is just a
working-class lad who works down the mine' or
'You know, the "posh" gentleman who called the
other day, they say he is the new chairman of the
board.' From a technical aspect, a 'class' is 'a social
group chiefly defined by its type of occupation
and its level of property ownership' (HMSO,
1987). The presence of classes in society is an
objective social phenomenon; it is an empirical
(based on experience) social fact. Sociologists,
however, are also aware that usage of the term
'class' is subjective. 'It concerns people's responses
to the objective facts of life: that is their consciousness of their class and of their common
interest with other members of their class'
(HMSO, 1987).

The concept of class is also associated with
the idea of 'stratification'. Stratification describes
'the division of a population into strata, one on
top of another' (Worsley, 1977), which leads to a
social hierarchy. With social class and its system of
stratification, Worsley argued, one can find or
identify the 'different strata in relationships of
inferiority and superiority, usually of many kinds:
political, social and even religious'.

Some authors, for example Marshall *et al.*
(1989), have explained the stratified nature of

class by focusing on the Marxist interpretation of class structure. Namely, that the inequality evident in the accumulation of capital and the division of labour, which conjointly impoverish the workers, polarises the classes. As Marshall *et al.* (1989) argued, with the distinction between ownership (which separates social classes) and the social division (which delineates strata or fragments within classes), the class hierarchy becomes more obvious.

Interpreting or analysing the concept of social class, therefore, cannot be done in isolation from other associated sociological terms, such as stratification, occupational structure, and 'social differentiation'. The last term was referred to by Nobbs (1987) when he noted: 'Social class is the most important term relating to social differentiation.' Like Worsley, he made an analogy with geology: just as geologists study the layers or strata in different rock formations, so the sociologist studies the strata in different societies:

> Each stratum will have its own peculiar 'thickness' depending upon its composition and age. Just as geological formations are piled on top of the other, so people in society are grouped in layers with some at the top of the social pile exerting pressure upon those unlucky enough to find themselves at the bottom.

Using a similar approach, Reid (1977) expressed the view: 'Social class is only one form of social stratification. Dictionaries define stratification as an arrangement of layers, or as the relative position of layers. Simply then, social stratification is an arrangement of society into layers.'

Reid, however, emphasised the need to exercise caution when attempting to clarify the concept of social class: 'Clearly, however, social class has a much more elusive character than age or sex. Indeed there appears to be a good deal of discussion, or even confusion, in sociological literature about the nature and meaning of social class.' The argument put forward by Reid (1977) relates to the multifaceted nature of social class.

To understand the meaning of social class requires an awareness of the 'partly invisible' categories in society and their effects on people. Reid's working definition of social class is the following: social class is a grouping of people into categories based on occupation.

Weeks (1982) considered the concept of class to be one of the most ambiguous in sociology and therefore one of the most difficult to define. He argued that class is sometimes used to refer to a 'category or collection of social phenomena', such as one-parent families or people who have retired from work. He acknowledged, however, that class is associated with social stratification.

▼ Types of Classes in Society and their Features

■ THE UPPER CLASS

This group occupies the uppermost echelon of the social system. Their distinguishing features are collectively described as an ethos of superiority. They possess distinctive social statuses; they exhibit separateness from the other classes (Bilton *et al.*, 1987); their sociocultural practices are different; they own properties [which, according to Bilton *et al.* (1987), is their 'fundamental and defining feature']; they have the power to invest their money in properties.

The history of the upper classes shows a consistent relationship of superiority in their dealings with the other classes, namely the middle and working classes; for example, the owning of land and the employing of farmers (the tenants), who subsequently hire the labour of the working classes to work the land. The upper classes, therefore, are in a position of control and ownership.

Land, industry, and finance are linked to the upper classes: they possess land, they own industries, and they are in close interrelationships with financiers and entrepreneurs. In this sense, one may say, they enjoy a degree of economic and political influence.

The tendency to maintain control and to preserve power as a group is seen in their transactions of passing on their 'productive property' to the next generation. There is also the practice of homogamy—marriage within a class or status group (Bilton *et al.*, 1987)—which evidently encourages the prevalence of group integrity. They also make use of educational provisions likely to develop scientific and managerial skills, the aim being to prepare offspring for the elite positions. Research findings have pointed to a preponderance of public-school boys in the higher echelons of the occupational structure (Bilton *et al.*, 1987).

It appears that the culture of the upper classes leads to 'strategic control of capital'. Their close partnership with key people in the industrial and financial worlds perpetuates the reproduction of power and elitism. Hamnett *et al.* (1989) argued how the aristocracy adapted to the industrialisation process by developing a 'rentier upper class'. By 'rentier' these authors mean the gaining of financial benefits through income from investments and various dividends from property.

■ THE MIDDLE CLASS

Middle-class people occupy an intermediate position in the social class structure: between the upper class and the working class. Hamnett *et al.* (1989) argued that, because of their 'intermediate' position and their heterogeneity (diversity), the middle class or classes have long been the main problem of class theorists. According to Hamnett *et al.* (1989), the city editor of the *Sunday Telegraph*, Patrick Hubter, used the phrase 'middle classes' as far back as 1976 to emphasise that there is not a homogeneous group, but great variety and diversity in middle-class patterns and groups. This diversity may be observed, according to Hamnett *et al.* (1989), in the proliferation of middle-class occupations

throughout the twentieth century. 'To make matters more complicated, this growth has involved new kinds of middle class occupation, for example, technical specialists and state employees like social workers. In both state and corporate sectors, larger organisations have seen the emergence of more differentiated hierarchies of power and responsibility' (Hamnett *et al.*, 1989).

- Levels of pay ('salary' rather than wages) and work conditions.
- The respective ownership of wealth-holding, for example owner-occupied housing.

The accumulation of wealth and the gaining of better working conditions in comparison with their working-class counterparts can only be achieved through a 'readiness to postpone satisfactions' (Hutber, 1976). To elaborate this concept, Hutber explained:

> Deeply imbued with the Puritan ethic, the middle classes in Britain have always been hardworking; in contrast to Germany before the Weimar inflation, the proportion of the population existing as 'rentier' on investment income has been tiny. But they have also been thrifty, and thrift represents no more and no less than a readiness to postpone a satisfaction today in order to enjoy a greater one at sometime in the future.

In the chase for a secure and financially rewarding future, the middle classes occupy positions of authority in organisations—much non-manual work and 'staff status' (Bilton et al., 1987)—noting the availability of opportunities for promotion and success in their careers. Successes of the middle classes are undoubtedly due to the 'cultural capital' assimilated in their years of higher levels of training and education. As discussed in Chapter 4, educational attainment is markedly higher among the middle classes compared with the working classes. According to Bilton et al. (1987), education has furnished them with a 'trained mind', a sense of independent judgement.

Bilton *et al.* (1987) argue that the middle class exercise a degree of social closure—that is, they prevent infiltration or encroachment from below (the working class)—although this is not strong enough to protect 'cultural unity'. This latter point was also explored by Hamnett *et al.* (1989) in their discussions about the 'embourgeoisement' theory. This theory states that affluence among the working class has moved them into effectively middle-class positions.

Another debate related to what constitutes the middle class centres around the latest term, 'service class'. This is used when referring to professionals and managers, such as bank managers and senior civil servants. These people are perceived to exercise some form of power, being in a position to demonstrate authority compared with, for example, a waiter or a postman. Hamnett *et al.* (1989) made the following comments:

> In general terms, we are dealing with groups which do not own amounts of property comparable to the bourgeoisie, though they may well own domestic property and industrial shares. However, they exercise a good deal of day to day control in industry or in bureaucracies, they tend to enjoy quite secure employment, and may find it possible to move jobs advantageously.

It is difficult to make clear-cut distinctions about the multitude of social factors, the life chances, and the variety of occupations people have that influence one's assessment of what makes up a middle-class person. The same may be said about the working classes.

■ THE WORKING CLASS

Writing about the tendencies and attitudes connected with the classes in society, Hutber (1976) commented on the differences between the working class and the middle class: 'The characteristic attitude of the working class starts from a different frame of mind, a reluctance to postpone satisfaction . . . the satisfaction is taken today . . .

there is a positive pride in spending every penny . . . there is much less belief in self reliance, much less desire for independence . . .' Although this statement contains an element of truth, it is inaccurate to generalise in this way because many working-class citizens are good savers and are prepared to work hard to achieve a secure and financially rewarding social position.

It is argued (for example, Hamnett *et al.*, 1989) that the position of the working class is changing. The change is noticeable in the expansion of the middle-class ranks as the working class become more affluent. It is said that the economy over the past 20 years has altered the material position of the working class: increased numbers of the working class are more able to develop technical skills and to afford to move into suburban areas to meet the demands of their jobs.

Although social change is affecting the class structure, the working class nevertheless maintain a high social profile and are a topic of great sociological significance. What are the distinguishing features of the working class group? Who are these individuals? These questions are now considered.

Sociologists often use the term 'proletariat' when alluding to the idea of the working class. The *Concise Oxford Dictionary* (1991) defines 'proletariat' as: 'Wage earners collectively, especially those without capital and dependent on selling their labour; in a derogatory way, the lowest class of the community especially when uncultured.'

Writing about the local class structures in the upland parish of Westrigg, a mainly rural county in the south of Scotland, Littlejohn (1963) commented:

> That the classes are viewed as superior and inferior to each other is soon apparent in conversation. When identifying a third party for me, informants would say, eg 'He's not a working man' or 'He's not a gentleman farmer, just a working farmer'. An upper-middle class man once remarked of agricultural labourers 'Of course some of

these people are hardly better than animals in intelligence and way of living . . . They are all alike these people, they just can't think'. A lower-middle class woman remarked of a working class neighbour 'You can see the lower element coming out even in her'. A view of the working class widely held among both the middle classes is that they are childish.

These are stereotypical images regarding evaluative judgements of the working classes. Another image that differentiates the working class is the identity created by their dialect—the way their speech is different to that of the middle classes. Littlejohn (1963) gave this example of a classroom interaction: 'During one lesson, for example, the children were asked to name various sorts of buildings shown to them in pictures of which there was a kennel. Asked to name it, one of the boys replied correctly in dialect "A dughoose". He was somewhat chagrined to be told he was wrong.'

This depiction is reminiscent of the work of Labov (1969), who supported the logic of nonstandard English. His study of black working-class children from the ghetto area confirmed his views that these children are not 'verbally deprived'; rather, contrary to common beliefs:

They receive a great deal of verbal stimulation, hear more well formed sentences than middle class children, and participate fully in a highly verbal culture; they have the same basic vocabulary, possess the same capacity for conceptual learning, and use the same logic as anyone else who learns to speak and understand English.

Still concerning language and speech, Bernstein (1970) argued that working-class individuals use 'restricted codes', which are based on condensed symbols, whereas the middle classes use 'elaborated codes', which have their basis in articulated symbols. According to Bernstein (1970), when working-class people speak they do not articulate the meanings of their communication; they do not make the information explicit. He explained this by saying: 'In these relationships the intent of the other person can be taken for granted as the speech is played against a backdrop of common assumptions, common history, common interests. As a result there is less need to raise meanings to the level of explicitness or elaboration.'

Another feature of the working class is the location of their housing: a high concentration of the working-class population lives in the inner cities: 'The population structures of the inner areas are therefore biased towards the manual working class . . . a higher proportion of accommodation in these areas being rented and less is owner-occupied than nationally.' (O'Donnell 1988).

Another sphere in which the working class are seen to demonstrate specific characteristics is concerned with their voting behaviour in relation to their political beliefs. O'Donnell (1988) argued: 'The influence of class on voting patterns has aroused considerable interest in that there is a presumed identity of interest between the Labour Party and the "working class" and between the Conservative Party and the "middle class".' Abercrombie and Warde (1988) made a similar observation in their statement:

[It was] frequently reported in the 1960s that manual workers voted consistently for the Labour Party because it was the party of the workers, of 'people like us' . . . Despite many claims to the contrary, recent sociological evidence suggests that this imagery and awareness remains predominant and is the only pattern consistently found among manual workers.'

It is true, however, to argue that many working-class individuals also vote Conservative; these are known as 'working-class Tories' (O'Donnell, 1988). As far as work or occupation is concerned, Persell (1990) argued that the working class 'have less occupational power and prestige, lower income and own little property'. The socio-economic position of the working classes in the social structure increases their vulnerability. Persell (1990) differentiates a type of working class as 'lower class'; these individuals are dominated by income or poverty, compared with the occupation-dominated working class who tend to be skilled labourers (electricians, plumbers, machinists, truck drivers). The 'lower class' work longer hours, suffer a higher rate of unemployment, and have poor financial resources.

According to Bennett *et al.* (1981), the working class is, by definition, a subordinate in relation to the upper-class structure's social and cultural formation. These writers went on to argue:

> Hegemony (the domination of one class over others, by a combination of political and ideological means) works 'primarily' by inserting the subordinate class into the key institutions and structures which support the power and social authority of the dominant order. It is above all, in these structures and relations that a subordinate class 'lives its subordination'.

The type of subordination experienced by the working class may be illustrated by citing examples from the shop floor of an industrial working environment, such as the following extract from Beynon's (1973) book *Working for Ford:*

> They take a terrible attitude to the men on the shop floor here. I don't know how they behave as they do. They tell you nothing. Look, we've been laid off this afternoon and we haven't even been told that officially. They tell you nothing. All your pay can be stopped and they tell you nothing. That's typical of this firm.

As Beynon explained: 'In their discussion of plant management the stewards continually made reference to the fact that an unpleasant job was often made intolerable by management's self-interested concern for production and their own careers.'

To some extent, these working-life experiences of the working classes match the theoretical perspective of Karl Marx: conflict in the work place, domination, and exploitation.

■ THE UNDERCLASS

Academics and politicians have recognised the existence of a group occupying the bottom social stratum, which they identify as the underclass. Close examination of this concept reveals a set of attributes consisting of social factors that form its ethos.

> At a very general level, one can perhaps detect three common features of most definitions; first, an underclass is a social stratum that suffers from prolonged labour market marginality; second, it experiences greater deprivation than even the manual working class; and third, it possesses its own distinctive subculture (Gallie, 1994).

The presence of the underclasses in cities is gradually becoming a common feature. In the United States, according to Selfe (1987), the underclass consists of members of ethnic minorities; they are the unemployed, 'trapped in a continuing web of poverty' and becoming 'a menace to people and property'. Selfe (1987) discussed how restrictive educational opportunities—as seen in some societies and evident in a 'closed stratification system'—could lead to the emergence of an underclass. The underclass has poor social mobility. Social inequalities in housing and employment could, according to Selfe, 'turn an underclass into a dangerous class'.

Regarding unemployment, one social problem experienced by the underclass, Nobbs (1987) commented: 'The degree of hardship experienced by the unemployed is closely associated with social class; the scales are tipped heavily against manual workers. Older manual workers may be downgraded or even sacked when they become less able to perform the work task.'

The underclass therefore forms a minority group sharing similar cultures: deprivation, social disadvantages, characteristics of low income, susceptibility to mental illness, and, above all, a feeling of 'stigma' associated with being unwanted by society (Nobbs, 1987).

▼ Theoretical Perspectives of Class

■ TRADITIONAL VIEWS

THE MARXIST PERSPECTIVE

Marx's view of class is based on his observations of the relationship that exists between the owners of production (capitalist entrepreneurs) and the proletariat. According to Marx: 'Private property, as the antithesis to social, collective property, exists only where the means of labour and the external conditions of labour belong to private individuals.' These private individuals are the capitalists who, because of their wealth, own the means of production. This position of power, according to Marx, leads to the 'expropriation of the great mass of the people from the soil, from the means of subsistence and from the means of labour'. This relationship rests on the 'exploitation of the nominally free labour of others, i.e. wage labour'. (*see* Worsley P. *The new modern sociology readings*, 1991).

To Marx, therefore, the concept of class is a system or network of domination and subordination; the exploiters (the capitalist class) and exploited (the working class or proletariat). He explained this system as follows: 'That which is now to be expropriated is no longer the labourer working for himself but the capitalist exploiting many labourers.' This exploitation, he stated, is the result of the capitalist mode of production and the growth of capitalist private property. The aim of the capitalist entrepreneurs is to accumulate as much wealth as possible, by control of the workers using a system of wage bargaining.

THE WEBERIAN PERSPECTIVE ON CLASS AND STATUS

Whereas Marx considered the economic relationship between capital ownership and the working classes, Weber, on the other hand, argued: 'Class has more to do with the distributional side of economic resources than the means of production'

(Weeks, 1982). Weber stated that market situations decide a person's class (class being a 'position in a pattern of inequality'). Weber's interpretation of class is based on specific factors:

- A group of people who have in common life chances of a similar nature.
- These life chances reflect a tendency towards economic interest seen in the possession of goods and the acquisition of financial rewards.
- The labour markets influence their life chances, their economic interests.

To Weber, 'class' refers to any group of people in the same 'class situations', which are related to 'market situations'. Thus, in society there are business people, entrepreneurs whose objective is to make use of commodities available to them, to maximise profits. These individuals form one class. On the other hand, there are 'those who have no property but who offer services [and] are differentiated just as much according to their kinds of services as according to the way in which they make use of these services.' These groups form a class also. (Weeks, 1982).

Weber also provides a clarification of the concept of 'status': 'Status describes a classification of social stratification in terms of social prestige or social honour' (Weeks, 1982). As a dimension of stratification, the idea of prestige and honour is analytically distinct from class. Weber gave the formula for 'social status' as follows:

- Mode of living (the life style of the individual; the financial resources that will have a bearing on his or her social status).
- Education (the quality of which may lead to a particular mode of life-economic opportunities that may enhance one's mode of living).
- Prestige of birth or of an occupation (here, Weber is alluding to the characteristics ascribed to those born within a particular social milieu, for example the caste system of India).

Although class and status are two different concepts, status is frequently linked to the economically determined class structure in society (Weeks, 1982).

■ MODERNIST PERSPECTIVES

The data gathered by the Oxford Mobility Survey of 1972 revealed that men, irrespective of their class origins, had become progressively more likely to move into professional, administrative, and managerial positions—the service class—of modern British society (Goldthorpe *et al.*, 1987). This survey and its findings highlighted the movement of the class structure (the gradual expansion of the service class and contraction of the working class); a social change that contradicts the Marxist prediction that capitalist societies will proletarianise the masses. The survey emphasised the constancy of the service class in maintaining its position, that there was no downwards mobility from that stratum.

Commenting on the occupational division of labour, Halsey (1986) remarked that whereas three-quarters of the employed and self-employed population were engaged in manual work at the beginning of the century, by the mid-century this proportion had fallen below two-thirds, and since then it has fallen still further, to about one-third. Halsey (1986) concludes: 'The first impression is of a gradual movement away from what might be called a proletarian society: and this transformation has been gathering pace in recent decades.'

Halsey's assessment is therefore congruent with Goldthorpe's findings. Hasley argued that the 'two-class model' of Marxism has to be adapted to take account of professional and managerial occupations, which Goldthorpe identified as the service class.

On a different theme, but still related to class analysis, Goldthorpe and Marshall (1992), in their discussions titled 'Why class analysis is still important—after Marx', commented on how their approach to class analysis differs significantly from that of Marxist sociology. They stressed that their understanding of the class debate does not encompass a theory of class exploitation

with underlying conflicts and a state of subjugation; their theory 'does not embrace a reductionist theory of political action'.

They found the service class of modern societies to be heterogeneous (diverse) in composition, whereas the working class were more homogeneous (of similar nature). In their consideration of social mobility (the upwards or downwards movement of the classes in the hierarchical structure, e.g. someone from a working-class background obtaining a middle-class occupation), they concluded: 'Different classes tend to be associated with specific "propensities" for immobility or mobility independently of all structural effects.' They also argued that classes will follow specific and distinctive trajectories, developing or contracting according to the demands the economies placed upon them.

Marshall *et al.* (1989) used the term 'labour aristocracy' when referring to the new working classes in contemporary Britain; those 'who have absorbed capitalist economic values'. They reported the move of the working class to better their social condition:

> The second half of the century sees the emergence of specifically artisanal housing areas as skilled workers moved away from the courts and alleys of the slums, where they shared facilities with unskilled and casual labour, to the often badly built but nevertheless self contained houses in superior suburbs.

This developing trend contradicts Marxist prediction of class revolution and 'class-based distributional conflict' (Marshall *et al.*, 1989).

▼ Social Stratification and Health Inequality

Social stratification is a particular type of social differentiation; it is related to hierarchy, how groups of people are ranked higher or lower than another in the admitted social order (Mitchell,

1979). Social stratification is best represented in diagrammatic form using the Registrar General Method of Classifications, as in the box.

SOCIAL CLASS

Class A Higher Managerial, administrative or professional

Class B Intermediate Managerial administrative or professional

Class C(1) Supervisory or clerical and junior managerial, administrative or professional

Class C(2) Skilled manual workers

Class D Semi and unskilled manual workers

Class E State Pensioners or undours (no other parents) casual or lowest grade workers, or long term unemployed

Source: Social Trends 25 Central Statistical Office, London; HMSO: 1995:242

The Registrar's classification demonstrates the socially structured hierarchy; one can identify the superior, middle, and inferior positions of the different classes. Some authors, for example Scambler (1991), consider that the term 'social stratification' refers generally to this type of socially structured inequality, and that the concept of social class describes the form that social stratification takes in modern societies. Hurd (1986) explained that as societies become more complex and advanced, 'so does an increase in the system of hierarchy or stratification, and the level of inequality'.

The caste structure of Hindu society provides the other extreme of stratification. Hurd (1986) commented how caste was a way of life in traditional India, and noted the existence of hundreds of castes, each of them broken down into subcastes. The stratification is evident in the demarcation of the various groups based on their social and occupational activities. For example, at the ultimate prestigious level of

the hierarchy are the Brahmins or priests, who personify purity, sanctity, and holiness and have expertise in law and ritual. At the other extreme is a group not even deemed worthy of designation within the officially recognised structure of Hindu society—the outcastes or 'untouchables'—whose associations with certain tasks, such as sweeping and butchery, were considered as 'unclean and polluting' (Hurd, 1986).

Therefore, as the caste system shows, stratification is concerned with social ranking and categorisation of individuals and groups. As Weeks (1982) pointed out: 'In this way social stratification is both a process (of differentiation and allocation) and the results of that process in terms of the unequal distribution of various scarce social resources, both material and symbolic.'

Social resources such as housing, education, employment, and healthcare provisions are not distributed equitably, with certain classes in the stratification system being at a disadvantage. Social issues such as inadequate housing, unemployment, and educational underachievement can all have implications for health.

The Black Report of 1980 pointed to the existence of widespread health inequalities in Britain, closely linked with class issues:

> There are marked inequalities in health between the social classes in Britain. Mortality tends to rise inversely with falling occupational rank or status, for both sexes and at all ages. At birth and in the first month of life twice as many babies of unskilled manual parents as of professional parents die, and in the next eleven months of life nearly three times as many boys and more than three times as many girls, respectively, die. (Townsend and Davidson, 1988).

The report documented evidence of a higher mortality rate among the lower classes, namely classes IV and V—comprising partly skilled and unskilled working-class people. It also identified other problems concerning the needs of older people from different social classes: class V elderly people neither received domestic help (from outside their family) nor felt the need of it; in comparison, social classes I and II already had privately paid or local-authority domestic help.

The report also distinguished marked differences in the utilisation of health services: again, the working classes were found to underutilise the provision. However, the services of both the hospital inpatient and outpatient departments were used more by working-class patients. The report reasoned: '[This] must imply that more working-class patients have illnesses requiring hospital admission, or that the working-class patient seeing his GP is typically sicker and/or that he or she is seen as less likely to receive adequate care at home.'

The report argued that working classes do not make use of available services (commonly known as 'public provision of domiciliary services') due to the interaction of two sets of factors: social and ecological. Services are not easily accessible to many working-class individuals. 'Reduced provision implied greater journeys, longer waiting lists, longer waiting times, difficulties in obtaining an appointment and so on.' Healthcare institutions are criticised for not meeting the needs 'of those who are less able to express themselves in acceptable terms'.

The Black Report provided a comprehensive assessment of the inequalities in health status from a broad perspective that is beyond the scope of this chapter. However, subsequent reports (Whitehead, 1988; Blank and Diderichsen 1996, Ford et al., 1994) have revealed that health inequalities still exist in society.

and so on. In particular westernised cultures, there are several divisions of social position, categorised as the upper class, the middle class, the working class, and the underclass. Each category possesses specific features based on modes of living, cultural practices, work circumstances, or unemployment situations.

The classic sociologists Marx and Weber considered social class from differing viewpoints. Marx saw social class as a two-model system: the bourgeoisie and the proletariat. In his view, these two classes are in a state of conflict, with the bourgeoisie exercising control and domination over the proletariat, the exploited ones. Weber, on the other hand, considered class from a 'market situation' viewpoint, which emphasises the relation to the distributional side of economic resources rather than the relationships between capitalists and workers. Weber also developed the term 'status' to describe a categorisation of social stratification related to social prestige or social honour.

The modernist approach to social class analysis, however, argues that there is evidence of social mobility in society, with the working classes being more upwardly mobile and a noticeable increase in the number of the service class. Contrary to the Marxist prediction of the proletarianisation of the masses, the working classes are seen to be enjoying a middle-class type of life style.

Society is characterised by a system of stratification and health inequalities. The Black Report of 1980 highlighted many issues concerning the link between occupational status and health problems. Working-class groups are more likely to suffer illhealth and die earlier than are the other classes (i.e. classes I and II). Social and environmental factors are possible reasons given for these disparities.

▼ Summary

Social class is a category, a type of grouping based on one's occupational status, as well as other issues such as ownership of resources, property,

▼ Application to Clinical Practice

It is imperative for nurses to have a thorough understanding of the relationship between social class, health, and illness. For example, failing to identify that the poor, unskilled, manual working-class person is more prone to ill-health is likely to create a situation that will undermine his or her remaining ability to cope with vulnerability to disease. Also, an awareness that the financial status of working-class individuals may make it difficult for them to afford a very nutritious diet, may have implications for health-promotion advice. As Brunner and Suddarth (1992) pointed out, it is not recommended to give excellent nutritional education to a person who cannot afford to buy the types of food promoted. 'Similarly,' the same authors argued, 'to advise a depressed, working class woman with young children to get out and meet more people by joining an evening class would be likely to arouse hostility rather than have a positive effect.'

Labov (1969) and Bernstein (1970) both discussed the meanings of language, its logic, and how it can be sometimes misinterpreted in its social context. Bernstein referred to the 'restricted code' of the working classes, and the 'elaborated code' of the middle classes. Labov, on the other hand, commented on the relevance and commonsense inherent in the dialect or language code of the working class. Knowledge of these theories should help the healthcare professional to gain insight into the meanings and content of the communication process when interacting with patients from different social backgrounds. For example, a working-class patient may express his psychosocial needs using the local dialect. Although it is unlikely that the professional can understand all the dialects used by patients from different parts of the country, he or she should be aware that important and relevant needs are being conveyed by the patient. Consequently, provision should be made to involve an interpreter to decode the communication.

Spending time with the patient, with the aim of developing a caring relationship, should help the care professional to reduce communication barriers. Listening and paying attention to the language code being used will not only enhance the relationship but will boost the patient's confidence. The dialect or restricted code of the working class is similar to a foreign language for the person with no knowledge of it: showing an interest and keenness to listen and learn can only boost morale and improve personal nursing satisfaction and self-esteem. Any form of language is important to the user. Whether the style used is restricted, elaborated, or simply in local dialect, the meanings conveyed are just as relevant and meaningful. As Porritt (1990) emphasised: 'Language is a powerful component of healthcare that can embrace or diminish the effectiveness of the interaction.'

Although the restricted code of the working-class person may present problems to healthcare professionals, elaborated codes may also cause communication difficulties. Because of the explicitness of middle-class conversation, and the ability of the middle classes to elicit information, care professionals may assume that such patients already have the necessary knowledge. To be articulate does not necessarily mean to be knowledgeable. Spending time listening and conversing with the middle-class patient will facilitate the interactive process and help to alleviate any fears or anxieties that may otherwise go unnoticed.

Molzahn and Northcott (1989), for example, suggested that discrepancies in the perception of health and illness are founded on social factors, such as socio-economic status. They commented that the socio-economic status of care professionals may influence their perception and interactions with patients: 'Healthcare professionals generally assume that their perception and assessments of their patients' health status are accurate and congruent with those of the patient and other healthcare providers.' Similarly, the patient's social status may affect his or her perception of information and lead to misunderstanding of medical and nursing roles. Molzahn and Northcott (1989) argued:

> Perceptions are known to vary between social classes. Stereotypes of persons in various classes persist, and interactions between individuals of different class groups can be affected. Because of the occupational prestige accorded to physicians in our society, physicians occupy a relatively high (upper middle class and upper class) social status.

Social status has implications for nursing care. The greater the social distance between the patient and the care professional (doctor or nurse), the harder it is to establish mutual trust, respect, and cooperation. Furthermore, referring to King (1962), Molzahn and Northcott (1989) noted how physicians, because of their status, may expect deference from the nurse. This could generate ineffective and conflicting interactions resulting in poor care delivery. The knowledge that one's social status in a clinical setting may affect one's perceptual skills should lead care professionals to be more objective in their contact with patients from any social class.

The role of the nurse in other care settings, such as in the community, must not be underestimated. In a study undertaken in Chippenham, Wiltshire, to assess parents' awareness of home-safety issues, social class differences in perception were noticeable (Colley, 1994). The higher socio-economic groups blamed individual responsibility for a lack of safety awareness and practice, whereas the lower socio-economic groups thought social and environmental factors were the cause. The role of health visitors, therefore, is to target groups with specific needs related to socio-environmental factors, as well as to increase information and health-promotion advice for all groups concerned.

Another area of concern in the field of health prevention is the poor uptake rate for cervical screening among working-class women. Smail and Smail (1989) found that a combination of skilled nurses and a flexible appointment system achieved dramatic improvements in the uptake rate. More working-class women attended the practice because the system introduced was more client-centred and based upon their individual needs.

Review Questions

1   Kingstown is an inner-city area with a population of 20,000, an area with a massive expansion of manufacturers and industrial processes. There is a predominance of manual working-class people, due to the types of industries and the manual-labour occupations available. A minority of the population is middle class; these people live on the outskirts of the city, mainly in the suburbs. The working class live in rented accommodation about three miles from their places of work; their dwellings are mainly high-rise flats.

Discuss the social and ecological issues a healthcare professional in this community should consider to ensure the health needs of the population are met.

2   'But I have since come to the conclusion that middle-classness is a state of mind, rather than status. Ours is a town of owner-occupiers. Terraces of good, stone-built houses that will last forever. My parents had paid off the mortgage during the 1920s. They had saved. They owed no one for anything. My mother was the best manager God ever made and we never went short of food or clothes and we were clean! "Soap and water cost nothing" was her motto! We were told to work hard at school and get out of "the mill"—too chancy altogether. We were also told that, although there was no money to help lame ducks, no one would ask us to leave school and go out to earn so long as we won scholarships and paid our way to 'college'.' [Comments from a professional class in *The decline and fall of the middle class* (Hutber, 1976).]

Discuss the above comments in relation to theories of class and status.

▼ References

Abercrombie N, Warde A. *Contemporary British society.* Cambridge: Polity Press; 1988.

Bennett T, Martin G, Mercer C. *Culture, ideology and social process. Dominant and subordinate cultures.* Milton Keynes: Open University Press; 1981:57–64.

Bernstein B. Social class, language and socialisation. In: Giglio P, ed. *Language and social context.* Harmondsworth: Penguin Books; 1970:157–178.

Beynon H. *Working for Ford.* Wakefield: EP Publishing; 1973.

Bilton T, *et al. Introductory sociology, 2nd ed.* Basingstoke: Macmillan; 1987:90–115.

Blank N, Diderichsen F. Inequalities in Health: *The interaction between socio-economic and personal circumstances.* Public Health 1996, **110**:157–162.

Brunner L, Suddarth D. *The textbook of adult nursing.* London: Chapman & Hall; 1992.

Colley L. Different backgrounds, different information needs. Home safety awareness among parents of pre-school children. *Professional Nurse* 1994, **9**:832–836.

Concise Oxford Dictionary 8th ed. Allen Red, *BCA*, London: 1991.

Ford G, Kate H, Russell E, *et al.* Patterns of class inequality in health through the lifespan: class gradients at 15, 35 and 55 years in the west of Scotland. *Soc Sci Med* 1994, **39**:1037–1050.

Gallie D. Are the unemployed an underclass? Some evidence from the social change and economic life initiative. *J Br Sociol Assoc* 1994, **28**:737–757.

Goldthorpe J, Llewellyn K, Payne C. Social mobility and class structure in modern Britain: (1987). In: O'Donnell M, ed. *New introductory reader in sociology, 3rd ed.* Walton-on-Thames: Nelsons & Sons; 1993:64–67.

Goldthorpe J, Marshall G. The promising future of class analysis: a response to recent critiques: (1992). In: O'Donnell M, ed. *New introductory reader in sociology, 3rd ed.* Walton-on-Thames: Nelsons & Sons; 1993:45–54.

Hamnett C, McDowell L, Sarre P. *The changing social structure.* London: Sage Publications; 1989.

Hasley A. Changes in British Society, 3rd ed. *A class-ridden prosperity.* Oxford: Oxford University Press; 1986:26–48.

HMSO. Divisions in Society. *Diploma in Nursing Block 2, Unit 2.* DLC. London: HMSO; 1987.

Hurd G. *Human societies. An introduction to sociology.* London: Routledge & Kegan Paul; 1986.

Hutber P. *The decline and fall of the middle class and how it can fight back.* London: Associated Business Programme; 1976.

Labov W. The logic of non-standard English: (1969). In: Giglioli P, ed. *Language and social context.* Hamondsworth: Penguin Books; 1972:283–307.

Littlejohn J. Local class structures 3: (1963) In: Butterworth E, Weir D, eds. *The sociology of modern Britain.* London: Fontana Collins; 1970:238–245.

Marshall G, Newby H, *Social class in modern Britain.* London: Unwin Hyman; 1989.

Marshall G, Newby H, Goodbye to social class. In: Worsley P, ed. *The new modern sociology readings.* Harmondsworth: Penguin Books; 1991:464–470.

Mitchell D. *A new dictionary of sociology.* London: Routledge & Kegan Paul; 1979.

Molzahn A, Northcott H. The social bases of discrepancies in health/illness perceptions. *J Adv Nurs* 1989, **14**:132–140.

Nobbs J. *Social Science for GCSE. Social Class.* Basingstoke: MacMillan; 1987:93–101.

O'Donnell G. *Mastering sociology, 2nd ed.* Basingstoke: MacMillan; 1988:202–203.

Persell C. *Understanding society—An introduction to sociology, 3rd ed.* New York: Harper & Row; 1990.

Porritt L. *Interaction strategies: an introduction for health care professionals.* Edinburgh: Churchill Livingstone; 1990.

Reid I. *Social class differences in Britain. A source book.* London: Open Books; 1977.

Scambler G. *Sociology as applied to medicine, 3rd ed.* London: Bailliere Tindall; 1991:115.

Selfe P. *Advanced sociology: underclass.* London: Pan Books; 1987:129, 140, 315.

Smail J, Smail S. Making the service suit the patient. *Nursing Times* 1989, **85**:49–51.

Townsend P, Davidson N. *Inequalities in Health The Black Report.* The Health Divide. Whitehead M, Harmsworth: Penguin; 1987.

Weber M. Social status. In: Worsley P, ed. *The new modern sociology readings*. Harmondsworth: Penguin Books; 1991:437–442.

Weeks D. *An introduction to sociology: glossary*. Milton Keynes: Open University; 1982:66–68, 74.

Whitehead M. The health divide. In: Townsend P, Davidson N, eds. *Inequalities in health*. London: Penguin Books; 1988.

Worsley P. *Introducing sociology, 2nd ed*. Harmondsworth: Penguin Books; 1977:395–396.

Worsley P, ed. *The new modern sociology readings*. Harmondsworth: Penguin Books; 1991: 431–433.

▼ Further Reading

Dahl E. Social inequality in health—The role of the healthy worker effect. *Soc Sci Med* 1993, **36**:1077–1086.

Consise Oxford Dictionary. *8th ed,* Allen Red. London: BCA; 1991.

Gift T, Barry M, *et al*. Social class and psychiatric disorder: the examination of an extreme. *J Nerv Ment Dis* 1988, **176**(10): 593–597.

Glendenning A, Shucksmith J, Hendry L. Social class and adolescent smoking behaviour. *Soc Sci Med* 1994, **38**:1449–1460.

Gomm R. *Sociology 'A' level. Sociological explanation for inequality—Unit 4*. Cambridge: NEC; 1990:60.

Pound A. The crisis of the inner-city family. *J Ment Health* 1994, **3**:143–146.

8

Social Construction of Behaviour: *Gender*

▼ The Meaning of Gender

The framework of gender involves two concepts: masculinity and femininity. These concepts involve the exhibition of socially determined personal and psychological characteristics associated with being male or female (Garrett, 1987). There is, therefore, a difference in the interpretation of 'masculinity' and 'femininity' compared with, respectively, 'male sex' and 'female sex'. Sex is biologically determined and denotes differences between males and females from a biological viewpoint—differences in sexual organs and the general physical characteristics that accompany being male or female.

Gender is of interest to sociologists because it is associated with many social factors that influence one's social position, progress, and advancement in society. People in society have specific expectations of how one should comport oneself. Garrett (1987), for example, summed it up concisely when she said: 'Whether you are born male or female will be of major consequence for all aspects of your life: for the expectations others in society will have of you, for your treatment by other people, and for your own behaviour.'

Thus, the social implications of gender are varied. We have seen in Chapter 7 how social class creates inequality; gender divisions in society are also linked with systems of inequality.

Sociologists have differing viewpoints concerning the developmental processes of gender. That is to say, how do gender characteristics develop? What factors influence their growth? There are two schools of thought on the subject: the 'nature-versus-nurture' debate. Nature, in this context, means the biological factors likely to predispose to either masculine or feminine type of behaviour; nurture considers the social factors leading to the formation of gender characteristics.

▼ The Nature Perspective on Gender

The biological arguments about how differences in gender develop rest on the following:

- **Physical differences**. These are noticeable in the external appearances and in the brain. Biologists argue that a female's brain is smaller.
- **Chromosomes**. 'Every human being has a special pair of chromosomes which is connected with sexuality' (Hayes 1994). Females have two 'X' chromosomes, males have one 'X' and one 'Y' chromosome.
- **Sex glands**: Ovaries in the female, testes in the males.
- **Hormones.** Although the same 'sex hormones' are found in males and females, the quantities produced by each sex vary; for example, males have higher levels of testosterone and females have higher levels of oestrogen. These differences result in different sexual characteristics.

According to Hayes (1994), biological theorists believe that the ultimate progression of an individual to be either male or female depends on these biological characteristics. She alludes to animal studies suggesting that sex-role behaviour (in this instance, mothering behaviour) can be induced in male rats by injecting them with the appropriate hormone, prolactin.

To use such biological factors to explain the development of gender characteristics is to adopt a deterministic approach, described by Mayes (1986) as 'Biology is destiny'. Mayes argued that this a popular idea that supposes that the anatomical differences between the sexes predispose them to different types of activity; for example, the maternal instinct, although ill-defined, is supposed to be common among women.

However, such a reductionist approach (the principle of analysing complex things into simple constituents) does not take into account the cultural variations and social factors that may influence gender formation.

▼ The Nurture Perspective on Gender

The role of culture in shaping feminine and masculine roles is an essential component in discussions on gender formation. Culture is undoubtedly closely interwoven with the process of socialisation. Socialisation therefore contains the elements that will shape the sexuality of the individual. Parents are the initial agents of socialisation. How parents respond to their child depends on its sex. For example: 'In western cultures parents' expectations of appropriate behaviour in teenage girls often exclude overt sexual activity, whereas for boys it is permitted or overlooked' (Garrett, 1992).

As soon as a sexual label is identified for the child, social behaviours specific to that label are put in motion for the development of gender roles and identity. Gross (1992) used the theory of social learning to explain this development. This theory is based on 'observational learning'. Children learn appropriate social behaviour regarding gender formation by observing 'models' in their environment. These models could be the parents. As Gross (1992) pointed out: 'Both fairly specific behaviours (e.g. nailbiting) and more general emotional states (e.g. fear of the dentist) can be modelled (the latter through facial expressions, body posture, etc.).'

Children therefore will observe and imitate the behaviour of their parents. According to Gross (1992), children are sometimes more likely to imitate a same-sex model than an opposite-sex model (even if the behaviour is sex-inappropriate). For example, a female child observing her mother putting on make-up or jewellery is likely to model herself upon her mother's behaviour; similarly, a male child observing his father chopping wood is likely to imitate this behaviour. The child therefore learns the adult perspective. This socialisation process is called 'identification'. Sex-appropriate behaviour is rewarded or reinforced by parents. Therefore, although children attend equally to all models, they imitate same-sex models more, because they are reinforced for doing so (Gross 1992). Activities within the home are divided according to sex stereotypes: wives organise the washing, bedmaking, hoovering, and the food preparation, whereas husbands will engage in do-it-yourself. Since these activities take place in the presence of children growing up, the social learning theory tells us that 'observational learning' takes place during this time. Consequently, girls will identify with their mother, and boys with their father: girls will play with dolls, and boys with chemistry sets or 'Action Man'. As Garrett (1987) went on to note, clothing can also denote the gender of a child; being dressed in pink or blue is a reminder for the appropriate gender-based approach to be used.

Reading material can have similar effects. The literature abounds with specific sex-appropriate images. Magazines for teenage girls, such as *Girls Talk, Girl about town,* and *My Guy,* revolve around boyfriends, love, and romance. These magazines endorse a particular kind of femininity: heterosexual femininity (Garrett, 1992). Boys, however, will read literature that covers areas such as fishing, soccer, and rugby; activities that tend to be outgoing rather than internal and nurturing. Therefore, masculine-type behaviour is socially structured. Mayes (1986), commenting on the ideology of children's toys and books, said: 'Educationalists stress the importance of toys, books, stories and songs when children 'rehearse' their adult roles and develop imaginative skills. By two years some children are aware that there exist sex differentiated ways of playing.'

Parental influences and the roles of reading material are not the only factors likely to reinforce masculinity and femininity. Gross (1992) referred to the effects of the media on gender role stereotypes: 'Social learning theorists are particularly interested in the way that males and females are portrayed on TV, in books, films, etc. Gender roles stereotyping is the belief that it is only natural and fitting for males and females to adhere to traditional gender role patterns.' Gross argued that exposure to the media (such as television and films) tends to strengthen gender identity. To assert that only biological factors or sociopsychological influences predispose and reinforce gender roles in society is to adopt a very constrictive perspective on the matter.

Rosaldo and Lamphere (1974) stated: 'Human activities and feelings are organised not by biology directly, but by the interaction of biological propensities and these various and culture-specific expectations, plans, symbols that coordinate our actions and so permit our species to survive.' These authors stressed the importance of using a biosocial approach to understand gender roles, 'since what is male and what is female will depend upon interpretation of biology that are associated with any culture's mode of life'.

Rosaldo and Lamphere (1974) discussed how studies of human behaviour from a biological perspective have reached similar conclusions as above: 'That biology constrains but does not determine the behaviour of the sexes, and that differences between human males and females reflect an interaction between our physical constitutions and our patterns of social life'.

▼ The Meaning of Feminism

Feminism is not an easy concept to define because there are many diverse interpretations. An immediate assessment of the term is its obvious link with 'feminine matters'—women, gender issues, and women's views on how they feel they are being treated in society and what should be done to improve their social position. This definition, however, does not fully explain the concept. Delmar (1986) expressed her understanding of the term to mean an attitude, a belief by women (feminists) 'that women suffer discrimination because of their sex, that they have specific needs which remain negated and unsatisfied, and that the satisfaction of these needs would require a radical change (some would say a revolution even) in the social, economic and political order'.

Feminism is linked with other images of self-presentation and with the movement of women to cause social change through political action. Self-presentation, Delmar (1986) argued, is to do with 'manners', and ways of behaving to men and women; it is about womanhood and the projection of femininity in one's behaviour. Political action is seen in the unified movement

exercised by women's groups. The feminist movement aims to fight 'economic oppression, commercial exploitation and legal discrimination' (Delmar, 1986).

Cott (1986), however, perceives feminism as aiming 'for individual freedoms by mobilising sex solidarity. It acknowledges diversity among women while positing that women recognise their unity. It requires gender consciousness for its basis, yet calls for the elimination of prescribed gender roles'. Women are seen as humans just like men, but, nevertheless, different, because of their 'reproductive biology' and 'gender construction'.

Rose (1986), on the other hand, argued: 'Feminism has been preoccupied with the distinctive activity of women—with our labour in the world. In bringing this labour out of nature and into history, feminism has uncovered both distinctive social relations around gender and a distinctive relationship to nature'.

The feminist, therefore, is deeply concerned with issues in society relating to the status of women; issues such as inequalities in health, employment, education, housing, and marriage.

▼ Gender and Social Inequality

Social inequality, often the consequence of belonging to a particular gender status, has been a perennial problem for more than a hundred years. Hibbert (1987), writing about the English in the ages of Shakespeare and Milton, commented:

> It was still generally considered, however, that to educate girls to the same standard as boys was unseemly, most people agreeing with Lady Newdigate who expressed a wish in her will that her sons should be brought up in 'good learning', and her daughters in 'virtuous and godly life'. The statutes of

some schools, Harrow for example, specifically excluded girls in accordance with the views of a commentator on female education who wrote in 1524, 'Many men put great doubt whether it should be expedient and requisite or not for a woman to have learning in books of Latin or Greek. And some utterly affirm that it is not only neither necessary nor profitable but also very noisome and jeopardus.'

Here is one of the possible root causes of discrimination between men and women. Such inequality, in thought and action, still pervades many spheres of social life in different parts of the world today. Calman (1992), in her examination of the status of women in India, remarked that the social framework within which women live can be blamed for the inequality they experience. Inequality is evident in the caste system. 'Community, class, and geographic setting create different problems for women of different spheres.' Calman also pointed out that the Hindu code and many Hindu social customs are not models of gender equality. The stereotypes of women in India are bluntly negative. 'A woman is called fickle-minded, sensual, seducer of men: given to falsehood, trickery, folly, greed, impurity and thoughtless action: root of all evil; inconsistent; and cruel.' Women are expected to look up to the male figure—the father, the husband, and the son. A state of subserviency is envisaged of her: 'A woman must never be independent.'

Neither is women's status improved in any way by the impact of religion. Calman (1992) argued that although the Qu'ran is filled with injunctions aimed at bettering the lot of women, the laws in India have been interpreted so as to legitimise the prevailing social norms that have put women in an inferior legal, social, and religious position. Nor is a woman's position in other aspects of her life, such as marriage, in any way much bettered. Whether she wants to or not,

a wife is expected to live with her in-laws; at the very least, her family loyalties are expected to change upon marriage. Men, on the other hand, have a much better deal: men are more valued than women, and boys more than girls. Calman (1992) illustrated this argument concisely when she said: 'Parent's investment of emotional and financial resources in their son is, therefore, an investment in their own future. Simply put, a son is an asset. A daughter is a liability.'

The worth (or lack of worth) of women is further reflected in their treatment as a source of financial reward. According to Calman (1992), the practice of dowry and 'bride price' is still intense. Furthermore, the pursuit to increase one's wealth status is so ardent that 'dowry deaths'—in which young brides are murdered by their husbands or in-laws—occur in their thousands every year. Death of the spouse gives the husband a rationale to ask for increased dowry payments.

Inequality of the sexes can be observed in other aspects of social life; for example, women are not always encouraged to participate in the educational process because this helps to limit the dowry. However, if education is likely to be financially rewarding—by increasing career prospects, for example—the woman is allowed to develop herself educationally.

Women in India do not always obtain occupation in sectors with a high status, such as industries and service fields; they often have to resort to low wages from the agricultural sectors. Calman (1992) argued that laws 'are in practice nearly useless' where equal rights for women are concerned.

In health, too, women are worse off. They are expected to ascertain that the male members of the family are served food first, and then eat what is left over (Calman, 1992);consequently, many women may suffer from malnutrition.

These inequities are not only prevalent in India. French *et al.* (1994) found similar social behaviour and attitudes in Pakistan. Their findings show female infanticide is the norm there. Female children are neglected, whereas males are the focus of benevolencey, respect, and caring. The mortality rate is also much higher among women. As happens in India, women in Pakistan have unequal chances regarding food, and their nutritional status is not satisfactory. Also, Pakistani women are still disadvantaged regarding career opportunities. French *et al.* (1994) argued that the patriarchal society upholds the status of males: education is not considered worthwhile for girls, and family influences (values, beliefs, socialisation control) and the government maintain the inequality.

In contrast, however, urban China seems to demonstrate a degree of gender equality (Stockman, 1994). This equality is, in principle, carried out by the 'danwei' system. Stockman stated:

> [A 'danwei' is] a unique form of
> organisation and is the basic building block
> in Chinese urban society. A 'danwei' can be a
> factory or factory complex, an
> administrative agency, a school or university,
> a hospital, a publishing house or any other
> of a host of apparently specialised
> organisations. Almost all urban Chinese
> belong to a 'danwei'.

Belonging to a 'danwei' means being a lifelong member, even after retirement. It has a multifunctional nature. It has sociopolitical, educational, regulatory (family planning and birth control, marriage counselling, etc.), and participatory (in local government) functions.

Stockman (1994) argued that the occupational structure of work units (within the 'danwei') lends itself to better equality for women than does the capitalistic structure of industrial societies. In China, he pointed out, nearly all women of working age work full-time; full-time or part-time housewives are almost nonexistent. Although inequality is evident in the earning dif-

ferences between men and women as age increases, Stockman concluded that 'Crude measures of gender inequality in urban China reveal no greater inequality than in industrial capitalist societies, in fact possibly greater equality, and a marked reduction in inequality over the period of the building of the communist regime, up to the mid-80s.'

Inequality of the sexes as discussed above is a generalised social phenomenon. It is noticeable in the Nordic countries too. Kaul (1991) recognised that although the Nordic countries, with their advanced rights for women, have come a long way down the road to achieving equality between the sexes, 'the fruits of patriarchal thinking' embodied in the laws perpetuate the implementation of gender segregation in the world of work. Kaul was mainly concerned with the links between parental legal rights (rights to leave-of-absence from work to care for children), and the preservation of the unequal sharing of economic parenting (man as the breadwinner) and practical parenting (caring for the sick, helpless child; feeding and keeping the child clean), through the gender-structured working world: 'Thus the gender structure of work moulds working conditions, which in turn influence a woman's possibility of combining a full working day with family responsibilities.' Lack of autonomy and flexibility at work reinforce the patterns of inequality.

Another factor that constricts women's opportunities for benefits to undertake equal parenting (practising the widely accepted ideology of equality between the sexes in caring) is their labour-market position. Kaul discussed, for example, how men with their 'recognised qualifications and their [male] sex manage to negotiate more autonomous jobs and more benefits for themselves'. Female workers, on the other hand, are excluded from participating in equal rights. The rationale for their exclusion seems to be based on the patriarchal organisation of work, although there is a school of thought, as Kaul pointed out, that their weak market position may be due to the 'family bond'. Staying at home provides women with more meaningful activities—childcare—because 'most women in the labour market work under conditions which do not strengthen their work attachment'. This has the effect of reducing the economic parenting role of women. Again they find themselves victims of their reproductive maternal role: childrearing. For men, however, the economic parenting role is enhanced, whereas the practical parenting aspect is undermined. Kaul concluded that equality in parenting is still a dream; the result of patriarchal laws that make women subordinate to men.

In southern Africa, the subordination of women is common (Akeroyd, 1991). Their role is underestimated and taken for granted; their productive labour is underevaluated; and their subordinate position constrains them in society. The subordinacy is evident in both the domestic and public domains. A case study (Crehan 1983) on 'Subsistence farmers in Mukunashi, northwest Zambia, 1979–81' described the inequality and prevailing attitudes: 'Women harvested grain and had exclusive rights over fields and granaries; a wife had to provide food for the husband and entertain his friends. Children were expected to help their mothers, though boys aged nine or ten became increasingly reluctant to perform 'women's work'.'

This extract highlights the attitudes and expectations about women. The attitudes of the boys probably reflect the influence of socialisation: that there is 'women's work' and 'men's work'. How one should behave as a woman—with reference to domestic and economic activities—is wrapped up in the single sentence: 'What are you doing just sitting there, do you think you are a man?' According to Akeroyd (1991), this was a common reproach by women to their

daughters; women had to be seen to endure their 'very heavy workload'.

In contrast, however, Akeroyd (1991) found that Msengezy women in Zimbabwe (11.5%) had direct management control over their work. Their participation in the running of the farms to some extent demonstrates the important role they play in productive labour. The husbands were criticised for their laziness and for being irresponsible, and women considered that it was only they who kept these men's farming enterprises from collapse. However, Akeroyd (1991) argued that although women recognised their importance in the labour market, this was not overtly acknowledged because they were 'caught up in the coils of 'customs''.

The position of women in southern Africa is perhaps best exposed in the following statement by a Malawian official, reported by Akeroyd (1991):

> Our custom is that women should be subordinate to men. This is how it always has been and it won't change easily. We have always been a male dominated society. Men were hunters but made most of the important decisions . . . Ask any women about decisions. They will talk but in the end they will say: you must ask the man. So this is a cultural thing. In this country men are always above women . . . Men's superiority here is customary—also it's Christian—it's in the Bible.

British women also seem to be caught up in the coils of custom. Lewis and Piachaud (1987), writing about women and poverty in the twentieth century, concluded: 'The persistence of female poverty can only be explained in terms of women's position in society. Women's work is rewarded less than men's and this affects their well being throughout their lives.' Callender (1987), using a different theme, criticised the disadvantaged position of women in the labour market and the resulting poverty, caused by the inadequacy of the social-security benefits system to meet their socio-economic needs. She argued: 'Neither redundancy payments nor social security benefits are rooted in the reality of women's working lives. Rather they are based on misplaced assumptions and upon male dominated notions of employment.'

Daly (1994), commenting on gender and its link with social policy, stated her viewpoint as follows:

> Different goals or objectives of policy can be identified for men and women. From the time of the new Poor Law, an over-riding goal of policy was to drive men to work . . . hence, the British income maintenance system is designed primarily around the need to compensate for the loss of male earnings in terms of the major risks covered: unemployment, illness, retirement from work.

For women, she argued, the aim of policy is to maintain their position in the family role, the caring and reproductive functions. This is achieved by making women more dependent on their husband or partner. However, in the United Kingdom, in spite of the stereotypical image of subordination described by feminists, there is evidence of women occupying prestigious positions: for example, Margaret Thatcher, who was Prime Minister for many years, and other female MPs; there are many female lawyers and solicitors, as well as female civil servants working in government. In addition, the number of female managers and executives is increasing. In the Health Service, for example, most unit managers and ward managers in general hospitals are female, and many more occupy positions of responsibility in community settings.

The dependency of women, their unequal position in society, and, to some extent, their domination by men, appears to be a common theme in social life. The social structures perpet-

uate the inequality between the sexes. The work of feminist writers has raised awareness of the status of women and explained how the status quo is maintained. On the other hand, women have been seen to show initiative and skills in their work and the will power to raise themselves above the stereotypical image of their feminine status.

▼ Summary

The concept of gender is associated with the social factors that make individuals masculine or feminine. Sex, on the other hand, is the biological interpretation of what makes a person male or female; it is therefore concerned with the physical characteristics of people in relation to the presence or absence of either female genitalia and breasts, or male genitalia. Social scientists and biologists have long debated whether gender is a social construction or the consequence of biological factors. The culture and/or nurture arguments rest upon the social influences that determine and produce masculinity and femininity. Social learning theories support this argument. Individuals learn and imitate the behaviour of same-sex adults during their lifelong development. Parents reinforce behaviour that matches their masculine or feminine orientation. On the other hand, biologists argue that the sex chromosomes determine maleness and femaleness, the basis for future femininity or masculinity. However, it is argued that such a reductionist approach is to be avoided; rather one should acknowledge that biosocial factors should be included in the discussions.

Feminism is a concept related to gender issues in general and the ways women are treated in society; it considers discrimination, and highlights the position and status of women. There are many social inequalities in society as far as the position of women is concerned. Various writers have exposed the social inequality, exploitation, and subordination of women in different parts of the world: in southern Africa, India, Pakistan, some Nordic countries, and Britain. This is evident in areas such as education, employment, and the home environment, as well as concerning social policy, which can be a cause of poverty.

▼ Application to Clinical Practice

Healthcare professionals in clinical practice sometimes encounter individuals whose sex and gender identities are ambiguous. The medical terms applicable in these circumstances are:

- Hermaphroditism: a state characterised by the presence of both male and female sex organs.
- Testicular feminisation syndrome: a condition due to lack of cellular receptors for testosterone and dihydrotestosterone, in which the subject is phenotypically female (phenotype: the entire physical, biochemical and physiological make-up of an individual), but lacks the nuclear sex chromatin and is of XY chromosomal sex: the uterus and tubes are absent or rudimentary, and the gonads are typically testes or may be abdominal or inguinal in position.

(*Dorland's Medical Dictionary*, 1988)

The psychosocial and sexual needs of individuals with ambiguous sex characteristics cannot be overemphasised. It is imperative that healthcare professionals make a thorough and empathetic assessment of the person, and identify any coun-

selling needs. Hermaphrodites and people with testicular feminisation syndrome experience intense emotional and psychological conflicts because of confusion about their sexual identity. As one sufferer expressed in the *British Medical Journal* (1994): 'I am chromosomally male, a pseudohermaphrodite. These two phrases pervaded my rational thought. I did not think I was female. I did not think I was male. I did not know what I was.'

Patients with testicular feminisation syndrome may consider themselves bizarre and unconventional; they may experience a state of 'freakishness'. They should be given time and encouragement to express freely their feelings, fears, and anxieties. The nature of their condition, and its manifestations, should be explained to them clearly and unambiguously, without using any technical jargon. It must be emphasised that although the patient is chromosomally male and their genotype is male, their phenotype is female (BMJ, 1994). The service of an experienced counsellor is recommended, with the patient's agreement. Helping patients to cope with their altered body image should include 'protection from the inevitable inquiries from fellow patients, family, and nursing staff' (*BMJ*, 1994). Some relatives and friends may be too inquisitive, thus adding to the distress of the patient. Anticipating and preventing such circumstances from occurring is possible by involving the patient in care intervention. Furthermore, members of the healthcare team should be thoroughly briefed as to their specific roles.

Ahlquist (1994) made a significant assertion when he said: 'To explain the diagnosis by telling the patient that she is fundamentally male but with abnormal sexual development may, to the purist, be embryologically correct but does nothing to help: it simply destroys a most fundamental part of a person's identity-gender. That is unecessary.' The focus of the explanation, he emphasised, should be on the understanding that the patient is female. Preserving the gender identity of the sufferer is an essential component of the care principle, and can be achieved by a tactful and empathetic approach. The patient, however, still needs unambiguous information concerning the physiological change (alteration in gonads, chromosomal sex, etc.).

Another suffer (*BMJ*, 1994) made reference to the parents' needs for support and appropriate counselling when the condition is first identified: 'Unless parents can talk openly at the time of diagnosis with a professional counsellor and are given information—on what and when to tell their child, contacts with other sufferers, sources of counselling or psychotherapy ...—they will become imprisoned by their own feelings.'

The feelings of shame and helplessness can traumatise both the patient and significant others. An atmosphere conducive to openness and support should be created by all professionals involved. Also, there are some patients, such as those reported by Dowdell (1983), for whom gender reassignment (trans-sexualism) becomes the ultimate personal goal. These patients experience the feeling of not wanting to be a man, and desire the adoption of female gender characteristics by undergoing surgery. Such individuals experience social traumas and are stigmatised for their 'unconventional' and 'bizarre' aspirations. Being a man and wanting to become a woman, or vice versa, creates tension and personal conflicts. As Rees (1993) pointed out: 'There was the conflict of my male identity, my self, with my abhorred female body: conflict with my family, whose expectations were never met; conflict with those around me; a society that taunted me— "he, she or it?".

Conflicts arise too from the dual roles the person feels the need to play. As Dowdell (1983) illustrated in her care study, Lesley (a man) had to work as a man during the day but went out as a woman at night. The risk of losing one's employment if discovered also creates increasing anxieties. Being called an 'it', or being branded a 'queer' or a 'freak' is a humiliating experience (Dowdell, 1983).

The role of healthcare professionals in the assessment and management of trans-sexual problems is comprehensively underlined by Schapira *et al.* (1979). They suggested a distinction should be made between transvestism—in which individuals (usually males) dress in the clothes of the opposite sex but do not regard themselves as belonging to that sex—and trans-sexualism. Trans-sexuals feel a sense of belonging to the opposite sex, of having been born in the 'wrong' sex, and need surgical remodelling of their genitalia. They experience a sense of estrangement from their bodies; all manifestations of sex differentiation are regarded as repugnant. They have a strong wish to be accepted and understood by society. The role of healthcare professionals is to understand all these characteristics.

Schapira *et al.* (1979) suggested a thorough and detailed assessment should be undertaken to identify the history as follows:

- The physical development (e.g. milestone development, illnesses, and operations in childhood).
- Psychological and psychosexual development (the patient's position in sibship, age of first cross-dressing, commitment for re-assignment, homosexual or heterosexual tendencies).
- Environmental factors (parental attitudes in relation to birth and sex of the patient, psychosexual problems in parents).

Employment records and a physical examination are other aspects to consider. A psychological and psychiatric profile is also required. The management of the trans-sexual should be based on an empathetic approach. As Thomas (1993) pointed out, trans-sexualism remains a much misunderstood condition, and continues to be sensationalised by the media. The professional's awareness of how stigmatised the patient may be should be sharpened. Rees (1993) wrote: 'Trans-sexuals often experience a great deal of tension in their lives, not only from their own dissatisfaction, lack of sexual wellbeing and difficulties in social adaptation, but also because of societal insensitivity, victimisation, ridicule and intolerance.'

A supportive and relaxed environment should be set up, in which the patient is given the opportunity to develop modes of behaviour and actions appropriate to his or her preferred gender role. Training in feminine or masculine skills is necessary to ensure the correct deportment is displayed. A multidisciplinary involvement is advised; for example, a beautician to suggest the best ways to apply make-up, a dressmaker to recommend the use of suitable clothes. Other professionals may include psychotherapists, counsellors and pharmacologists (for medication). Throughout the treatment, the role of the healthcare professional is to give continuing support: active listening, unambiguous communication, and the seeking of specialised advice when necessary. Professionals in a variety of healthcare settings must participate in the caring process to ensure patient care needs are met optimally. The sociolegal and personal implications of the new gender identity are wide-ranging. After treatment, the patient will still need continuing and objective support to cope with the new image. Thomas (1993) expressed the following viewpoint: 'The majority of trans-sexuals suffer from problems such as anxiety and depression, which is not surprising considering the profound psychological disturbance they experience in their gender identities and roles. Unresolved gender identity often leads to suicide attempts, alcoholism or drug misuse.' The role of the nurse in preventing unnecessary distress and stress in the patient cannot be overemphasised.

Caring for people who are gay or lesbian is another area that has stimulated many discussions in the nursing arena. The role of healthcare professionals in recognising the humanity of individuals who are lesbians or gay men should be affirmed. Platzer (1993) uncovered the attitudes of nurses and doctors in their interactions with gay men and lesbians. She asserted: 'There is evidence that a significant number of nurses and doctors are prejudiced towards, and fearful of, lesbians and gay men.' Platzer (1993) went on to argue that there is also evidence of 'hostility, distancing rejection, voyeurism, inappropriate psychiatric referral, and not allowing the partner to visit or accompany the patient'. These observations have implications for nursing practice. To provide clinical care for gay men and lesbians requires a nonjudgemental approach and much empathy. Neglecting to do this may result in patients failing to disclose crucial information related to health practices. There may be a fear that confidentiality will not be maintained, the long-term consequences of which could endanger factors such as employment and housing, custody of children, and the freedom to emigrate (Platzer, 1993).

Assumptions and stereotypes about gay men and lesbians tend to restrict their care needs. As Platzer pointed out, it is often assumed that   family life and relationships in the lesbian and   gay community are somehow less serious. Professionals should give sensitive care to the patients and their loved ones, whatever the circumstances.

To many people, being a gay man or a lesbian means an association with humna immunodeficiency virus (HIV) and acquired immunodeficiency syndrome (AIDS). This unfortunately leads to homophobia, an irrational fear and distorted view of homosexuality and homosexuals. Many lesbians and gay men, therefore, experience rejection from their families, friends, and health-care professionals. Mental ill-health, social isolation, suicidal tendencies, and unwanted pregnancies are some of the possible results. It is important in clinical practice, therefore, to show empathy and to provide a supportive and therapeutic environment in which the patients may regain self-confidence, self-esteem, and self-worth.

When trans-sexuals, gay men, or lesbians are admitted to the ward environment (either mental health or general nursing settings), they may suffer harassment and hostility from other patients and some members of the ward team. The role of the healthcare professional is to discuss the patient's needs in private, paying regard to their feelings about interactions with other patients and staff. The issue of confidentiality should be considered. The use of a side-room should be offered to patients who so wish. Caring for patients with conflicting gender identities can be challenging in clinical practice; nurses often find it difficult to decide upon which approach to use, and in which type of ward the patient should be nursed.

■ GENDER DIFFERENCES IN CONFLICT MANAGEMENT IN CLINICAL PRACTICE

Men and women use different strategies to manage conflict, in both clinical and non-clinical settings. For example, Valentine (1995) referred to Rahim's 1983b study of the conflict management style used by 50 female and 50 male managers in business and industry, which found that women were 'more integrating, avoiding, and compromising, and less obliging than men'. Valentine found that other studies in non-clinical settings had drawn similar conclusions: women avoided 'destructive competition, made greater concessions, and tried to find accommodating solutions if the other player was cooperative from the

beginning'; women tended to ignore competition and aggression issues, preferring to discuss subjects such as loving others, home, and family.

Valentine's study (1995) found that avoidance was also a strategy used by nurse educators. Female nurse managers, however, were seen to be less competitive and collaborative, and more avoiding than their male counterparts. Valentine argued that the avoidance strategy of women is probably the result of socialisation processes. Women are seen to prevent the disruption of interpersonal relationships. To be dominant and assertive seems to be contradictory to the nurturing and caring approach that is expected of nurses. Valentine (1995) argued: 'There is a need to understand conflict management from women's (nurses') perspectives. This understanding would help nurses better evaluate how to handle conflictual situations.'

■ THE INTEGRATION OF MALE AND FEMALE PATIENTS ON THE WARDS

Although there is a high predominance of female personnel in the nursing profession, the trend is gradually changing, with an increase in the number of male nurses. This has implications for clinical practice. Female nurses havetraditionally worked on both female-patient and male-patient wards. Male nurses, on the other hand, need chaperoning by a female member of staff whenever they attend to female patients' needs. Male nurses contribution to care delivery, however, is just as relevant, and becomes more so on mixed-sex wards. Burgess (1994) suggested that before integrating male and female patients in hospital settings, account should be taken of their values and beliefs, as well as their customs.

Swan (1994) pointed to the beneficial effects of gender integration: a marked reduction in the amount of major tranquillisers used by patients compared with that used by the same patients when they resided in other wards at the same hospital; a reduction in the amount of seclusion and in self-injurious behaviour.

Thomas *et al.* (1992) noted that most patients (57%) at the Maudsley Hospital preferred to be in a mixed ward. Reasons given were that it would be an opportunity to develop relationships and that it would provide a more balanced atmosphere. However, some women (27%) disagreed with integration because of reports of some women being harassed by men walking into their room, particularly at night, while others felt nervous in the company of men and thought they would benefit from mixing exclusively with other women.

Review Questions

1 'Teenage boys, particularly if they are in a group, are registered by adults as threatening and treated accordingly. Of course their loud, physical, swaggering behaviour contributes to this perception . . . It is the reaction to his behaviour that will begin to teach him he has the power to frighten people—a power which he may not actually want at all or which, on the other hand, he may enjoy' (Phillips, 1993).

Discuss the social influences likely to predispose to masculine behaviour in boys.

2 Lesley is a 40-year-old male-to-female trans-sexual. She works in a supermarket in the day time. At night she works as a barmaid in the local pub. She lives on her own in a village, a few miles out of town.

(i) Examine the social and psychological implications of being a trans-sexual in a westernised society.

(ii) Discuss the assessment and management profile of Lesley prior to gender re-assignment.

▼ References

Ahlquist J. Gender identity in testicular feminisation. Phenotypically, anatomically, legally and socially female. *Br Med J* 1994, **308**:1041.

Akeroyd A. Gender, food production and property rights: constraints on women farmers in southern Africa. In: Afshar H, ed. *Women development and survival in the third world.* Harlow: Longman; 1991:139–171.

Anonymous. Once a dark secret. *Br Med J* 1994, **308**:542.

Anonymous. Be open and honest with sufferers. *Br Med J* 1994, **308**:1041–1042.

Burgess L. Mixed responses: gender, patient choice. *Nursing Times* 1994, **90**:30–33.

Callender C. Redundancy, unemployment and poverty. In: Glendinning C, Millar J, eds. *Women and poverty in Britain.* Brighton: Wheatsheaf Books; 1987:137–158.

Calman L. *Toward empowerment. Women and movement politics in India.* Oxford: Westview Press; 1992.

Cott N. Feminist theory and feminist movements: the past before us. In: Mitchell J, Oakley A, eds. *What is Feminism?* Oxford: Basil Blackwell; 1986:49–62.

Crehan K. *Women and development in north western Zambia: from producer to housewife.* Review of African political economy. 1988, **27/28:** 51–66.

Daly M. A matter of dependency: gender in British income maintenance provision. *Sociology* 1994, **28**:779–797.

Delmar R. What is feminism? In: Mitchell J, Oakley A, eds. *What is Feminism?* Oxford: Basil Blackwell; 1986:8–33.

Dorland's Illustrated Medical Dictionary 27th ed.: no. 27. Philadelphia: W.B. Saunders & Company; 1988: 617.

Dowdell P. Sex change operation. Nursing care study. *Nursing Mirror* 1983, **156**:46-49.

French S, Watters D, Matthews D. Nursing as a career choice for women in Pakistan. *J Adv Nurs* 1994, **19**:140–151.

Garrett S. *Gender.* London: Routledge; 1992.

Gross R. *Psychology, the science of mind and behaviour,* *2nd ed.* London: Hodder & Stoughton; 1992:675–699.

Hayes N. *Foundation of psychology. An introductory text.* London: Routledge; 1994:749–751.

Hibbert C. *The English. A social history 1066–1945.* London: Book Club Associates; 1987:272.

Kaul H. Who cares? Gender equality and care leave in the Nordic countries. *Acta Sociologica* 1991, **34**: 115–125.

Lewis J, Piachaud D. Women and poverty in the twentieth century. In: Glendinning C, Millar J, eds. *Women and poverty in Britain.* Brighton: Wheatsheaf Books; 1987:28–52.

Mayes P. *Sociology in focus. Gender.* Harlow: Longman; 1986.

Phillips A. *The trouble with boys.* Hammersmith: Pandora; 1993.

Platzer H. Nursing care of gay and lesbian patients. *Nursing Standard* 1993, **7**:34–37.

Rahim A (1983b). Measurement of Organisational Conflict. *Jrnl of General Psychology,* 109(**4**):189–199.

Rees M. He, she or it? Transsexualism. *Nursing Times* 1993, **89**:48–49.

Rosaldo M, Lamphere L. *Women, culture and society.* California: Stanford University Press; 1974:5.

Rose H. Women's work: women's knowledge. In: Mitchell J, Oakley A, eds. *What is feminism?* Oxford: Basil Blackwell; 1986:161–183.

Schapira K, Davison K, Brierley H. The assessment and management of transsexual problems. *Br J Hosp Med* 1979, July **22**:63–69.

Stockman N. Gender inequality and social structure in urban China. Sociology. *J Br Sociol Assoc* 1994, **28**(**3**):759–777.

Swan T. Living together—specialist hospitals—gender. *Nursing Times* 1994, **90**:34–36.

Thomas B, Vearnals S, *et al.* Involuntary cohabitees. *Nursing Times* 1992, **88**:58–60.

Thomas B. Gender loving care. *Nursing Times* 1993, **89**:50–51.

Valentine P. Management of conflict: do nurses/women handle it differently? *J Adv Nursing* 1995, **22**:142–149.

▼ Further Reading

Corea G, *et al. Man made women. How new reproductive technologies affect women.* London: Hutchinson; 1985.

Figes E. *Patriarchal attitudes. Women in society.* London: Faber & Faber; 1970.

Figes K. *Because of her sex. The myth of equality for women in Britain.* London: Macmillan; 1994.

Fuller T, *et al.* Gender and health: some Asian evidence. *J Health Soc Behav* 1993, **34**:252–271.

Weiner G. Feminist education and equal opportunities: unity or discord? *Br J Sociol Educ* 1986, **7**:265–274.

Social Construction of Behaviour: *Ethnicity and Race*

9

▼ Towards a Definition of Ethnicity and Race

Classification in every life does not follow the same principles as classification in the laboratory. People give to themselves names which show who they claim to be rather than who they actually are. They give to others names which show how they perceive these others, and which may differ from the names the others have for themselves. The names show they identify themselves by religion or nationality more often than by race (Banton, 1988).

Minority groups, such as the Afro-Caribbeans in Britain, identify themselves not only by their nationality and religion, but also by their sociocultural beliefs, values, and practices. These attributes become apparent among a society in which practices are sharply different, for example in the British culture. Banton (1988) regarded ethnicity as an attribute of minorities. The minorities, such as Hindus, Muslims, Chinese, are the ethnic groups. Ethnicity is the sum of cultural characteristics: language, history, customs, religious beliefs and practices, art, music, type of food, type of clothing, etc. Banton pointed out that the English have not regarded themselves as an ethnic group because being the largest (i.e. majority) group and the dominant element in the population, there has been no pressure on them to ask what makes them distinctive. They do, however, become a minority group when they are abroad.

O'Donnell (1991) argued that ethnicity should be seen as a 'real' social and cultural 'phenomenon', in comparison with race, which is sociologically interpreted as an 'ideological invention and myth'.

Posing the question 'What is ethnicity?', Eriksen (1993) presented a contrasting viewpoint:

> Contrary to a widespread commonsense view, cultural difference between two groups is not the decisive feature of ethnicity. Two distinctive, endogamous groups, say, somewhere in New Guinea, may well have widely different languages, religious beliefs and even technologies, but that does not necessarily mean that there is an ethnic relationship between them. For ethnicity to come about, the groups must have a minimum of contact with each other, and they must entertain ideas of each other as being culturally different from themselves.

Eriksen (1993) identified the main ingredients of ethnicity to be the social relationships between 'agents who consider themselves as culturally distinctive from members of other groups with whom they have a minimum of regular interaction'. His argument is founded on Michael Moerman's fieldwork on ethnic relations in Thailand, among an ethnic group called the Lue. Although the Lue's culture as described by themselves was no different to other groups, the researcher concluded that their ethnicity is substantiated by the perception of themselves as distinctively different to other groups. Eriksen referred to the technical term 'emic category of ascription', which means the native's point of view rather than the observer's assessment or analysis of the social situation.

Eriksen (1993) argued that ethnicity can also be expressed by using stereotypes. He stated: 'Used analytically, the concept of stereotyping refers to the creation and consistent application of standardised notions of the cultural distinctiveness of a group.' Eriksen gave examples of such stereotyping to explain his argument, citing experiences gained on the polyethnic, Indian Ocean island society of Mauritius: for example, Creoles are stereotyped as 'lazy, merry, careless', whereas Hindus are considered to be 'stingy, dishonest, hardworking'. He stressed that stereotypes may not depict a realistic picture of ethnic groups, but do serve the purpose of 'defining the boundaries of one's own group'.

From a contrasting viewpoint, Rex (1986) argued that the terms 'race' and 'ethnicity' are used in a variety of ways 'in popular and political discourse'. This makes it difficult to provide a clearcut definition, since the terms sometimes blend into each other. He explained that ethnic differences are perceived to be related to racial differences, for example between blacks and whites. On the other hand, there is a school of thought that considers all minorities who are immigrants as ethnic. In the United Kingdom, he pointed out, in a 'peculiar popular usage', black and Asian people are regarded as immigrants, whereas actual immigrants from Europe, Ireland, and the white Commonwealth are not. From being called immigrants at an earlier period, the blacks and Asians later become known as ethnic minorities. Rex also evaluated the tendency to use a phenotypical approach in the elucidation of the concept of race, whereas ethnicity is seen to be more founded on cultural differences.

One cultural aspect that denotes ethnic differences and boundaries is language. Modood et al. (1994) recognised the importance of linguistic heritage in showing the distinct feature of ethnicity, which, they stressed, 'is widely regarded as the central element of peoplehood'.

In their fieldwork exploration of ethnic identity, Modood *et al.* (1994) reported their findings on community languages in the maintenance of ethnicity. The Asians interviewed were more keen to maintain their linguistic heritage: 'Moreover, they had brought up their children to speak in the relevant community language and believed that this was an important part of their children's upbringing and cultural identity.' A similar finding was highlighted among the second-generation Caribbean population: 'There is no doubt of the desire amongst the Caribbean second generation for a revival of the Creole and the Patois linguistic heritage.'

Marriage, family, social contacts, and religion are also factors likely to enhance one's ethnic exclusivity. These varying social tendencies will make a distinct ethnic group. Ethnicity is related to an ethnic group's relationships with the society as a whole and with other groups in it (Sills, 1968). Cashmore (1984) stated that ethnicity is a term applied to 'a group possessing some degree of coherence and solidarity composed of people who are at least aware of their common origins and interests'. Whatever the interpretations given to the notion of ethnicity, it is founded on distinct, exclusive, social practices of a minority group, whose subjective awareness of themselves as a group must be taken into consideration.

The *Concise Oxford English Dictionary* (1991) defines race as each of the major divisions of humankind, having distinct physical characteristics; a tribe, nation, regarded as of a distinct ethnic stock. To define race in physical or biological terms is, according to O'Donnell (1991), unsuccessful as a basis for categorising people and of explaining differences in behaviour. The concept of race in sociology, he argued, is concerned with the social interpretation and construction of 'myths' in connection with 'superiority and inferiority around notions of racial difference'. In society, therefore, people will use the term 'race' in connection with groups of people, for example the Chinese race, the English race, the African race, and so on. The members of these groups, biologists argue, are distinguishable by the physical characteristics they possess, such as skin colour and type of hair. If specific races are linked with concepts of superiority and inferiority (as in Nazi Germany), these are social constructs, myths created by one race to undermine the integrity of another race. On the other hand, one can argue that there is only one race in the world: the human race.

Banton (1988) asserted that there is a social process by which individuals are assigned to categories. This categorisation, he stated, is founded on 'people's consciousness of such differences' according to circumstances. He gave this example:

> A person may not remember whether the bus driver to whom he or she paid a fare two hours ago was black or white because colour does not signify very much in the relationship between a bus driver and a passenger. But if that same person's sister had brought home a new boyfriend the previous week, he or she would remember whether the boyfriend was black or Asian or white, and a lot more about him.

As Watson (1977) explained, 'Definitions of race, like 'colour', vary widely according to the perceptions and social expectations of the beholder.' When black and white children play together, they only notice the differences in their complexion. There is no subjective feeling of racial differences, a 'them-and-us' situation. However, parental attitudes and socialisation processes may soon alter the children's perceptions.

Although physical differences, evident in skin

colour and hair type, are used to categorise a race, the social construct is seen to be an influential factor. Social processes, perceptions, and circumstances are linked in the framework.

▼ Ethnic Minorities in Society

Most of the literature on ethnic minorities tends to focus on immigrants such as the Africans, Chinese, Polish people, etc., but somehow fails to consider one ethnic minority that for more than 500 years has made its presence felt within the British Isles: the gypsies.

■ THE GYPSIES

Gypsies are diverse groupings of travelling people who lead a nomadic type of existence. Hawes and Perez (1995) made a distinction between gypsies and new-age travellers, stating that the latter form a quite different group of nomads; they are a phenomenon mainly of the south and south-west of England, of younger families with no generational history of travelling, whose ranks have been increased in the 1990s by many younger homeless people for whom the shortage of social housing has left no alternative but to take to the road. Gypsies, in contrast, have been in existence since well before 1500. Although they probably originated from India (Hawes & Perez, 1995), the term 'gypsies' is a corruption of 'Egyptian'. Hawes and Perez stated that Henry VIII's 'Egyptian Act' reflected the generally held belief that gypsies came from Egypt. The name they apply to themselves is Rom, which may be derived from Romanoi (Horsley, 1987).

The wandering or nomadic life style of the gypsies has been a perennial social issue. To the authorities and to the majority, this minority group represents a source of interference 'for new and higher standards of urban and rural development, transportation, conservation and social development' (Hawes & Perez, 1995). Their overcrowded living conditions in tents or caravans, as Hawes and Perez pointed out, are classed as 'a statutory nuisance if prejudicial to the health of inmates or giving rise to nuisance'.

Another social issue is in relation to their camping on unauthorised land, forced by a shortage in the number of appropriate caravan sites provided by local authorities. Hawes and Perez (1995) stated that the Caravan Sites Act of 1968 was 'in fact flawed and inadequate; it was ignored by recalcitrant authorities and by unenthusiastic ministers'.

Hawes and Perez highlighted the many facets of the social conflicts that arise between gypsies and the state. They underlined how the specific social needs of gypsies are not adequately met. The provision of caravan sites is not sufficient in itself, since the travelling population have other basic needs: water supply, health facilities, education, a place of safety for families to live, and freedom from harassment and prejudice as well as discrimination. Being a gypsy does not limit one's confrontation to only the authorities and the law, but also includes the residents of the area where one is living as well. Conflicts arise between town dwellers and gypsies due to misunderstandings of each other's practices and beliefs, and are compounded by stereotyping, the result of many years of misperception as well as fears of gypsies.

Intervention to minimise the plight of gypsies by local government is seen in the Local Government Planning and Land Act of 1980. This gave local government access to implement services for gypsies and to provide more sites.

■ THE CHINESE, MUSLIMS, WEST AFRICANS, AND POLES

In this section are outlined some social facts relevant to the ethnic minorities listed above. It is emphasised, however, that these are just some of the minorities to be found in society.

The Chinese are well known for their ubiquitous presence in almost every British county, where they have established a niche for themselves in the catering trade take—away outlets and various restaurants. Watson (1977) saw the Chinese as being in control of the economic aspect of their lives. This 'economic niche', he said, 'allows the migrants to live, work, and prosper without changing their way of life to suit British social expectations.'

British social expectations are not contradicted because this hard-working minority group are in competition with other minorities in the food trade. Watson argued the Chinese 'do not compete directly with English workers for jobs in commerce or industry'. Their interests in food processing and the high profile of their restaurants are developments to meet the increasing competition from other immigrants in catering.

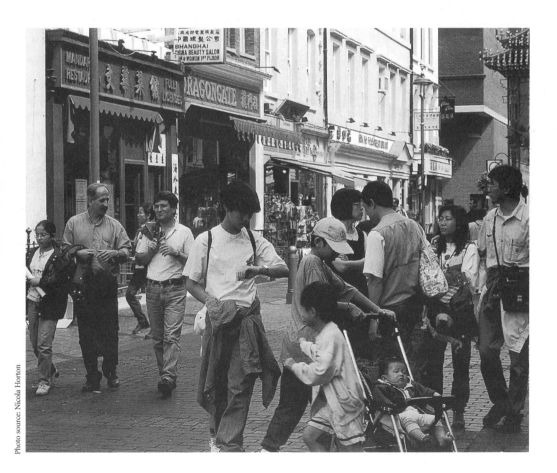

Photo source: Nicola Horton

▲ *London's China Town.*

'The Chinese compete vigorously with the Cypriots and the Bengalis in the catering trade but they do not carry the same spirit of entrepreneurial adventure with them into the wider society' (Watson, 1977).

Catering is not the only forte of the Chinese; there are many Chinese professionals—doctors, solicitors, teachers, bankers, and business executives—too. However, in these situations they form the minorities, in comparison with their position in catering.

As is the case in certain other countries (e.g. the United States, India, Mauritius, and Thailand), some major cities in Britain have their own China Town. In China Towns, Watson (1977) pointed out, such as that in the West End of London, the Chinese congregate. Restaurants, gambling halls, shops, and travel agencies constitute some of the economy-oriented establishments.

Many Chinese have learned to speak the English language, and Chinese children in Britain often play an indispensable role in the family as interpreters (Watson, 1977). Failing to communicate adequately has implications for health and illness matters. As Watson pointed out, many Chinese resort to Chinese doctors for help.

According to Watson, the industrious, quiet, and hard-working Chinese in the catering trade have acquired a new stereotype, the effect of sensationalised news from the media: heroin trafficker and 'Triad' member.

Muslims form another ethnic minority in Britain and elsewhere. Jansen (1994), commenting on Muslims in the Netherlands, acknowledged the strength of their religious conviction, to the extent that the Dutch public experienced shock when Muslims held public demonstrations supporting the death penalty on Salman Rushdie. To Muslims, religion is law and law is religion. In Dutch society, as Jansen pointed out,

'religion may be marginal . . . but to Muslims religion is not marginal; it is one of the central facts of life'. The Dutch consider Muslim communities in the Netherlands as 'ethnic communities' (Jansen, 1994). The problem identified by Jansen is related to what constitutes a priority for the Dutch and Muslims. According to Jansen, both the general public and the authorities interpret these communities according to a variety of social factors, not according to religious criteria; conversely, the Muslims define many of their problems as religious. The conflict arises when Muslims, guided by their religion, demand acceptance of their practices from Dutch authorities. Jansen gave some examples: 'Should polygamous marriages be recognised by Dutch laws? Should Dutch rules be bent to accommodate Muslim law on parental custody after divorce?' Another issue that causes debate is the Islamic method of animal slaughter, which involves the cutting of the animal's carotid arteries, a practice not totally accepted by the Dutch public. Other issues concern whether provision should be made for mosques to be built and whether Dutch education authorities should allow girls to wear head-dresses as prescribed by the Qu'ran.

Other ethnic minorities living in Britain include the Polish immigrants. These people left Poland as political exiles following the war in the 1940s, or later because of economic reasons. Patterson (1977) noticed the degree of integration of Polish people after many years of exile. She commented: 'With their large proportion of urbanised, educated members, such exile groups are more adaptable and ultimately more acceptable to the receiving society in social and cultural spheres than are most groups of economic mass migrants.'

In contrast to the Poles, West Africans have come to Britain to acquire professional qualifications and to develop technical skills that will be used subsequently on their return to Africa (Goody & Groothues, 1977). To achieve this objective, according to the researchers, this ethnic group arrange fostering for their children to help the parents cope with the demands of their studies and the part-time work they have to do to survive financially.

Ethnic minorities bring with them diversified cultures. In most cases, their ties with their homelands remain strong. Their ability to adapt to their new social environment has helped them to maintain a good economic position.

▼ Manifestations of Racism in Society

Racism may be defined as the belief of superiority of one race over another. Solomos (1993), however, argued that the term 'race' does not exist in any scientifically meaningful sense. He defined racism as a broad term encompassing 'those ideologies and social processes which discriminate against others on the basis of their putatively different racial memberships'. Racism, he asserted, should be viewed in its wider social context—not as a 'static phenomenon', but as a process in continual motion, 'being produced and reproduced' by the media, the legal system, and other institutions in society.

The approaches and strategies used by institutions in their dealings with groups of migrants expose the attitudes and concerns that their presence stirs in society. For example, Solomos' 1992 article on the 'Politics of immigration since 1945' revealed a common theme of social uneasiness and increased concern about immigration of black people. However, as Solomos stressed, concern was not so overtly evident in relation to other migrants from Europe: 'What recent research has made clear is that even at this early stage black migration and settlement was politically perceived in a different way from European migration.' From 1945 to 1962, the political debate was 'racialised', concern being expressed regarding the social problems of 'having too many black migrants and the question of how they could be stopped from entering given their legal rights in the 1948 British Nationality Act'. While the racialisation of immigration policy was taking place, there were immigrants from the Republic of Ireland 'retaining the right of unrestricted entry and settlement', while the state was also encouraging the use of migrant labour from Europe (Solomos, 1992).

Solomos argued the same process of discrimination was also evident during the 'Thatcher Years'. The British Nationality Act of 1981 was criticised by the public and parliamentarians for reinforcing racial discrimination. 'The power of immigration as a political symbol', as Solomos put it, wields more tightening measures of control, in the form of visa controls introduced in 1986 for visitors from India, Pakistan, Bangladesh, Nigeria, and Ghana. The riots of 1981 and 1985 were perceived by many of the public and some politicians as the consequence of black immigrants in the country. Nobody seemed to have expressed it more forcefully than Enoch Powell, when in 1968 he talked about the 'rivers of blood' and the 'enemy within'.

Immigration control and the role of the state in the debate concerning immigrants and the black communities represent one aspect of a complex phenomenon. Other issues are related to the labour market and the racial disadvantages associated with it; the housing situation; and the relationship between the welfare state and the black people.

Brown (1992) discussed how the employment of racial minorities is a complicated issue, with the institutions in society and the media being partly responsible for the complexity. He stated: 'The underlying processes are racial exploitation and exclusion, economic migration and community consolidation.' In his comments about black immigrant workers in the 1950s and 1960s, Brown remarked how the quality of their jobs was poor compared with that of non-black people: 'Migrants moved into public service employment which was falling behind private industry in wage levels, and into industrial jobs with long hours, shiftwork, or unpleasant conditions.'

Skellington and Morris (1992) argued that the trends of the 1950s and the 1960s concerning work and the black immigrants have not altered, since there is still a high concentration of black people employed in the manufacturing and manual work for which they were recruited originally. These authors described how, in 1988, 53% of men from the ethnic-minority groups in general were employed in the distribution, hotels, and catering sectors, where wages are low, compared with 36% of white men.

Therefore, segregation and exclusion, as far as ethnic black minorities and employment are concerned, have hardly been annihilated, despite the three Race Relations Acts of 1965, 1968, and 1976. 'The lack of substantial improvement in the general position of blacks and Asians within the labour market is all the more disappointing because the past decade has been a period of apparent political breakthrough for Britain's minorities' (Brown, 1992).

The employment sector is not the only arena where racism prevails. For instance, Ginsburg (1992) referred to studies conducted during the 1970s and 1980s on race and council housing. Research in a number of local authority housing departments—including Nottingham, Liverpool,Hackney, Tower Hamlets, Bedford, and Birmingham—mostly documented institutional processes by which black applicants for council housing waited longer than white people and, once rehoused, received inferior accommodation to white people. Nor is the situation limited to council housing. Skellington and Morris (1992) highlighted how evidence at the beginning of the 1990s suggested that racial bias still persisted in the private rented sector, although at more subtle levels.

Catering for the housing needs of Asians and the black minorities is marginal, and becomes even more so when one considers women in the minority groups (Watson & Austerberry, 1986). A similar feeling is expressed by Ginsburg and Watson (1992) on the issues of race and gender: 'A second key aspect of housing and race in Britain is the growth of official homelessness over the past decade which has differentially affected black people, while their right and their treatment under the Homeless Persons Act have been inferior.' Ginsburg and Watson (1992) argue that increased homelessness can be seen among black women: 46% of Brent's officially homeless were single mothers in 1986.

Even if the hurdles to obtain accommodation are overcome, Asians and black minorities may then encounter more problems. Skellington and Morris (1992) reported the dilemmas faced by the minorities who are the victims of racial harassment by other tenants on the estates where they live.

Social dilemmas for the ethnic black and Asian minorities encompass the bulk of problems they have to tackle: how to maintain their culture in spite of racial inequalities; how to cope with socio-economic eventualities; and how to exercise self-control in spite of adversity and numerous types of social rule. Racism, unfortunately, is firmly embedded in the social structure and is expressed in many subtle ways.

▼ Summary

Ethnicity is interpreted to mean the sum of cultural characteristics—such as language, history, customs, religious practices and beliefs, art, music, type of food, and type of clothing—of a group. A group is perceived to be ethnic when these characteristics do not match those of the dominant or majority culture: for example, Muslims are ethnic groups in British and Dutch societies. Ethnicity therefore shows distinctiveness. It is a sociocultural phenomenon. It should also be seen from the ethnic group's subjective interpretation of what makes them different to other groups, a term called 'emic category of ascription'.

The terms 'race' and 'ethnicity' are sometimes used synonymously, which complicates clarification of their distinctiveness. Some scholars have explained the meaning of race from a phenotypical approach, whereas ethnicity is understood to be culturally founded. Race, however, is still the product of a combination of social processes.

There are many types of ethnic minorities in society, such as gypsies, Africans, Chinese, Poles and Muslims. Each ethnic group displays individual sociocultural needs and socio-economic adaptability away from their home origins.

Racism is defined as the belief of superiority of one race over another, although 'race' is a social construct. Racism is expressed institutionally when various forms of social control are implemented, as in immigration restricting black people and Asian minorities from entering a country. It is also evident in the labour and housing markets. To be black or of Asian origin and female will further reduce one's life chances for social success.

▼ Application to Clinical Practice

Health status is related to ethnicity and race. Krieger and Fee (1994), for instance, posited: 'Whatever the specific categories chosen, reports agree that white men and women, for the most part have the best health, at all ages.' This demarcation, they observed, can also be seen in care settings within the occupational structure:

> The work of looking after sick people follows the same categories. Simply walk into a hospital and observe that most of the doctors are white men, most of the registered nurses are white women, most of the kitchen and laundry workers are black and Hispanic women, and most of the janitorial staff are black and Hispanic men.

One's socio-economic position has implications for one's health. A poorly paid occupation, the causation of poverty and a source of stress for the worker, will undermine his or her health status. Nor is this the only factor impinging on the health status of ethnic minorities. Krieger and Fee (1994) recognised how racism shapes people's environment: 'Several studies, for example, document the fact that toxic dumps are most likely to be located in poor neighbourhood of colour.'

The many healthcare inequalities evident in society seem to be racially based (Funkhouser & Moser, 1990). These workers noted that in American society, when compared with their white counterparts, black people are 1.3 times as likely to die of heart disease, twice as likely to die of stroke, 2.2 times as likely to die of diabetes, 3.2 times as likely to die of kidney disease, and six times as likely to be murdered.

Unequal access to healthcare facilities, as well as the inability to obtain adequate healthcare, contribute to the situation. Although healthcare professionals are unable to alter directly policy machinery to counteract the social and health inequalities, their roles in preventive measures—both at ward level and in community settings—must not be underestimated. For example, they can undertake blood pressure monitoring and the teaching of self-examination (breast and testicles), which will aid early detection of carcinoma and the implementation of treatment and counselling at a very early stage; they can provide good advice about nutrition, early and continued prenatal care, and adequate postnatal care to 'reduce the alarming maternal and infant mortality rates among blacks' (Funkhouser & Moser, 1990). However, professionals must remember that ethnic minority groups may have limited financial resources and therefore may be unable to afford a highly nutritional diet.

Ethnic diversity and cultural variations are integral in the conceptual framework comprising these groups. During their careers, nurses and other staff in care settings are expected to 'work with culturally diverse patients who need to be appreciated as persons with cultural beliefs and values' (Fong, 1985). A nurse who is unable to comprehend the rationality behind the ethnic patient's behaviour is likely to fail in meeting the holistic needs of the individual. As Fong (1985) postulated: 'The nurse must be cognizant of both the patient's and the nurse's cultural orientation. Treating all patients alike with disregard for diverse cultural needs is unsafe.' There is also the tendency for ethnocentric behaviour (the beliefs that one's culture is 'superior' to other cultures) to develop in response to ethnic group diversity. Recognising such an attitude could prevent conflicting interpersonal relationships and foster a more positive patient response to the health services.

Fong pointed out that certain cultural components are present in every ethnic group, with subtle as well as obvious similarities and differences existing among them. To formulate a cultural profile, Fong (1985) suggested the 'Fong's CONFHER model', which lists the following components:

- Communication style, e.g. dialect and language preference.
- Orientation, e.g. ethnic identity, acculturation.
- Nutrition, e.g. symbolism of food.
- Family relationships, e.g. structure and roles, life styles, etc.
- Health beliefs, e.g. alternative healthcare, health crisis, and illness beliefs.
- Education, e.g. learning style, socio-economic level.
- Religion, e.g. preference, beliefs, rituals, and taboos.

The communication process is a fundamental aspect of care. It stimulates interaction between healthcare professionals and patients. It is essential to assess the communication style of the individual. Failure to achieve this goal could lead to a stereotypical attitude, such as Bowler's (1993) finding of the 'they're not the same as us' opinion held by British midwives about maternity patients of south Asian descent.

Fong (1985) suggested a patient-centred approach to orientation, allowing them to 'identify their own identity'. The role of the healthcare professional is to ask specific questions that will lead the patient to explain his or her identity. The patient's identity could be a complex framework of beliefs. The Chinese, for example, believe in the concept of 'Yin' and 'Yang', the two opposing forces or elements in the universe (Chan, 1995); the balance of Yin (cold) and Yang (hot) forces sustains their health and wellbeing (Lea, 1994).

Nutritional habits, Fong (1985) argued, are symbolic and meaningful to ethnic groups. Orthodox Hindus believe in the doctrine of 'ahimsa' (non-violence) and the sanctity of the cow (McDonald, 1985). Haitian Americans believe that not all foods are good at all times for the human body; the use of food must be in harmony with the individual's life-cycle (Laguerre, 1981). Cambodian women avoid eating hot food such as pepper during pregnancy, as they believe it causes spontaneous abortion of the fetus (Kulig, 1988). Neile (1995) suggested a careful assessment of the postnatal dietary needs of Chinese women, since they do not all eat beef and pork. However, it is essential not to assume that ethnic groups will automatically require ethnic food while under care.

Family relationships should be explored to gain insight into the dynamics of social action and integration: the respective roles of women and men, how they cope with any problems within the family, the strategies they use to maintain health equilibrium, and their priorities and goals.

Health beliefs also require adequate consideration. Dula (1994), in a narrative account of an elderly black woman, pinpointed the patient's particular health belief 'to cool down and thin the blood if you take a little bit of garlic water, or lemon juice, or vinegar'. Health beliefs may be focused on the magical effects of plants, the belief that the Creator is the source of all plants used for medicine and healing (Gregory, 1987).

There is no one way of looking at health or health beliefs. Individuality in the expression of ethnic group health beliefs needs exploring. Asking the right questions may elicit appropriate responses. For example: 'How does the patient generally respond to pain?—with stoical endurance, with loud cries, or with quiet withdrawal?' (Fong, 1985). Healthiness according to ethnic perspectives among some groups may be perceived in ways markedly contrasting with the official, modern, biomedical perspective. According to Aggleton (1990), some ethnic

majority groups (e.g. elderly people from Aberdeen) consider themselves or others healthy although they may be badly diseased; and some societies explain the onset of illness by recourse to supernatural forces—wrathful gods or ancestral spirits who inflict suffering on those who have broken moral codes. The ethnic French view many ailments as a by-product of liver disfunction. Consumption of mineral water, such as Badoit, Evian, and Perrier, is believed to restore the balance. In contrast, some Germans believe many ailments to be the cause of cardiovascular disruption (Qureshi, 1994).

Education and religion should be included in the assessment procedure because they form part of the overall framework of the patient as a social being. Identifying the patient's preferred method for learning (e.g. talking, reading, audiovisual aids) will facilitate the role of the nurse as a health educator and promoter. Religious beliefs may strongly influence a patient's mental and physical health (Fong, 1985). Rassool (1995) postulated that religion and language have profound effects on patients' perception and recognition of their health problems.

Application of the above formula will ensure that patients' needs are identified within a structured framework. However, care professionals must be adaptable in their approach. For example, the nomadic existence and high mobility of gypsies creates difficulties in the implementation of a constant and regular health surveillance. Streetly (1987) reported a low uptake of antenatal care, family-planning facilities, developmental screening, and immunisation among gypsies and travellers. Vernon (1994) concluded that gypsies and travellers often have minimal contact with non-travellers and, of more relevance, with healthcare agencies. This causes a disruption in care continuity and fragmentation of medical profiling. Gypsies, therefore, are exposed to a similar situation of unequal access to health-care facilities as Hayes (1995) found among non-English-speaking Asians.

The provision of culturally and ethnically sensitive care is paramount in care settings. Socio-economic and environmental constraints prevent many ethnic minorities from reaping the benefits of the health resources available to them. Although it is impossible for healthcare professionals to be knowledgeable about every aspect of cultural practices and beliefs of all ethnic populations, some realistic and practical measures can be taken in appropriate circumstances, such as:

- Extending the role of interpreters and/or linkworkers to facilitate effective, accessible, and acceptable care (Hayes, 1995).
- Affording respect for religious practices and privacy for prayer to those who wish it and recognising the ethnic status of groups such as the Irish (Tilki, 1994) and gypsies.
- Focusing on ways in which racism, racial prejudice, and racial discrimination can be abolished (Alleyne et al., 1994).
- Recognising that for some ethnic minorities the demand is for more personal care, with greater emphasis on continuity and improved access (Rashid & Jagger, 1992).
- Encouraging the individual to express their understanding of what 'their ethnicity means to them and their condition in terms of health care', since this is 'central to the concept of dealing with the whole person' (George, 1994).

Review Questions

1   There are various ethnic groups in Britain, living in different parts of the country: in London there is China Town; a few miles from Heathrow Airport, in Southall, there is 'Little India', where many Asians live and work; Irish ethnic groups are scattered in other locations in London and elsewhere in the country; the gypsies migrate throughout the year to the cities or rural areas

Discuss the sociopolitical implications and problems a polyethnic society has to consider.

2   Culturally sensitive care is paramount in any healthcare setting. Healthcare professionals within the hospital and community framework are expected to implement care to suit the needs of ethnic groups.

Examine and discuss the nursing measures that should be taken to ensure that the holistic needs of individuals from ethnic minorities are met.

3   There is a group of gypsies living in caravans on an unauthorised site not far from the town. The local residents have been complaining to the local authorities about their presence in the area.

(i)   Examine the social and environmental factors that have led to the development of hostility towards the gypsies.

(ii)   Describe the role of healthcare professionals as agents of health education and promotion for the ethnic minority gypsy group.

▼ References

Aggleton P. *Health*. London: Routledge; 1990.

Alleyne J, Papadopoulos I, Tilki M. Antiracism within transcultural nurse education. *Br J Nurs* 1994, **3**:635–637.

Banton M. *Racial consciousness*. Harlow: Longman; 1988.

Bowler I. 'They're not the same as us': midwives' stereotypes of South Asian descent maternity patients. *Sociology of Health and Illness* 1993, **15**:159–172.

Brown C. Racial disadvantage in the employment market. In: Braham P, Rattansi A, Skellington R, eds. *Racism and anti-racism. Inequalities, opportunities and policies*. London: Sage; 1992.

Cashmore E. *Dictionary of race and ethnic relations*. London: Routledge & Kegan Paul; 1984:97–102.

Chan J. Dietary beliefs of Chinese patients. *Nursing Standard* 1995, **9**:30–34 .

Consise Oxford Dictionary 8th ed., Allen R, ed. London: BCA; 1991.

Dula A. The life and death of Miss Mildred: an elderly black woman. *Clin Geriatr Med* 1994, **10**:419–430.

Eriksen T. *Ethnicity and nationalism. Anthropological perspectives*. London: Pluto Press; 1993.

Fong C. Ethnicity and nursing practice. *Top Clin Nurs* 1985, **7**:1–10.

Funkhouser S, Moser D. Is health care racist? *Adv Nurse Sci* 1990, **12**:47–55.

George M. Accepting differences. *Nursing Standard* 1994, **8**:22–23.

Ginsburg N. Racism and housing: concepts and reality. In: Braham P, Rattansi A, Skellington R, eds. *Racism and anti-racism*. London: Sage; 1992.

Ginsburg N, Watson S. Issues of race and gender facing housing policy. In: Birchall J, ed. *Housing policy in the 1990s*. London: Routledge & Kegan Paul; 1992:140–162.

Goody E, Groothues C. The West Africans: the quest for education. In: Watson J, ed. *Between two cultures*. London: Basil Blackwell; 1977:151–180.

Gregory D. Nurses and traditional healers: now is the time to speak. *The Canadian Nurse* 1987, **83**(8):25–27.

Hawes D, Perez B. *The gypsy and the state: the ethnic cleansing of British society*. Bristol: SAUS Publication; 1995.

Hayes L. Unequal access to midwifery care: a continuing problem? *J Adv Nurs* 1995, **21**: 702–707.

Horsley E. Gypsies. In: Horsley E, ed. *Hutchinson 20th Century Encyclopaedia, 5th ed.* London: Hutchinson; 1987:581.

Jansen J. Islam & Muslim civil rights in the Netherlands. In: Lewis B, Schnapper D, eds. *Muslims in Europe*. London: Pinter; 1994:39–53.

Krieger N, Fee E. Man-made medicine and women's health: the biopolitics of sex/gender and race/ethnicity. *Int J Health Serv* 1994, **24**:265–283.

Kulig J. Childbearing Cambodian refugee women. *The Canadian Nurse* 1988, **84**(6):46–47.

Laguerre S. Haitian American. In: Harwood A, ed. *Ethnicity and medical care*. Cambridge: Harvard University Press; 1981:180–209.

Lea A. Nursing in today's multicultural society: a transcultural perspective. *J Adv Nurs* 1994, **20**:307–313.

McDonald R. Cultural exchange. Community issues 2. *Nursing Mirror* 1985, **160**:32–35.

Modood T, Beishon S, Virdee S. *Changing ethnic identities*. London: Policy Studies Institute; 1994.

Moerman M, *Who are the Lue?: Ethnic Identification in a Complex Civilisation*. American Anthropologist; 1965, **67**:1215–1229.

Neile E. The maternity needs of the Chinese community. *Nursing Times* 1995, **91**:34–35.

O'Donnell M. *Race and ethnicity*. Harlow: Longman; 1991.

Patterson S. The Poles—an exile community in Britain. In: Watson J, ed. *Between two cultures*. London: Basil Blackwell; 1977:214–241.

Qureshi B. *Transcultural medicine, 2nd ed.* London:

Kluwer Academic Publishers; 1994.

Rashid A, Jagger C. Attitudes to and perceived use of health care services among Asian and non-Asian patients. *Br J Gen Pract* 1992, **42**:197–201.

Rassool H. The health status and health care of ethno-cultural minorities in the United Kingdom: an agenda for action. *J Adv Nurs* 1995, **21**:199–201.

Rex J. *Race & ethnicity*. Milton Keynes: Open University Press; 1986.

Sills D. *International encyclopaedia of the social sciences, Vols 5 & 6*. New York: McMillan Co & Free Press; 1968:167–172.

Skellington R, Morris P. *'Race' in Britain today*. London: Sage; 1992.

Solomos J. The politics of immigration since 1945. In: Braham P, *et al.*, eds. *Racism and anti-racism. Inequalities opportunities, and policies*. London: Sage; 1992:7–29.

Solomos J. *Race and racism in Britain, 2nd ed*. Basingstoke: Macmillan; 1993.

Streetly A. Health care for travellers: one year's experience. *Br Med J* 1987, **294**:492–494.

Tilki M. Ethnic Irish older people. *Br J Nurs* 1994, **3**:909–913.

Vernon D. The health of traveller-gypsies. *Br J Nurs* 1994, **3**:969–972.

Watson J. Migrants & minorities in Britain. In: Watson J, ed. *Between two cultures*. London: Basil Blackwell; 1977:1–20.

Watson S, Austerberry H. Housing & homelessness, a feminist perspective. London: Routledge & Kegan Paul; 1986.

▼ Further Reading

Diosi A. Learning from each other—professional gypsy foster parents in Hungary. *Adoption and Fostering* 1994, **18**:38–42.

Donald J, Rattansi A. *'Race', culture and difference*. London: Sage; 1992.

Geary R, O'Shea C. Defining the traveller: from legal theory to practical action. *J Soc Welfare Family Law* 1995, **17**:167–178.

Kim M. Cultural influences: depression in Korean Americans. *J Psychosoc Nurs* 1995, **33**:13–18.

McMillan I. Tribal quest (delivering culturally sensitive care to North American Indians). *Nursing Times* 1995, **91**(1):34–35.

Sugirtharjah S. The notion of respect in Asian traditions. *Br J Nurs* 1994, **3**:739–741.

Uehara E. Race, gender and housing inequality—an exploration of the correlates of low-quality housing among clients diagnosed with severe and persistent mental illness. *J Health Soc Behav* 1994, **35**(4):309–321.

10

Social Construction of Behaviour:
Deviance

▼ LEARNING OBJECTIVES

The reader will be able to:
- Define the term 'deviance'.
- Describe common theories of deviance.
- Explain the functions of deviance in society.
- Evaluate the social processes causing deviance.

▼ What is Deviance?

Society has rules. These rules have been formulated by groups within society and, according to Becker (1963), define situations and the type of behaviour appropriate to them, designating some actions as 'right' and prohibiting others as 'wrong'. Here, Becker was stressing the influences of groups in deciding which actions are compatible with the norms of society. In other words, Becker was restating the traditional sociological viewpoint that deviance and its causes are located in social forces (Cochrane, 1983).

Becker's perspective is founded on groups, the rules they make, and how breaking such rules causes deviance. The person breaking the rule is the deviant, as defined by the groups who formulated the rules. The social groups make moral judgements about people whose behaviour has deviated from the rules (Gomm, 1990). Downes and Rock (1988) defined deviance as a 'product of the ideas which people have of one another'. Deviance therefore is related to meanings (Gomm, 1990), meanings that social groups give to other people's behaviour. The interpretation of people's behaviour is left at the mercy of society (social groups), 'which determine, as with normality, how it [deviance] should be patterned' (Littlewood & Lipsedge,

1989). The same authors also pointed out how insanity can invert the basic rules of society.

As Becker (1963) argued, once a person has broken the rules, he or she becomes an 'outsider', not to be trusted to live by the rules agreed by the group. To break the rules goes beyond what society considers normal. Normality is, according to Thompson and Mathias (1994), rather like reasonableness; it largely depends on the person who undertakes the defining. Deviant behaviour does not match the 'shared reality' and the 'mutual value system' a community has developed.

Defining deviant behaviour includes the use of 'labels'. As Beck *et al.* (1988) discussed, labels are the product of 'norm deviation'. People in society use a variety of labels in their interpretation of behaviour that deviates from the norm, such as 'bizarre', 'crazy', and 'insane'. The emphasis is on the social meaning attached to a particular behaviour that is incongruent with social expectations.

When social expectations are not met, the group exhibiting the deviant behaviour form a subculture. The members of the group, who have a number of countervalues in common, do not accept the normal rules (O'Donnell, 1993). However, their behaviour must be evaluated within the context in which they find themselves, as it is the context that determines whether their behaviour is deviant (Power *et al.*, 1986). For example, a man who picks up a sledgehammer and suddenly starts breaking the coffee table in front of his guests is being a deviant . . . until, that is, one notices a film director and his crew capturing the scene; the man is, in fact, demonstrating the latest sledgehammer on the market to the guests for an advertisement!

In an interesting discussion about nature and culture, Bauman (1990) used an analogy to explain the concept of order and disorder, or norm and deviation from the norm. He referred to the farmer and gardener 'weeding out the unwelcome guests, the "uninvited" plants which have grown "on their own initiative", and therefore spoiled the neat design of the plot, diminished the planned profitability of the field, or detracted from the aesthetic ideals of the garden'. It is the farmer and the gardener, he argued, who set the criteria and who conjure up the 'visions of things'. Similarly, society sets the criteria for what should be orderly, non-deviant, and normal behaviour.

What constitutes social order is the result of decisions made by groups in society, the consensus of values. 'Undersocialised' individuals, who are unable to integrate into society, will need coercion (Worsley, 1987). What is correct behaviour and what is reprehensible, Worsley stated, has been agreed by the vast majority of people. Deviance in society, he posited, helps us to understand why people conform and how social disorder is interpreted. Deviance is a cultural concept with a symbolic function. It functions by 'defining the norm and delineating that which is beyond the scope of normal behaviour' (Gerbner, 1978). Gerbner argued too that the socialisation process, by making us behave in 'socially functional ways', plays a role in influencing our interpretation of what is normal and what is deviant. However, socially functional behaviour, and how it is interpreted, can change with time; thus, deviance and its social definition change with time.

In the early 1900s, many middle-class American women used laudanum, an opiate, to relieve menstrual cramps and other pains. Many of these women were addicted to the drug but they were not classified as deviant much less criminal. A few decades later, when the law made narcotics use and possession punishable, the social definition of opiates users changed; it was still not illegal to be an addict, but it was illegal to possess or use opiates such as laudanum or heroin (Conklin, 1984).

The social character of deviance is not only influenced by time but also by place. As Baldridge (1980) noted, acts acceptable in large urban areas are often unacceptable in small towns; for example, the behaviour of the police in the ghettoes of New York, where pimping and prostitution are ignored, is very different from the aggressive response of the law to similar deviant acts in a small town.

▼ Theories of Deviance

■ BIOLOGICAL THEORY

The attempt to explain deviance in terms of biological or genetic attributes has been the pursuit of biologists for many years. In the nineteenth century, certain physical characteristics—such as a large skull, forehead or jaw, or high cheek bones were thought to indicate criminal attributes (Baldridge, 1980). One proponent of this biological theory was Cesare Lombroso, who thought that criminals were 'biological reversions to a more primitive stage of humanity' (Conklin, 1984).

Some researchers argue that physiological differences, the results of chemical imbalances in the body, predispose to conditions such as schizophrenia. Gelder *et al.* (1994) suggested that the predisposing factors in the aetiology of schizophrenia are genetic: 'Schizophrenia is more common in the families of schizophrenic patients than in the general population (where the life time risk is a little less than 1%).' They argued that twin studies have shown that a major part of this familial loading is likely to be

due to genetic rather than environmental factors. Biochemical studies of disordered brain functioning, and the fact that patients with schizophrenia respond to antipsychotic drugs, they concluded, suggest a biochemical basis for the condition. Rose (1994), however, although acknowledging the importance of genetic inheritance in the aetiology of schizophrenia, referred to the uncertainty as to what the genetic mode of inheritance is.

Concerning personality disorder, studies have suggested a link between criminal behaviour and some inherited component (Rees, 1982; Dally, 1982; Rose, 1994).

To consider the aetiology of deviant behaviour from a purely biological perspective, however, is to be a reductionist; there are other factors (environmental, social, and psychological) that interplay with biology.

■ PSYCHOLOGICAL THEORY

Sigmund Freud's explanation of human behaviour from a psychoanalytical stance has helped to explain partly the causation of deviance. His theory of the 'id' (the primitive impulse) explains the instinctual impulses that might be associated with violence, uncontrolled sexual behaviour, and other forms of deviance (Baldridge, 1980). O'Donnell (1992) explained how personality traits such as extroversion and a predisposition to criminal behaviour may be linked. Gibbons and McNicol (1983) detailed how some personalities are more likely to develop adult psychiatric disorders. Rose (1994), however, identified some personality disorders (such as cycloid and schizoid) that may be partial expressions of a mental illness (such as manic depression and schizophrenia, respectively).

It is argued (Baldridge, 1980; O'Donnell, 1992) that psychological interpretations and explanations of deviance are more popular than biological perspectives among sociologists. An assessment of the aetiology of deviance, nevertheless, should always adopt an eclectic (deriving ideas from various sources) approach.

■ SOCIOLOGICAL THEORIES

The study of social deviance by sociologists is portrayed as a fertile ground in comparison with crime. The richness of social deviance has been identified by sociologists to encompass 'mental illness, bestiality, voyeurism, lying, stripping, homosexuality, blackmail, sectarianism, blindness, radicalism, stuttering, prostitution, murder and physical illness' (Mann, 1983). Deviance, therefore, extends to any 'other sanctionable straying from the path of convention' (Outhwaite & Bottomore, 1994). The sociological theories developed over the years have similarly shown a highly productive array of perspectives to attempt to explain the meanings of deviance and, what is more important, to emphasise the social context of deviance and its social definition.

Who are the deviant or abandoned groups of society? Forster and Ranum (1978) answered this question by listing the underprivileged groups in society: vagrants and tramps, prostitutes, abandoned children, convicts, arsonists, the insane. Where do the terms for deviant behaviour come from? From 'law codes, learned works on medicine and jurisprudence, and works of piety exhorting the faithful to charitable activities, and in novels plays and etchings' Forster and Ranum (1978). As Connor (1972) noted, the legal definitions of deviance are enacted indirectly by legislators. This all goes to underline the social and human context of deviance—'Behind these terms for behaviour are people' (Forster & Ranum, 1978).

It is therefore people who identify, label, and categorise other groups according to their behaviour. Social behaviour is extremely complicated. Sociologists have mainly used the following perspectives in their attempt to explain the complex nature of social deviance: the demonic perspective, anomie, functionalism, and the labelling (societal reactions) perspective.

▼ Perspectives on Deviance

■ DEMONIC PERSPECTIVE

'According to the demonic perspective the human world is but a battleground for the forces of another more powerful world, the world of the supernatural. . . . When we succumb to the influence of evil forces we are drawn into deviant behaviour' (Pfohl, 1985).

The demonic perspective is, as Pfohl described, the oldest of all known perspectives. The essence of this approach is founded on the examination and understanding of social deviance as the consequence of supernatural forces—possession by devils and transgression 'against the will of God' (or gods). It is no wonder that contemporaries in early modern Europe 'saw in the poor not only Christ but sometimes the Devil himself' (Jutte, 1994). Poverty, crime, and deviance were closely related. Deviance was equated with sin (Pfohl, 1985), whereas crime and sin always accompanied poverty (Jutte, 1994).

Pfohl (1985) argued that demonic explanations remain the only true explanations for many people: 'Evangelical preachers fill football stadiums and amass large radio and television audiences with sermons suggesting that behind the rising crime rate and the spread of sexual immorality lies the malicious hand of the devil.'

The demonic perspective is limited, however, because it is founded on superstitious beliefs of supernatural forces, an abstraction that is very hard to verify. Scientific progress has helped by formulating more naturalistic explanations of deviance (e.g. hysteria, depression).

■ ANOMIE

Anomie—derived from the Greek words *anomos* and *anomia*, and the French word *anomie* meaning lawless—describes a lack of the usual social or ethical standards in an individual or group.

Sociologists often make use of this term when they refer to Durkheim's assessment of social change and normlessness in society. O'Donnell (1992), for example, stated:

> Durkheim was in no doubt that social pathology tended to increase during times of great social change. In such times people are often left without clear rules or normative guidelines, and so become more prone to deviance. In particular the decline of religious certainties could undermine security and confidence in traditional morality. Durkheim referred to this state of 'normlessness' as 'anomie'.

According to Hester and Eglin (1992), this concept has been employed by the sociologist Merton in a different way:

> [Merton] linked deviant behaviour with the disjunction between institutionalised aspirations and the availability of access to legitimate opportunity structures. The prime candidates for criminal behaviour such as property theft, for example, were those whose class position prevented them from realising material success through school, work and other legitimate opportunity structures.

Using Merton's perspective, Power *et al.* (1986) argued that when legitimate means to gain educational qualifications and achieve success are not at the disposal of some, 'a condition of anomie is created in which we experience a sense of hopelessness that eventually leads to a moral collapse in society and an increasing unwillingness to obey laws'.

At the nucleus of the anomie theory is the understanding that deviance develops from the thwarting of human aspirations; a constrictive social network that disadvantages the minorities, the future deviants. The theory, nevertheless, has been the focus of some criticisms. For example, Pfohl (1985) pointed out that Durkheim's argument of the link between normative deregulation and suicide is 'vague and occasionally contradictory'. Other criticisms are laid against the notion that only lower-class persons are susceptible to deviancy, as a result of exposure to their social conditions. As Pfohl (1985) explained, members of the middle and upper classes are similarly exposed to 'certain deviant adaptations . . . as owners of highly competitive corporations'. Similarly, Taylor *et al.* (1973) argued that deviance is far more widely distributed than Merton would allow, and that, in particular, the lawbreaking activity of the 'well-to-do' (those with no obstruction on their opportunity) is much more widespread.

Downes and Rock (1988) too acknowledged that the anomie theory has flaws, since there is evidence that criminality and deviance perspectives are 'reproduced in police practices which focus far more on working class than on middle or upper class criminality'.

■ FUNCTIONALISM

To explain that deviance and deviant behaviour have functions in society does not appear to follow commonsense, until one 'puts a different pair of theoretical spectacles on with lenses which sharply focus our attention on some features of society [so that] the previously indistinct features of the world are now highlighted' (Holdaway, 1988). These indistinct features are the positive aspects of deviance, which do not always come to the forefront of people's minds.

'In the first place crime is normal because a society exempt from it is utterly impossible' (Durkheim, 1964). To Durkheim, deviant behaviour, as a social phenomenon, functions to maintain social order. It is deviance, in the form of crime, that raises people's consciousness and collective sentiments to reassess social order. Clinard (1974), on the other hand, argued that deviance both strengthens community spirit among the conforming group and enhances the importance of conformity within the group. Social deviance and society's response to it clarify the boundaries and the rules of normality. Deviance is seen to function as a 'safety valve': 'For example, it may be argued that prostitution performs such a safety valve function without threatening the institution of the family, and without involving the emotional attachments outside marriage that might arise from premarital or extramarital relations' (Clinard, 1974).

In this context, one may point out that deviance has essential functions in society by Pfhol (1985):

- Establishing control of internal social tensions.
- Allowing for adaptive innovation.
- Setting moral boundaries.
- Strengthening group solidarity.
- Symbolising what is right and wrong, by reminding us of the penalties we face if we deviate from expected conventional behaviour.
- Providing a 'moral map of do's and don'ts of everyday life'.

The uniqueness of functionalism lies in its positive evaluation of deviance as a concept serving society by maintaining stabilisation and integration. However, the theory has been criticised for its inadequacy in explaining for whom deviance is functional (Downes & Rock, 1988). One group may see deviancy as functional, whereas others may perceive it as dysfunctional (although it may not be always so). As Downes and Rock (1988) put it: 'Institutions may be functional for very large numbers. If deviance is functional, how functional is it for the victims of rape, mugging and burglary?' The circularity of functionalism (logic of reasoning depending on a vicious circle) can provide and 'identify the positive consequences of virtually any aspect of social life' (Pfohl, 1985). The problem with the functionalist explanation of deviance, however, is its failure to consider historical circumstances and personal meanings. It has a mechanistic interpretation of social life. Is deviance more positive for some than others? Functionalism does not analyse how sanctions against the deviant are functional. Deviance may be functional, yet in an unequal society its functions will not be equally distributed (Pfohl, 1985).

■ LABELLING PERSPECTIVE

The labelling perspective, also known as the societal reactions perspective, has been a notorious theory in the field of understanding deviance, in particular its nature. It considers the question of *how* social actors (people in society) become defined and treated as deviant, rather than *what* makes social actors commit deviant acts (Filstead, 1972). Thus, the societal reactions of groups of people— onlookers observing a social behaviour—will identify certain acts as deviant. Acts are identified as deviant by the nature of the reactions to them (Gibbs, 1972). As Hester and Eglin (1992) argued, society's reaction is to control socially the person seen as deviant. Once labelled as criminal, the person 'internalises that label and comes to see him or herself as essentially criminal'.

Douglas (1984) asked: ' How do we get social values and rules that can be used to define who is and who is not deviant?' He proposed that the more powerful people in society make the rules that the less powerful have to abide by. According to Douglas, there are social rules of ancient origins that are rarely violated and that are taken for granted, for example, those against public nudity and 'insanity'. 'In general, we can expect that the more powerful official bureaucracies of control are, the less problematic will be the construction of official deviance categories and of concrete cases of deviant identities' (Douglas, 1984).

Society does not only react to deviant behaviour, but also interacts with the individuals labelled as deviant. 'It is what happens in the life of the deviant after the social definition has been made that is the focus of interactionist analysis' (O'Donnell, 1992). The process of socially defining a behaviour as deviant depends much less upon what he does or what he is, than upon what others do to him as a consequence of his actions (Thorsell & Klemke, 1979). The interactionists, as Thorsell and Klemke pointed out, interpret deviance as the product or result of the interaction between the individual who performs the deviant act and those who respond to it by labelling the individual as a deviant person.

A school of thought developed by Howard Becker (1963), which has become an often-quoted classic statement, is as follows: 'Social groups create deviance by making rules whose infraction constitutes deviance, and by applying those rules to particular people and labelling them as outsiders.' These actors (the delinquents, homosexuals, alcoholics, individuals with psychological and physical disability, and so on), thus labelled, become the 'victims'; the definers, the 'victimisers'. In the process of being labelled, people are isolated, compartmentalised, categorised, and stigmatised (Fitzgerald, 1983). A stigma is used to refer to 'an attribute that is deeply discrediting' (Goffman, 1970) or any 'persistent trait of an individual or group which evokes negative or punitive responses' (Susman, 1994).

Susman explained: 'If one accepts that experiences of disability have been influenced, up to the present day, largely by perceptions of negative difference (deviance) and their evocation of adverse responses (stigma), then any work which says something about the social construction of disability's meanings necessarily also says something about stigma and deviance.' Susman referred to research showing that society views a disabled person as 'damaged, defective, and less socially marketable' than able persons. The disability smothers any personal identity of the individual; it becomes the 'master status' attached to the features of the person. The defining characteristic of stigmatisation projects a deviant characteristic to the person as a master status (Braithwaite, 1989).

As Williams (1994) posited:

If people know about the criminal label it is likely to affect the way in which they treat the individual. For many, the criminal label is likely to be the overriding identifying label. A person previously known mainly as a parent or a school child, or whatever, is now primarily known as a thief.

The thief, the delinquent, or the homosexual now becomes differentiated from others, segregated, and 'may eventually be excluded from conventional society' (Balch & Kelly, 1979).

Deviance only exists in the eye of the

beholder; that is, a person only becomes a deviant when his or her deviance is noticed by other people. As Williams (1994) pointed out, if an offence is committed in the street, agents of social control and the public are more likely to see it and to respond or react to it than if the act takes place out of sight in private. Many deviant acts do not reach the attention of the public. It is argued that acts carried out in secrecy, for instance within a group, are not labelled as deviant since there are no definers of the act.

The labelling theory helps us understand the social process that leads to the formulation of a category negative in character, a category to be applied to certain groups in society that deviate from conventional approaches. The theory has some flaws, however. Williams (1994) pointed out that the labelling theory appears to protect the offender (the deviant), by classing him or her almost as the victim, and fails to consider that there are 'real' victims of his or her crimes. By removing the 'normative element' of the deviant act, supporters of the labelling theory make it appear morally neutral. Furthermore, the theory does not match empirical testing, as it is not easy to test in social life how a label can make someone become a criminal.

Gibbs (1972) argued that it is not clear whether the theory is about deviant behaviour or about reactions to deviation. He stated that if Becker's focus is on the latter, then his focus on reactions rather than deviants is puzzling. Gibbs criticised the lack of specification from theorists regarding the kind of reactions that identify deviation. What makes homosexuals deviants? It is the reactions of the public, he argued, what type of reactions should we be looking at? Does a 'mild' response to homosexuals from the public suggest a lack of deviance? These are some of the questions asked in relation to the relevance of reaction as a criterion of deviation, and the use of labelling.

■ OTHER PERSPECTIVES

Besides the perspectives detailed so far, there are others that, although often used in attempts to explain deviance, are beyond the scope of this section. Consequently, these are given below in outline only.

CULTURAL TRANSMISSION THEORY

This theory is based on the understanding that deviance is the product of cultural factors, and is learned. Sutherland and Cressey (1979), concerning criminality, stated that this learning takes place 'in interaction with other persons in a process of communication' and 'within intimate personal groups'. Sutherland and Cressey use the term 'differential association' to apply to their theory. It is purely a theory of learning, which means that an individual learns how to be a criminal by association with others (Williams, 1994).

SOCIAL DISORGANISATION THEORY

This theory, based on a school of thought originating from Chicago in the United States, emphasises the social causation of deviance, rather than biological and pathological processes. Deviance is viewed as a natural by-product of social change (Pfhol, 1985). Proponents argue that social change fractures the normative structure until reorganisation occurs. Before reorganisation, conflict and competition within the social structure cause an increase in the incidence of deviant behaviour. Periods of intense disorganisation lead to tendencies towards nonconformity and deviance.

▼ Summary

Deviance is said to occur when a person behaves in an unconventional way. This unconventional demeanour has fractured the sets of rules that powerful groups in society have laid down. Deviance, as argued by theorists such as Becker, is defined from an evaluation of the person committing the deviant act. This evaluation is context-based, meaning that the social context in which the behaviour is seen by others, followed by their interpretation, will decide whether it is categorised as deviant or not. It is therefore a product of the ideas people have of one another; it is related to the meanings that people give to the actions they observe and to the moral judgement that they subsequently make.

Norm deviations lead to the formation of 'labels'. To describe someone as 'an eccentric', 'a slag', or 'a whore' is to apply a label to the person concerned. Labels have negative connotations that cloud the other identities of the individual and become the master status.

In their attempts to explain deviance, sociologists have developed a plethora of theories. The **demonic perspective** focuses on beliefs that the supernatural causes the deviant behaviour due to possession by the devil. In a sharp contrast, the **anomie theory** considers the social context and the state of normlessness that encourages deviance. Anomie has been interpreted differently from a Mertonian perspective to mean the disjunction that exists between the societal goals of aspirations and the means to attain them. Failure to reach such goals due to one's social position may cause deviance. The individual deviates by breaking the rules of society to achieve certain ends. **Functionalism**, on the other hand, tends to explain the positive aspects of deviance, that deviance has functions in society. It helps to clarify boundaries between good and bad behaviour; it serves as a reminder to society that rules exist and nonconformity will lead to official sanctions. The **labelling perspective** provides us with an insight into the social processes that cause deviance; it concentrates mainly on societal reactions to conformist and nonconformist behaviour. As such, it studies the interactions among persons or groups and what meanings are attached to demonstrable behaviour. Other theories employed in the sociology of deviance are the **disorganisation and differential–association approaches**. The disorganisation theory explains that deviance occurs when society is in state of social change which fractures the normative elements binding the structures together. Differential–association explanations are based on the learning of deviance from association with groups likely to be indulging in deviant activities.

▼ Application to Clinical Practice

In this section we shall identify some broad categories of deviance in clinical practice: nursing staff's perceptions of patients' illnesses and their attitudes to them; the stigma attached to having a particular illness or disability; patient compliance and noncompliance (deviation and/or deviance); deviancy among nurses in clinical practice; mental disorders causing deviant behaviour; and the perception of AIDS and homosexuality as aspects of deviance.

The very education of nurses that aims towards the creation of an effective practitioner may, in subtle ways, impede professional practice and interfere with professional awareness regarding an objective assessment of the actions and behaviour of others. Baxter (1992) detailed how 'blind obedience' and 'paramilitary organisation of nursing staff' still prevail in nursing education. The implementation of traditional nursing doctrines in disguised form, such as the use of concepts like 'accountability for obedience' creates an environment in which students who challenge such approaches 'may be labelled as troublemakers and quickly stamped upon to restore order'. Baxter argued: '[The] social processes, interpersonal relationships and climate of a college of nursing may serve to distort individuals' perception of events and their judgement of the actions and characteristics of others.'

If one side-effect of education is to cause negative perceptions of social events and behaviour, this may partly explain nurses' attitudes in clinical practice towards stigmatised individuals with physical or psychological disabilities.

■ MENTAL ILL HEALTH

Mental ill health causes changes in a person's behaviour. To behave differently can often lead to rejection by others in the community; this is the 'penalty' mentally ill people have to pay for 'being different' (Philipps, 1979). Philipps described how the seeking of psychological support by those in need can be perceived by others as deviant:

> Although it is probably true that the public does not hold negative attitudes toward clergymen and physicians, I suggest that an individual consulting either of these help-sources may more often lose face, and more often be regarded as deviant, than an individual exhibiting the same behaviour who does not consult one of these professional sources.

This has implications for healthcare delivery. If individuals with mental illnesses or psycholog-

ical problems are reluctant to disclose information because of the fear of stigmatisation and being classified as deviants, their holistic needs are less likely to be met. Healthcare professionals must therefore exercise tact and sensitivity, and instill confidence in the patient that confidentiality will be maintained. It is important that professionals know about the processes that lead to the labelling of patients as deviants, since this will help them to gain an understanding of the patients' mental states. This knowledge should also help to raise the professional's awareness of the negative effects of labelling.

According to Kelly and May (1982), a number of studies have shown that practitioners in healthcare settings respond negatively to certain illnesses, such as mental disturbance and all kinds of psychiatric conditions. Some psychiatric patients (e.g. those with schizophrenia) are likely to exhibit deviant or rule-breaking behaviour due to cognitive and emotional changes, which may result in staff perceiving the patients as 'bad' (Kelly & May, 1982). Mental illness is therefore socially represented as a type of deviancy.

Studies on lay people's assumptions about mental illness indicate, according to Johnson and Orrell (1995), the persistent prevalence of 'magical' and 'morally deviant' representations of the mentally ill, alongside a 'medical' representation. Sometimes, an extreme attitude is expressed towards the mentally ill, such as that observed among people in a French village: '. . . a fear of contamination which, though not openly voiced by the villagers, was evident in their strict separation of the cutlery and laundry of the mentally ill from their own, and carefully enforced taboo against sexual contact with the mentally ill' (Johnson & Orrell, 1995). This behavioural expression is situated within a particular culture; a condition whereby 'psychologically disturbed people are perceived or dealt with differently at different times and in different social situations' (Cochrane & Carroll, 1991). In contrast to the French example, however, Pretorius (1995) described how mental disorders and disability in South Africa are viewed in a distinguishable way. He pointed out that an individual with psychological problems is sometimes expected to live at the healer's home for months or even years.

These two contrasting pictures of attitudes indicate the sharply distinctive perception of the same problems between the two cultures. Patients should be cared for with these differentiated cultural beliefs in mind. It must be remembered, firstly, that patients' responses to healthcare intervention may be strongly influenced by their social background, and, secondly, that the social functioning of some patients, such as those with schizophrenia, is likely to be impaired. Nurses must also recognise that the judgements they make about the 'moral fitness' of patients can affect the treatment given to them (Grief & Elliott, 1994). In a study undertaken by these authors, in a Canadian setting, it was found that nurses in the emergency department identified and accordingly labelled certain patient characteristics:

> Nurses do not differ from the rest of society; they evaluate patients according to how they perceive that patient's moral judgement and subsequent behaviour differ from or coincide with the societal norm. Patients may be negatively evaluated if they breech social rules that are merely customs or conventions as well as those that must be followed to prevent others from being hurt (eg, operating a vehicle while under the influence of alcohol) (Grief & Elliott, 1994).

The authors argued that, from a negative angle, this evaluative attitude caused nurse–patient communication and relationships to be jeopardised. Patients with psychological problems who had overdosed were classified as 'repeat offenders' exhibiting 'attention-seeking behaviour', who should 'learn to do it right'. Overweight patients were labelled as having an 'attitude problem', whereas regular patients were not popular because they were considered 'abusers of the healthcare system'. Such attitudes have serious implications for nursing practice; the exhibition of negative tendencies towards specific patient characteristics means that sensitive and empathetic nursing care is not being delivered. Grief and Elliott (1994) argued that there is a lack of self-awareness among nurses regarding the negative attitudes they display: 'None of the respondents volunteered that they morally evaluated their patients in an attempt to increase control in the emergency department.'

To ensure that the delivery of care to patients with mental illhealth is not jeopardised, Grief and Elliot (1994) suggest that healthcare professionals need to be made aware of the dynamics, consequences, and inherent risks of labelling patients and to improve their understanding of patients identified as 'unfavourable'.

McKeown and Clancy (1995) emphasised the importance for nurses engaged in the promotion of health and the support of clients with mental-health problems in the community to develop an 'interest in the mechanisms by which popular notions and images of mentally ill people are generated, and how these impinge on people's lives'. They pointed out that the media do not always portray mental ill health from a positive viewpoint:

> A distinction can be drawn between those which offer negative, stereotypical, stigmatising images and those which promote more positive images, or purport to be more 'accurate'. The former include images in fiction and news reporting of mentally ill people as homicidal maniacs,

narcissistic parasites, monsters, dangerous, and in need of containment; a danger to themselves and in need of asylum; open to ridicule or affording titillation; raving mad, bad or evil.

They explain that the positive aspect, although more realistic, tends to be less extreme.

Therefore, mental-health workers should, as pointed out already, take note of the social context of how 'negative representations may operate to restrict the quality of life of people with mental illness, particularly in community settings' (McKeown & Clancy, 1995).

Patients' social functioning in the community is reliant on the standards of the social environment; how the clients are perceived and accepted is dependent on the societal norms and beliefs of the community settings. Gamble and Midence (1995) noted that social functioning is an important concept in the diagnosis of schizophrenia and the assessment of patients with this condition. They explained how an assessment of social functioning should focus on the patient's social skills in meeting the demands of basic daily-living activities, but consideration must also be given to the client's particular community, as social functioning varies greatly from one culture to another.

■ THE NONCOMPLIANT PATIENT

Healthcare settings have set rules and norms that give workers a framework within which to operate. Patients are expected to abide by these rules and set expectations. A demonstration of noncompliance may attract such labels as 'undesirable', 'bad', or 'deviant'.

In his editorial, Papper (1970) explored briefly how some patients may be classified as 'socially undesirable'. The personal characteristics of the patients may contribute to the 'apparently irreconcilable differences between the patient and the physician'. To be dirty or uneducated, Papper argued, may lead to being patronised and denigrated by the physician. The expectation that patients should be grateful is another type of personal bias, with a failure to show gratitude leading to strong negative responses. Similar attitudes were found among nurses in a qualitative, nonexperimental study by Breault and Polifroni (1992): patients who asked too many questions, who wanted to know too much, were also viewed negatively. Papper (1970) postulated that undesirability may be based on physical grounds too:

> To some physicians the absence of physical illness is sometimes cause for negativism rather than an opportunity to share the patient's sense of relief with his good fortune; he may even be labelled a 'crock'. In other instances the presence of physical illness may be grounds for rejection especially if the data prove the physician's initial assessment to be in error.

Donovan and Blake (1992) referred to the presence of an ideology that portrays non-compliance as deviant behaviour and ensures that the blame for it is directed largely towards patients. They pointed out that the influence of medicine as an expression of dominance in relation to compliance should not be ignored: 'An historical analysis has shown that what clinicians now refer to as compliance used to be presented more overtly as physician control.'

Compliance does not necessarily apply only to drug taking, but includes following advice on exercise, diet, and other care issues. As Donovan and Blake (1992) asserted: 'Non-compliance exists on different levels and is expressed in different ways. It is also not just concerned with drugs, although this is the most commonly studied form.'

According to Donovan and Blake (1992), to avoid categorising patients as deviant on the basis of noncompliance with the prescriber's instructions, care professionals should look at compliance from the patient's perspective; for example:

- Assess the patients' ways of thinking and feeling about their illnesses and treatments.
- Attempt to recognise how these illnesses impact on their behaviour.
- Acknowledge the patient as an individual able to make decisions and to choose. Patients are not, on the whole, 'passive or powerless . . . they are quite capable of making choices about treatments and lifestyles rationally within the context of their beliefs, responsibilities and preferences' (Donovan & Blake, 1992).

Wade and Bowling (1986) referred to some studies indicating that noncompliance may be a reflection of patient dissatisfaction. They expressed the view that the term 'compliance' has 'coercive connotations'. They also argued that a distinction should be made between noncomprehension and noncompliance—if patients do not know the reasons why they need to take specific medications and the side-effects of such treatment, they are least likely to comply (Wade & Bowling, 1986; Donovan & Blake, 1992).

When patients deviate from compliance expectations, more frequently their behaviour is guided by beliefs and fears that the medications they are taking are causing them more harm than good. Establishing a better therapeutic relationship with the doctor and other members of the care team should help to alleviate the problem, with the effective provision of information on the medications they are prescribed.

■ AIDS AND HOMOSEXUALITY

AIDS, as well as being an epidemic (Breault & Polifroni, 1992), is perceived and considered to be a stigmatised disease (Peate, 1995). As gay men continue to be the largest group developing this condition, AIDS is often associated with homosexuality (Getty & Stern, 1990). According to Peate, homosexuality, AIDS and HIV are seen as expressions of deviance because the behaviour of this minority group (homosexuals, gay men) is incongruent with the accepted norms and beliefs of society:

> Homosexual people, with or without HIV or AIDS, are often considered deviant, as homosexual sex is often thought 'abnormal'. Intimate homosexual behaviour is seen by some as departing from the accepted 'norms', which is fundamentally rooted in a belief system in which penetrative sex is acceptable only within a heterosexual relationship.

This deviation from the belief system predisposes to what Getty and Stern (1990) called 'social death' (rejection, alienation, and ostracism from the family). Homosexuals are hence stigmatised. Punitive responses evoked by this trait are not only exhibited by the lay people in society (Peate, 1995; Taylor & Robertson, 1994; Getty & Stern, 1990), but also by healthcare professionals. Melby *et al.* (1992), for example, list some studies that highlight the poor attitudes of care professionals towards people with HIV and/or AIDS. Speight (1995), in his article on homophobia, stated: 'The truth is that the medical establishment has failed to combat negative attitudes toward gays and lesbians, and I argue that it is time for medical schools, medical associations, and individual physicians to begin to fight these injustices.'

To understand the homosexual as an individual should be the main focus in the sphere of professional interactions. Berger (1994) argued for a psychodynamic approach towards the care of homosexuals, recommending that such patients should be understood and can be cared for successfully.

NURSING MEASURES THAT CAN BE TAKEN TO ENSURE THE NEEDS OF HIV – AIDS PATIENTS ARE MET

- Understand that the patient's behaviour is influenced by antihomosexual behaviour from various sources.
- Be nonjudgemental and empathetic to alleviate the fears patients with AIDS have regarding the consequences of being open about their sexuality (Taylor & Robertson, 1994) and to provide an atmosphere conducive to a therapeutic relationship.
- Reassure the patient that confidentiality will be maintained among staff delivering the care, as patients may worry that a breach of confidentiality will have negative consequences for them in relation to housing and employment (Taylor & Robertson, 1994).
- Recognise and acknowledge that many problems faced by gay people centre around their requirement to cope with prejudice and to forge for themselves a worthwhile identity in the face of stigmatisation (Anderson, 1992).
- Develop health-education programmes that will help gay men to unlearn the myths about homosexuality by including information about and positive acceptance of homosexuality (Getty & Stern, 1990). Healthcare professionals should also undergo a similar programme to help them to

foster a more positive acceptance of homosexuality and to deliver sensitive and empathetic care.

■ DEVIANCE AMONG NURSES IN CLINICAL PRACTICE

The conflicts in our social world lead all of us to construct fronts to hide our private realities from public observation. Certainly individuals differ in how much they do this. Even more they differ in the kind of fronts they construct, the success they have in doing this, and the kinds of private realities they are involved in that they want to hide by frontwork (Douglas, 1984).

The private realities referred to above have been investigated in connection with nursing practice among a small group of nurses (25) in one hospital in the United States (Dabney, 1995). Dabney exposed the behaviour of 23 of the 25 nurses engaged in deviant practices consisting of drug theft and drug use. He stated that deviance in the workplace is common. Nurses steal drugs as a result of the influence of workgroup norms. He argued for an understanding of employee deviance by distinguishing 'two substantive subcategories—property deviance and production deviance'. Property deviance, he pointed out, means the stealing of money, supplies or merchandise; pilferage and embezzlement are terms used for this category. Production deviance, however, is related to 'counterproductive behaviour on the part of employees: slow, sloppy work and deliberate restrictions in output, and on the job substance use'.

Dabney (1995) referred to literature focusing mainly on the individual from a medical perspective; substance use is viewed primarily as a disease, neglecting external social factors. Dabney acknowledged, however, that an interaction of social and psychological factors is at play. Nurses steal drugs to increase their coping mechanisms. The results of semistructured interviews by the author revealed the following:

- Overall, 92% of the nurses admitted to stealing supplies.
- All 25 respondents were aware of other nurses stealing supplies.
- Of the nurses, 21 agreed that an estimated 100% of nursing staff engaged in supply theft.
- The nurses interviewed agreed that drug theft was a norm.
- The nurses were aware of their deviant behaviour.
- The drugs stolen were mainly non-narcotics.
- Various strategies were used by the nurses to cover up their deviancy and

thus ensure a regular supply of drugs. As Dabney (1995) explained: 'Nurses were able to circumvent controls by stockpiling excess medications that resulted from overprescribing or the death or transfer of patients.'

- There was evidence of 'on-the-job' use of stolen drugs, with the rationale that quality of nursing care would be enhanced.

If deviant behaviour among some staff is the accepted norm, particularly regarding drug theft, administrators and hospital managers are faced with an alarming and dangerous situation. As Dabney (1995) asserted, this form of deviancy threatens the delivery of quality nursing care and raises a host of legal and ethical questions.

▼ Review Questions

1 Richard is in his early 30s, gay, and has AIDS. Although he decided not to tell his father he was gay, his mother, Maggie, has known for a long time. She also knew when Richard was diagnosed as HIV-positive, and worried when he started to lose weight and became progressively more exhausted. In the summer of 1986, her worst fears were confirmed: Richard developed pneumocystis and was taken into hospital. It was there that he told his mother that he had AIDS (Richardson, 1989).

Examine the social issues that Richard and significant others will have to face following the disclosure.

2 A lesbian presents in hospital with abdominal pain, which is diagnosed as an ectopic pregnancy, although the woman repeatedly tells the doctor she is a lesbian and has never had sex with a man. Although she comes with her lover and identifies her as such, the nurse records 'friend' beside the partner's name on the intake sheet and the doctor will not examine the patient until her 'real' next of kin, her mother, arrives. The woman and her partner, upset at their treatment, do not see a doctor again for years (Speight, 1995).

(i) Evaluate the healthcare professional's interaction with the patient and her partner.

(ii) Discuss the factors that may have led to the inadequacy of nursing and medical intervention in this case.

3 Discuss the concept of deviance with reference to the theory that it is socially constructed.

▼ References

Anderson C. Coping with illness. In: Anderson C, Wilkie P, eds. *Reflective helping in HIV and AIDS.* Milton Keynes: Open University Press; 1992.

Balch R, Kelly D. Reactions to deviance in a junior high school: student views on the labelling process. In: Kelly D, ed. *Deviant behaviour: Readings in the Sociology of Deviance.* New York: St Martin's Press; 1979: 24–41

Baldridge V. *Sociology: a critical approach to power, conflict and change, 2nd ed.* New York: John Wiley; 1980:146–180.

Bauman Z. *Thinking sociologically.* Oxford: Blackwell; 1990.

Baxter R. Labelling students in nursing. *J Adv Nurs* 1992, **17**:971–974.

Beck C, Rawlins R, Williams S. *Mental health psychiatric nursing—A holistic life cycle approach.* St Louis: CV Mosby; 1988:38.

Becker H. Outsiders (1963). In: Gomm R, ed. *'A' level sociology. 'Deviance'.* Cambridge: NEC; 1990.

Berger J. The psychotherapeutic treatment of male homosexuality. *Am J Psychother* 1994, **48**:251–261.

Braithwaite J. *Crime, shame and integration.* Cambridge: Cambridge University Press; 1989.

Breault A, Polifroni E. Caring for people with AIDS: nurses attitudes and feelings. *J Adv Nurs* 1992, **17**:21–27.

Clinard M. Sociology of deviant behaviour (1974). In: Holdaway S, ed. *Crime and deviance.* Basingstoke: Macmillan; 1988:67–68.

Cochrane R. *The social creation of mental illness.* Harmondsworth: Longman Group; 1983:148–152.

Cochrane R, Carroll D. *Psychology and social issues.* London: Falmer Press; 1991.

Conklin J. *Sociology an introduction.* New York: Macmillan; 1984:99–123.

Connor W. *Deviance in Soviet society. Crime, delinquency and alcoholism.* New York: Columbia University Press; 1972.

Dabney D. Workplace deviance among nurses. The influence of work group norms on drug diversion and/or use. *JONA* 1995, **25**:48–55.

Dally P. *Psychology and psychiatry, 5th ed.* London: Hodder & Stoughton; 1982.

Donovan J, Blake D. Patient non-compliance: deviance or reasoned decision making? *Soc Sci Med* 1992, **34**:507–513.

Douglas J. *The sociology of deviance.* Massachusetts; Allyn & Bacon: 1984:98–101.

Downes D, Rock P. *Understanding deviance. A guide to the sociology of crime and rule breaking.* Oxford: Oxford University Press; 1988.

Durkheim E. The rules of sociological method (1964). In: Holdaway S, ed. *Crime and deviance.* Basingstoke: Macmillan; 1988:65–66.

Filstead W. *An introduction to deviance.* Chicago: Markham Publishing; 1972:1–5.

Fitzgerald M. *An introduction to sociology.* Milton Keynes: Open University Press; 1983:24–27.

Forster R, Ranum O. *Deviants and the abandoned in French society.* London: John Hopkins University Press; 1978.

Gamble C, Midence K. The assessment of social functioning—conceptual and methodological difficulties. *Psychiatric Care* 1995, **2**:52–54.

Gelder M, Gath D, Mayou R. *Concise Oxford textbook of psychiatry.* Oxford: Oxford University Press; 1994:172–174.

Gerbner G. Deviance and power, symbolic functions of 'drug abuse'. In: Winick C, ed. *Deviance and mass media.* Beverley Hills: Sage; 1978:13–30.

Getty G, Stern P. Gay men's perceptions and responses to AIDS. *J Adv Nurs* 1990, **15**:895–905.

Gibbons J, McNicol G. *Psychiatry.* London: Heineman Medical; 1983.

Gibbs J. Reaction as a criterion of deviation. In: Filstead W, ed. *An introduction to deviance.* Chicago: Markham Publishing; 1972:229–231.

Goffman E. *Stigma. Notes on the management of spoiled identity.* Harmondsworth: Penguin; 1968.

Gomm R. 'A' level sociology. 'Deviance'. Cambridge: NEC; 1990.

Grief L, Elliott R. Emergency nurses' moral evaluation of patients. *Emergency Nursing* 1994, **20**:275–279.

Hester S, Eglin P. *A sociology of crime.* London: Routledge; 1992.

Holdaway S. *Crime and deviance.* Basingstoke: Macmillan; 1988.

Johnson S, Orrell M. Insight and psychosis: a social perspective. *Psychol Med* 1995, **25**:515–520.

Jutte R. *Poverty and deviance in early modern Europe.* Cambridge: Cambridge University Press; 1994.

Kelly M, May D. Good and bad patients: a review of the literature and a theoretical critque. *J Adv Nurs* 1982, **7**:147–156.

Littlewood R, Lipsedge M. *Aliens and alienist. Ethnic minorities and psychiatry, 2nd ed.* London: Unwin Hyman; 1989:200–206.

Mann M. *'Deviance'. Macmillan student encyclopaedia.* London: Macmillan; 1983.

McKeown M, Clancy B. Media influence on societal perceptions of mental illness. *Mental Health Nursing* 1995, **15**:10–13.

Melby V, Boore J, Murray M. Acquired immune deficiency syndrome: knowledge and attitudes of nurses in Northern Ireland. *J Adv Nurs* 1992, **17**:1068–1077.

O'Donnell G. *Sociology today.* Cambridge: Cambridge University Press; 1993.

O'Donnell M. *A new introduction to sociology.* Walton-on-Thames: Nelsons & Sons; 1992.

Outhwaite W, Bottomore T. *Blackwell dictionary of twentieth century social thought.* Oxford: Blackwell; 1994.

Papper S. The undesirable patient. *J Chron Dis* 1970, **22**:777–779.

Peate I. A question of prejudice stigma, homosexuality and HIV/AIDS. *Professional Nurse* 1995, **10**(6):380–383.

Pfohl S. *Images of deviance and social control. A sociological history.* New York: McGraw-Hill; 1985.

Philipps, D. Rejection: A possible consequence of seeking help for mental disorders. In Kelly D. ed: *Deviant behaviour readings in the sociology of deviance.* New York: St Marbus; 1979: 425–439.

Power R, Robinson D, Popowicz A. *Discover sociology.* London: Pitman Publishing; 1986.

Pretorius H. Mental disorders and disability across cultures: a view from South Africa. *Lancet* 1995, **345**:534.

Rees L. *A short textbook of psychiatry, 3rd ed.* London: Hodder & Stoughton; 1982.

Richardson D. *Women and the AIDS crisis.* London: Pandora Press Unwin Hyman; 1989.

Rose N. *Essential psychiatry, 2nd ed.* Oxford: Blackwell Publications; 1994.

Speight K. Debating point: homophobia is a health issue: True Stories. *Health Care Analysis* 1995, **3**:143–156.

Susman J. Disability, stigma, deviance. *Soc Sci Med* 1994, **38**:15–22.

Sutherland E, Cressey D. Differential association theory. In: Kelly D, ed. *Deviant behaviour. Readings in the sociology of deviance.* New York: St Martin's Press; 1979:93–99.

Taylor I, Robertson A. The health needs of gay men: a discussion of the literature and implication for nursing. *J Adv Nurs* 1994, **20**:560–566.

Taylor I, Walton P, Young J. *The new criminology.* London: Routledge & Kegan Paul; 1973.

Thompson T, Mathias P. *Lyttle's mental health and disorder, 2nd ed.* London: Bailliere Tindall; 1994.

Thorsell B, Klemke L. The labelling process: reinforcement and deterrent? In: Kelly D, ed. *Deviant behaviour. Readings in the sociology of deviance.* New York: St Martin's Press; 1979:654–664.

Wade B, Bowling A. Appropriate use of drugs by elderly people. *J Adv Nurs* 1986, **11**:47–55.

Williams K. *Textbook on criminology, 2nd ed.* London: Blackstone Press; 1994.

Worsley P. *The new introducing sociology.* London: Penguin Books; 1987:407–450.

▼ Further Reading

Goffman E. Characteristics of total institutions. In: Kelly D, ed. *Deviant behaviour. Readings in the sociology of deviance.* New York: St Martin's Press; 1979:354–367.

Hall G. Using group work to understand arsonists. *Nursing Standard* 1995, **9**:25–28.

Mays J. *Crime and the social structure.* London: Faber & Faber; 1963.

Newton J. *Preventing mental illness.* London: Routledge; 1988.

Szasz T. *The myth of mental illness.* London: Paladin; 1972.

Walters J, Canady R, Stein T. Evaluating multicultural approaches in HIV/AIDS. Educational Material. *AIDS Education and Prevention* 1994, **6**:446–453.

11

Social Anthropology

▼ The Nature of Social Anthropology

The word 'anthropology' is derived from the Greek words *anthropos*, meaning humankind, and *logos*, meaning word or study. Anthropology therefore means the study of man or humankind. Cheater (1989) pointed out, however, that this transliteration is too broad as an academic definition because the 'study of man' is undertaken by many other disciplines, one way or another. She argued that the study of man came to focus on the contemporary organisation of society (social anthropology) and the differences among cultures (cultural anthropology). Similarly, Coleman and Watson (1990) explained how social and cultural anthropology is related to the practice of ethnology, which is often defined as the comparative study of cultures.

When anthropology emerged as a formal science at the end of the nineteenth century, it was concerned exclusively with 'primitive' (i.e. illiterate) people (Foster & Kemper, 1974). Similarly, Lewis (1969) referred to anthropology as the study of the way of life of primitive people as they can still be found today, not too much altered by contact with civilisation.

However, as Foster and Kemper (1974) noted, anthropological fieldwork has gradually expanded to include human societies in cities too. 'Anthropologists today study more than just primitive societies. Their research extends not only to village communities within modern societies but also to cities, even to industrial enterprises' (*Encyclopaedia Britannica*, 1992).

▼ Social Anthropology and Other Sciences

To gain further insight into the concept of social anthropology, it is necessary to discuss some other sciences, and how they compare with and complement social anthropology.

■ HISTORY

It has already been highlighted that social anthropology is the study of humankind,

social cultures, and social living conditions. History, on the other hand, is concerned with people's state of living. According to Beattie (1964), historians are chiefly interested in the past, remote or recent. Social anthropologists may make reference to the past too, but their approaches tend to be comparative in nature, in an attempt to understand sociocultural practices as they are today, and how they differ between societies. For example, does the practice of sorcery and witchcraft differ from one African tribe to another? Historians emphasise the sequence of social events, the dates these events happened, in an attempt to 'reconstruct a record of human activities and to achieve a more profound understanding of them' (*New Encyclopaedia Britannica*, 1992).

This does not mean, however, that anthropologists do not aim at a profound understanding of human cultures. They gain a thorough understanding of other societies' lives by living with the people under study and by asking pertinent questions: How do they live together? How do they associate with each other? Not 'What ought to be done?', but 'What is done' (Carrithers, 1992). To the anthropologist, therefore, the interrelationships that exist among humans are essential aspects of study. As Carrithers argued: 'We cannot know ourselves except by knowing ourselves in relation to others.'

Kuper (1983) commented on the function of history in relation to anthropology by referring to the opinions of two eminent social anthropologists, Radcliffe-Brown and Evans-Pritchard. Radcliffe-Brown believed that 'proper' history might illuminate social studies and that, perhaps more importantly, one can always analyse societies from a historical viewpoint. Evans-Pritchard increasingly stressed the use of history, arguing that there was little essential difference between history—particularly social history— and social anthropology.

Beattie (1964) reaffirmed the importance of history in anthropological research by pointing out that the two disciplines, although different, are very closely related. According to Beattie, an anthropologist who aims to achieve as complete an understanding as possible of the present condition of the society under study can hardly fail to ask how it came to be as it is. Beattie explained that while the anthropologists's central interest is in the present, not in the past for its own sake, often the past may be directly relevant in explaining the present.

The importance of the past, and its relevance to the present, cannot be overemphasised. Ohnuki-Tierney (1995) explained: 'Under the rubric of, for example, "The past in the present" and "The uses of the past", historical anthropologists interested in the role of agency have often examined how historical actors use the past.' By 'historical actors' Ohnuki-Tierney meant 'real individual or event subjects who are members of a social group and who thus are not free from the constraints of culture. They are not always cognizant of their intentions, and yet contribute to make changes in the society, but usually not directly, immediately, and as intended.' Anthropologists, therefore, will make considerable efforts to interpret the thinking processes a particular group has about the past and how their ideas are related to the present. It is a form of 'historical consciousness', a 'synchronic mode of thought' (Ohnuki-Tierney, 1995)—meaning a mode of thought that exists at one point in time.

Associated with history is the concept of myths. Myths are 'people's beliefs about their remote and sometimes not so remote past' (Beattie, 1964). The history of a society may contain myths that could explain the current attitudes of the culture under study. For example, Kuper (1977) referred to the social organisation of an Australian clan by interpreting their systems of customs and beliefs in an attempt to explain the relations between the society and the animals and plants and other natural objects that were socially important.

Historians are interested in the historical nature of the institutions they study, their particularity, and what make them unique at certain point in time. The anthropologist may use historical documentation to evaluate some aspects of his or her work. Having recourse to history simplifies the task of making the way of life of the subject under study intelligible (Beattie, 1964). As such, it is a valuable asset for the anthropologist, whose study approach is mainly based on the interpretation of cultural variations among groups and their way of life.

■ PSYCHOLOGY

Psychology is mainly concerned with the nature and functioning of individual human minds (Beattie, 1964). Sutherland (1991) argued that it is a systematic study of behaviour and the mind in man and animals. The goal of psychologists, Roth (1990) pointed out, is to gain an understanding of the functions of the mind and what experiences people are having, based on observations of human behaviour. Psychologists therefore examine 'all aspects of how the mind and behaviour function ranging from mental processes such as thinking, memory and attention to complex social behaviour such as speaking a language, making friends or helping someone across the road' (Roth, 1990). It can be argued that social anthropology is a different field of study because it concentrates on the sociocultural relations of people. The fact is, however, that historians, social anthropologists, and psychologists all deal with people, but use different perspectives.

Psychology, like history, does play a part in anthropological knowledge. Anthropologists who use psychology in their research may call their field 'psychological anthropology'. As far back as 1967, Robert Hunt, an assistant professor of anthropology, argued:

> The psychological anthropologist by definition works with what can be called 'psychological variables' and 'socio-cultural variables'. He is interested in the relationships between them, and one of the most important questions he can ask in this context is what are the effects these two kinds of variables have upon each other. Does one determine the other, and if so, which? Or, if they are not dependently related, what is the nature of their relationship?

Although gradually gaining in importance, the application of psychological concepts to anthropological studies has not always been seen in a favourable light. Beals (1982) described how psychological anthropology had not appealed to him, particularly in its early form of culture and personality studies. His earlier rejection stemmed from a belief that the psychology of the time, including the shortcomings of psychoanalysis, was inadequate. Beals acknowledged that psychological anthropology is an important and developing specialisation in anthropology, but nevertheless argued strongly that 'cultural and social institutions are part of the phenomenal world and may profitably be studied independently of the psychological problems of the actors involved'.

Crick (1982) affirmed the relevance of psychology to anthropology, in particular concerning 'enculturation and cognition' (culture assimilation and thought processes)

Nevertheless, he expressed considerable doubt as to the crosscultural validity of much psychological anthropology. According to Crick, psychologists and anthropologists are often analysing very different subject matters, so that there is no agreed framework for making the connections between the disciplines. Even when the terms they use are the same, Crick (1982) noted, their interests may not be identical.

Psychology is applied by many anthropologists during fieldwork, however. Tambiah (1990), for instance, remarked how anthropologists such as Tylor, Fraser, and Malinowski organised their research materials by resorting to observations of 'the mental aptitudes of the individual actor, i.e. to individual psychology and biology as providing the ultimate explanation of human thought and action'.

A good example of the application of psychology in fieldwork, and its relevance to the understanding of behaviour, is evident in the field studies of Levine (1963) on witchcraft and sorcery in a Gusii community (East Africa). Levine argued that the fear associated with witches and witchcraft is a learned behaviour, a learning that took place during the primary socialisation process.

> How does the Gusii individual learn fear of the dark in general and of witches in particular? There are some clear-cut childhood antecedents to this fear. If a child of three or four years is intrepid enough to leave the house at night, he is reprimanded by his parents, explicitly instructed in the dangers of the night, and specially warned about hyenas that are waiting to devour him. Some parents also mentioned witches at this time. . . . Some children who cry at night are threatened with being thrown out to the hyenas and witches if they do not stop.

Although the above extract does help to explain the behavioural features among some groups in other cultures, psychology, according to Kuper (1983), is seen to create ambivalence among some anthropologists. He referred to Radcliffe-Brown's concern about 'the integrity of social anthropology'. The argument was founded on the basic premise that social facts cannot be explained in terms of individual psychology, although it is possible that some forms of psychology might help sociology (anthropology).

■ SOCIOLOGY

Sociology is the study of society and of groups within it. Anthropology is also concerned with the study of groups within society. So what are the features of sociology that make it distinct from the field of anthropology?

The famous anthropologist Radcliffe-Brown distinguished between the two disciplines based on the relative importance of the comparative method (Srinivas, 1958). According to Radcliffe-Brown, this method is used by social anthropologists but not by sociologists. He was prepared to apply the term 'sociology' to social anthropology as long as the word 'comparative' (used here in the sense of comparing one culture with another) was added.

Gellner (1987) pointed out that the distinction between sociology and anthropology is a social rather than a logical one: there is no 'neat dividing line' as such, but observable differences may result from factors operating at various times and in various places that caused people to class themselves as sociologists or as anthropologists. The goal of anthropology, however, remains 'the understanding of human behaviour, both the similarities and the differences across cultures' (Rubel & Rosman, 1994).

One distinction that is often used in marking the boundary between the two fields is their comparative interest in 'advanced' and 'primitive' societies (Gellner, 1987). By 'advanced'

one means the modern, technological societies that interest sociologists; in contrast, 'primitive' ('preliterate') or 'traditional' cultures are the customary objects of study by anthropologists. However, as Gellner pointed out, anthropologists do not cease to be anthropologists—in their own opinion or that of others—when they study, for example, middle-class kinship in London or Chicago. Many cultural anthropologists undertake fieldwork among western populations and among modernising, formerly colonial populations (*Encyclopaedia Britannica*, 1992).

Another point that is often used to demarcate the differences between the two sciences is in relation to the sociologist's interest in large, complex, European societies, whereas the anthropologist analyses small, simple, non-European ones (Koentjaraningrat, 1964). Gellner pointed out, however, that so-called small and simple societies can be disconcertingly complex. This was also recognised by Radcliffe-Brown, quoting Fraser (Srinivas, 1958): 'Indeed compared with man in his absolutely pristine state even the lowest savage today is a highly developed and cultured being.' Complex sociocultural behaviour, therefore, can still be found in cultures studied by anthropologists. The complexity may be increased due to the fact that social anthropologists immersed in non-European cultures have to decipher the language of the people they are studying. Beattie (1964) argued that the problem of translation is less acute for sociologists, although it certainly exists for them too.

Other differences between sociology and anthropology may be outlined as follows:
- The methodological approach in anthropology is mainly, if not above all, fieldwork.
- Sociology uses research in an extensive way rather than intensively (Gellner, 1987).
- Sociology developed from dramatic effects

of social change within Europe; the interest in European society and the changes associated with it. Anthropology, on the other hand, found its source from European contact with non-European cultures (e.g. the Trobrianders of New Guinea, the Nuer of southern Sudan).

Whatever different features may be identified between the two disciplines, there is no clear boundary that separates them. Both the sociologist and the anthropologist investigate humans in society. Their methods or approaches may differ— one—may undertake his study intensively rather than extensively—but this is not always the case.

▼ Anthropologists and their Methods of Study

■ FIELDWORK

The study of other cultures cannot be undertaken in its fullest extent by perusing the literature or by reading ethnographic (descriptive accounts from fieldwork) material written by other social scientists. Consequently, social anthropologists believe the best method of study to be fieldwork analysis and interpretation. The fieldwork method is also known as participant observation. The participant observer is a researcher who immerses himself or herself as thoroughly as possible in the life of the community he or she is trying to understand (Lewis, 1985).

Fieldworking involves commitment and dedication by the anthropologist, who has to infiltrate the culture being studied. Such involvement can present difficulties for ethnographers, who may be initially unprepared for the environment that they have chosen to research (Seymour-Smith, 1986). The anthropologist is seen to go through a process of 'rite of passage', a cultural-socialisation set of stages, as he or she experiences disorientation. The researcher has to adapt to the codes of conduct and values of the people being studied. There is another problem: language. To acquire knowledge from a remote culture, the local language must be grasped, so that interpretation of the social scenes may be analysed and compared 'with accuracy and subtlety' (Lewis, 1985).

To gain valuable knowledge, the dedicated anthropologist must disregard any ethnocentricity and his or her own inhibitions and scruples, and be prepared to participate in the local society and become 'the life and soul of the party' (Lewis, 1985). Cheater (1989) contradicted this viewpoint by expressing the view that 'participant observation is often romanticised and misunderstood'. According to Cheater, a stranger very rarely becomes fully part of the society he or she is studying; more often, the anthropologist is in, but not fully of, that society—a privileged outsider, even when participating in its social activity.

It is the social differentiation between the observer and the observed that creates a 'social distance' and makes the task so much more difficult. Race, class, education, culture, language, and power are key characteristics that impinge on the interactions between anthropologists and informants (Cheater, 1989). The aim of fieldwork is to study people and their cultures in their natural settings. The anthropologist may, for example, spend two to three years living with some remote tribe on some Pacific island, with the goal of achieving a thorough understanding—from an inside perspective—of the natives, to obtain the holistic view of the social scientist (*International*

Encyclopaedia of the Social Sciences, 1968).

The decision to do fieldwork may be a personal one, as well as at the instigation of an official authority (a colonial government, for example). Before commencing fieldwork, an anthropologist will do a literature search to find out as much as possible about the people he or she is going to study—their language, customs, and so on if such information is available.

The activities of fieldworkers were aptly described by Lewis (1985):

> They rush about from place to place and function to function, attempting to record all aspects of the local scene, trivial as well as tragic; their range of interests encompasses all aspects of life—births, marriages, deaths, quarrels, reconciliations, rhetoric, religion, cultivation, animal husbandry, homecrafts, and politics; as they hasten here and there, their notebooks become filled with an amazing collection of miscellaneous information.

Some anthropologists may do fieldwork unaccompanied—for example, Bronislaw Malinowski (1884–1942) spent three years in the Trobriands on his own—whereas others may have their families living nearby. The length of time is crucial (2–3 years) if 'immersion' in the cultures under study is desired, since it is considered 'a scientific investigation' (Beattie, 1964). Total immersion, however, is not an easily achievable goal.

Seymour-Smith (1986) explained how fieldwork involves problems for the ethnographer, including those associated with establishing a role within the community and a rapport with informants. According to Seymour-Smith, anthropologists sometimes find it difficult to explain their presence or the nature of their investigations to the people concerned. Consequently, some have found it easier to invent a false identity, which the local community more readily accept. Immersion in other distant cultures exposes the researcher to periods of loneliness, frustration, and concerns for one's health. Sometimes, one is unable to extract the desired information from informants (Coleman & Watson, 1990), who may be constrained by their own beliefs. In the early stages of contact, the fieldworker may experience anxieties about his or her lack of knowledge of the etiquette and taboos of the social group under study:

> He likewise has to cope with his own emotional problems, for he often experiences anxieties in a strange situation. He may be overwhelmed by the difficulties of really getting 'inside' an alien culture and of learning an unrecorded or other strange language. He may wonder whether he should intrude into the privacy of people's lives by asking them questions (International Encyclopaedia of the Social Sciences, 1968).

Foote Whyte (1984) reported his feelings during his fieldwork study of an Italian–American slum district in 1936: 'The strain is greatest when you are a stranger and are constantly wondering whether people are going to accept you. Much as you enjoy your work, as long as you are observing and interviewing, you have a role to play, and you are not completely relaxed.'

With reference to etiquette and taboos, Foote Whyte stressed that caution should be exercised during immersion into another culture, to avoid jeopardising relationships with the community and informants:

> The next morning the fellows on the street corner were asking me: 'How's your steady girl?' This brought me up short. I learned that going to the girl's house was something that you just did not do unless you hoped to marry her. . . . However, this was a useful

warning. After this time, even though I found some Cornerville girls exceedingly attractive, I never went out with them except on a group basis, and I did not make any more home visits either.

This extract gives some indication of the dilemmas and difficulties anthropologists may experience during fieldwork. Participation in another culture is not an easy task outsiders who want to study the lives of other people possess drastically different cultural expectations (Foote Whyte, 1984).

■ CULTURAL COMPARISONS

Let us now consider some findings of fieldwork research, to compare the cultural behaviour of some nonwestern societies with westernised cultures.

Writing on folk religion in Japan, Hendry (1987) described how the time and place of birth is thought to influence the character and destiny of a person, as is their chosen name. Parents, therefore, often consult a specialist before choosing a name for their child. Hendry explained how the issue centres on the number of strokes it takes to write the chosen characters, and how a problem may be alleviated by retaining the pronunciation of a name but choosing a different character to write.

Leakey and Lewin (1979) described how endocannibalism (eating the bodies, or parts of the bodies, of dead relatives or members of the tribe) is practised in many parts of the world:

In the Dieri, an aboriginal people of southeastern Australia, when someone died an old man who was a relative cut all the fat from the face, belly, arms, and legs, and then handed it round to eat. These people believe that a person's fat contains unusual powers which may be acquired by those who eat it.

In some South American tribes, the people say that the home of the soul is in the bones, not the fat. These people burn their dead and then mix the ashes of the bones with their drinks. In this way the soul takes up residence in the people who drink the mixture.

The same authors reported how, in the Cubeo tribe, a dead enemy's penis is offered to the wife of the chief to be eaten at the end of a meal, to increase her fertility.

Concerning westernised cultures, in contrast, Gannon (1994) described how most travellers expect to find the British 'stuffy and starched'. Although, as Gannon pointed out, there are examples of such stereotypes—the gentleman wearing pinstripes and a bowler hat and carrying a furled umbrella, and the 'oh-so-proper' lady shopping and having afternoon tea at Harrods—one may also find 'punks' with orange or green, spiked hair, as well as other less-noticeable eccentrics.

In American culture, Gannon noted, football is not only a sport but also an array of common beliefs and ideals; 'a set of collective rituals and values shared by one dynamic society'. The intensity of involvement in their favourite sport reflects typified American culture, Gannon asserted.

If the wearing of pinstripes suits, the taking of tea at Harrods, and sport such as American football embody some aspects of westernised culture, it is not surprising that anthropologists undertaking fieldwork away from home-base find that their cultural expectations are in conflict with the cultures they encounter. Thus, it is not unusual for them to experience 'culture shock'.

Powdermaker (1968), however, believed that culture shock is not as problematic to the trained anthropologist, because he or she has prior general knowledge of the people and their culture, through having immersed themself in the literature. In this way, Powdermaker explained, the researcher gains gradual access into the culture, and this prepares him or her for the anticipation of unexpected modes of behaviour.

▪ OBSERVING, RECORDING, AND PARTICIPATING IN THE CULTURE

In order to record all actions of the people being studied, the anthropologist must have accurate observational skills and a certain detachment and objectivity.

Observing cultural life becomes a learning situation for the researcher. The researcher quickly comprehends the appropriate behaviour to adopt by inspecting the group or the gang, their actions, their interactions, as well as their interrelationships. Researchers have to understand their own actions and activities as well as those of the people they are studying (Burgess, 1982). The purpose of having self-awareness is to be able to recognise one's own cultural beliefs and attitudes, which may not be compatible with the behaviour or attitudes of those being observed. Participation by the anthropologist requires conscious self-discipline, to avoid as much as possible the pitfalls of ethnocentrism. The field researcher must maintain 'an outsider's perspective' (i.e. detachment) to obtain 'an insider's view' (i.e. involvement). This objective can only be reached by the development of self-criticism and self-awareness (Burgess, 1982).

Burgess (1984) underlined some other facts about the role of the fieldworker:

> Participant observation facilitates the collection of data on social interaction; on situations as they occur rather than on artificial situations (as in experimental research) or constructs of artificial situations (as in survey research). The value of being a participant observer lies in the opportunity that is available to collect rich detailed data

based on observations in natural settings. Furthermore the researcher can obtain accounts of situations in the participant's own language which gives access to the concepts that are used in everyday life.

To participate in the culture and to be accepted, the anthropologist relies on his relationship with informants. Informants provide the bridge between the sociocultural group under study and the ethnographer.

▪ ANTHROPOLOGISTS AND THEIR INFORMANTS

It is a daunting experience for any fieldworker to find himself or herself amid some remote and unfamiliar cultures. To achieve the goals of observation of activities (such as cooking, eating, drinking, talking, and so on) and accurate data collection, the anthropologist needs the help of local people. The task of the fieldworker is an intensive one. The anthropologist becomes more and more dependent on other workers (Beattie, 1964). It is not unusual, therefore, for the researcher to befriend some local members of the community. These recruited individuals become the advisers or informants.

Informants have an important role to play during fieldwork: they know the local dialect or language, consequently they can translate more specifically the meanings and moods of the interviewee; they can make useful local contacts, as well as collect information and carry out surveys under the anthropologist's supervision (Beattie, 1964).

The relationship between an anthropologist and his informant is evident in the following extract:

> When I went away from the village for a month in the summer of 1966, I asked Mohammed and one or two other men to

keep a diary of the events which I would miss. I did not ask any women to do so, mainly because the ones I knew best, like Mwahadia, were illiterate. Mohammed's was the longest diary, and it proved so rewarding that I asked him to continue to keep it up during the remainder of my stay in the village, and after I left Kanga to work in the south of the island (Caplan, 1992).

The ethnographic material in an informant's diary is a valuable asset for the anthropologist, since a record of activities—births, rituals, deaths, possessions by spirits–provides—the cultural richness required to make sense of other people's social world.

The informant is the observer's observer (Burgess,1982). The investigator substitutes the observations of a member for his own observations; it is the use of informants as if they were colleagues. Burgess noted how there has never been a participant-observer study in which the observer gained full knowledge of all roles and statuses through his or her own direct observation. It is impossible for any anthropologist to see the whole of any society or to be in many places simultaneously. Furthermore, the informant can report events that the fieldworker may not be able to, because of other commitments, for example, or social taboos that restrict the fieldworker's involvement. As Burgess registered, the value of the informant used in this way is to increase the accessibility of the group to the investigator.

Crick (1992), for instance, found his relationship with his informant, Ali, 'crucial' during his fieldwork study in Sri Lanka in 1982. Crick relied on his informant to help him gain access to districts, such as the slum area in which Ali lived, where it would have been difficult for him to be accepted.

Ali and Mohammed are examples of what anthropologists call 'key informants'. The fieldworker's systematic observations may need

exploration and scrutiny, and so rely on the support of the informant. Hastrup and Hervik (1994) argued that anthropologists and informants act as catalysts to each other's efforts to make sense: the anthropologist's keen interest in what to the informants may be only trivia, may speed up the informant's own reflections, which in turn become subject to the anthropologist's analysis.

The interactions between the anthropologist and the informant lead to a situation in which both learn about each other. Informants must 'interpret both their own culture and that of the anthropologist, which they do by first becoming self-conscious about it and objectifying their own life-world, and then by presenting it to the anthropologist' (Caplan, 1992).

Fieldwork is the most important tool of the anthropologist. It is only by immersing himself or herself into other cultures that the anthropologist can achieve realistic interpretations and comparisons of the cultural landscape.

▼ The Concept of Culture in Anthropology

A question often asked is, 'What is culture?' It is certainly a broad concept, open to different types of interpretations. Mitchell (1979), for example, defined it as the amalgamation of human action (and its products), in comparison with the biological or genetic aspects of humankind. In this sense, 'culture' is interpreted to mean all the social aspects of human life. According to Mitchell (1979), anthropological definitions of 'culture' originated from the writings of one anthropologist, E B Tylor: 'Culture or civilization is that complex whole which includes knowledge, belief, art, morals, law, custom, and any other capabilities and habits acquired by man as a member of society.'

Pelto and Pelto (1976) gave the following definition: 'The systematic patterns of explicit and implicit concepts (ideas) for behaviour and for behaviour settings (environments) learned and used by individuals and groups in adapting to their environments.' Culture is therefore seen to represent the core concept that deepens the anthropologist's understanding of people's methods of adaptation.

According to Helman (1990), anthropologists have provided a combination of definitions of culture; for example, it is a representation of ideas, a conceptual framework comprising social meanings and the rules by which people abide.

Hamnett et al. (1989), on the other hand, argued that the term is used by anthropologists to mean 'material culture', that which relates to the collection of objects such as tools and various devices used by people in daily living.

Professor Malinowski (1937) explained the meaning of culture in this way:

Culture, in fact, is nothing but the organised behaviour of man. Man differs from animals in that he has to rely on an artificially fashioned environment: on implements, weapons, dwellings and man-made means of transport. To produce and to manage this body of artifacts and commodities, he requires knowledge and technique. He depends on the help of his fellow beings. This means that he has to live in organised, well ordered communities. . . . All this artificial equipment of man, material, spiritual, and social, we call technically culture. It is a large scale molding matrix; a gigantic conditioning apparatus. In each generation it produces its type of individual. In each generation it is in turn reshaped by its carriers.

Culture, therefore, is not a fixed and stagnant body of knowledge created and used by people in society; it is subject to change and redesign by the people. However, culture as a social concept possesses powerful influences. Humans are controlled by their cultures from birth onwards. Man's attitudes, values, ideals, and beliefs, as well as his overt motor activity, are powerfully influenced by the culture that surrounds him (New Encyclopaedia Britannica, 1992).

Let us look at some examples of human sociocultural behaviour.

Wood (1979) documented how the fear of 'pollution' slants the attitudes towards menstruating females in many societies. He cited the Gururumba of New Guinea as a striking example. A girl at the menarche is considered a menace not only to men—and in this example to the society's valued pigs as well—but also to herself. She is isolated in her mother's house, where she may not touch her body or eat with her fingers. During her seclusion, she is constantly cautioned about how dangerous her sexuality is to men and pigs at this time. At the end of her isolation period, she is welcomed back into the public domain, where, for a while, she is the centre of happy attention at a food exchange.

With reference to Turkish people, Gannon (1994) illustrated what Holfstede (1980) described as their 'feminine' nature—the extent to which they value care for others, quality of life and people—by noting their response to a traffic accident: within moments, everyone who witnessed the collision, along with those who did not, was on the scene. Gannon stated that if a vehicle breaks down at night, Turkish passers by usually do not hesitate to stop and offer assistance to the driver. To ignore someone in distress is considered indecent in this culture. In contrast, Gannon pointed out, many Americans would not dare to stop for fear of their own safety. 'In Turkish culture, involvement and interdependence are the ideal' (Gannon, 1994).

Rodman (1993) gave the following account from his ethnographic studies on the island of Ambae in Vanuatu (New Hebrides):

Margaret and I found out about 'vugivugi' (Ambaeans believe in kinds of spirits that are corporeal manifestations of certain kinds of mental processes). Over the course of our study, we came to perceive vugivugi as unbidden instruments of self -destruction. Immoral thoughts liberate vugivugi. These thoughts may arise from jealousy or envy or lust. We understood the process of unleashing vugivugi to be entirely reflexive, a person's mind turned against his or her own body with often fatal results.

Cultural beliefs such as these, direct and control human behaviour. Keesing (1981) expressed the view that culture—'the realm of ideas, the force of symbols' is—'centrally important in shaping human behaviour'. To study the cultures of social groups, therefore, is to gain knowledge of the meanings expounded and transmitted by them in regard to their ideas and beliefs and their interpretations.

All humans have cultures. Each culture possesses differentiated patterns, as evidenced in the above examples. To understand cultural variations, one should attempt to penetrate the meanings attached to the behaviours under study.

▼ Family and Kinship in Nonwestern Societies

■ THE DEFINITION OF KINSHIP

Kinship, a subject of interest to the anthropologist, has been a dominant theme since the nineteenth century. It is not unusual to find groups of people in society who derive a sense of belonging, identity, and individuality from the mere fact of being members of a family and kinship group. But what is kinship? From an anthropological perspective, kinship means the social rela-

tions—not the blood relationships—that exist among groups (Coleman & Watson, 1990). Kinship is founded on the strong affinity among members of a particular social structure, which is in turn based on the social relationships or cultural ties that bind people together. The kinship concept is influential in guiding the social behaviour of groups in all social situations, be they economic activities, birth and marriage, or competing for political power. As Coleman and Watson (1990) explained, the actions and decisions of people are likely to be influenced by ideas of kinship. The kinship relations may be based initially upon biological ties, but their meanings established social and cultural factors (Rogers, 1993). The foundation of social organisation in societies that have inequalities in authoritative power distribution—so-called rank societies (Pearson, 1974)—is reliant on kinship.

The powerful influence of kinship is illustrated by Pearson's observations of the Arunta of central Australia. On the rare occasions that these people are compelled to seek blood revenge, blood has a deep 'magico-kinship' significance. Pearson (1974) described how the men first rub themselves with the hair of the slain kinsman and then cut their own veins and smear each other with their blood, to dedicate themselves more deeply to the common task of revenge. Hence, this 'bond' of kinship is associated with the allegiance to customs that guide and constrain social behaviour. These features, Pearson posited, command compliance and enforce social pressures, so that a consensus and harmony are easily maintained.

Fox (1991) argued the bonds between kin are potentially the most fundamental of all social bonds because they are based on irreducible biological facts, the features that make humans human. Kinship, according to Fox, only develops from the urge to classify and categorise objects in nature, including people. Kinship, therefore, is socially constructed from what is biologically available and in existence. Fox (1991) pointed out that all animals have their uncles, aunts, and cousins, but—with perhaps the rare exception of some primates—they do not recognise these relationships or utilise them in building their societies. Fox went on to describe how human societies range from those that make a minimal use of kinship ties, such as our own, to those like the tribes of aboriginal Australia, where the whole society is a large kin group in which everyone is a relative of everyone else. Among the Arunta of central Australia, for example, every child has its legitimate (biological) parents, and social (kinship) provides the key to both the economic and social structure (Pearson, 1974).

In the social structure, for instance, kinship is the framework with all the armoury of rights and obligations that ensure the cohesiveness of the group. 'It defines systems of inheritance and the duties of exchange or sharing' (Rogers, 1993). The pervasiveness of kinship is clearly noticeable in many aspects of social organisations, such as farming, manufacturing industries, and the ways goods are distributed (Rogers, 1993).

Bell (1986) illustrated the importance of kinship in African society by commenting on the writings of President Nyerere. Nyerere claimed that the traditional African economy and social organisation were founded on socialist principles of communal ownership of the means of production in which kinship and family groups took part in economic activity and were jointly responsible for welfare and security. Nyerere's view is based on the power of the extended family, where the bonds of kinship can be found. According to Nyerere, the African socialist considers all men as his brethren, as members of his ever-extending family. Such family and kinship networks have an important role to play; for example, as Bell (1986) explained, the acquisi-tion of rural housing and cattle in Africa is made easier through these networks.

■ THE SIGNIFICANCE AND IMPORTANCE OF KINSHIP

In tribal societies, kinship places the individual in the scheme of things (Keesing, 1981). Belonging to a particular kinship group means the expectation from other members of the group of certain obligations, duties, specified ritualistic behaviour, and participation in economic activities. The behaviour expected throughout the lifespan of the person may even extend beyond death: for example, the rituals performed to please the ancestral spirits.

As well as the many social activities that operate within the kinship framework to strengthen the cultural bonds among members, kinship has a powerful force in providing emotional wellbeing. Peoples and Bailey (1994) referred to how, in most societies, people depend heavily on their relatives for emotional support and turn to their kinsfolk in times of crisis and need.

The kinship group, hence, is a milieu of intense social, spiritual, economic, and psychological activities. The kin groups and the complex network of relationships are regarded as multifunctional (Peoples & Bailey, 1994), because they organise many kinds of activities. The aims of these activities are to ensure the accomplishment of tasks and to solve common problems. Keesing (1981) explained that even when individuals in a tribal society are competing for economic advantage or political power, they are liable to talk about what they are doing in terms of kinship.

Kinship provides the model of the framework—or, as Keesing pointed out, the 'template'—on which relationships are based. Relationships between relatives are morally binding. The kinship ties have symbolic meanings. They demonstrate the collective philosophy rather than an individual belief.

▼ Summary

Social anthropology is the study of the culture and social organisation of living people. It is a social science that uses comparative approaches. Although it is said that anthropology focuses on primitive or preliterate cultures, it is also well known that anthropologists study western cultures too.

For academic purposes, attempts have been made to compare and contrast anthropology with other sciences. History, for example, is seen to examine the sequences of events that have occurred in the past. Anthropologists use history to make sense of sociocultural practices and how they differ from one society to another. Psychology, the study of mental life, is also used by some anthropologists (psychological anthropologists) who work with both psychological and sociocultural variables to identify the relationships between them. There is, however, no valid framework to connect the two disciplines. The application of psychology helps the anthropologists to assess the mental aptitude of the actor. Sociology, it is argued, studies human groups in European cultures, whereas social anthropology is to do with preliterate non-European societies. There are anthropologists who do study human groups in cities, however.

Fieldwork, also known as participant observation, is a popular method of study in anthropology. It is regarded as important since it allows the investigator to gain close access to groups from other cultures. It is this involvement, face-to-face interactions with the community, that provides the researcher with a wealth of information on the daily cultural activities of people. Immersion into other cultures is the main goal of the anthropologist, but is not an easy task. A period of adaptation and a rite-of-passage stage are needed. It may take time before the anthropologist feels accepted by the people he or she is studying. Loneliness, frustration, misunderstandings, and illhealth are some of the perils of fieldwork.

To obtain valuable knowledge, the dedicated researcher has to disregard any ethnocentrism and his or her own inhibitions and scruples, and be prepared to participate in the local society. Participation requires care and sensitivity about the taboos and etiquette of the social group under study. A degree of awareness regarding one's own cultural beliefs and attitudes is expected, to ensure objectivity. Informants are used to help the investigator in his or her fieldwork. The role of informants is to bridge the gap between the researcher and the community being studied.

Anthropologists' main focus of study is the 'culture' of humankind. Culture means the systems of ideas, beliefs, and customs of people in different societies, their methods of adaptation, and the devices they use to survive in their environment. Culture is thus used to refer to the social aspects of human life, in comparison with the genetic perspective of humans. Culture is, however, in a state of fluidity; it is changed over time by the people who are under its powerful influences. The power of culture can be seen in the social behaviour of various groups throughout the world. It is argued that culture both shapes the behaviour of people and directs them.

Kinship is considered to be a social construct that is based on biological facts. It is the meanings a group gives to the social relations they have. Kinship provides the member with a sense of belonging. It guides behaviour; it increases group cohesiveness; it reinforces the economic obligations of the group, the duties and responsibilities they have towards each other.

▼ Application to Clinical Practice

Anthropology is relevant to nursing care. It has begun to appear as a topic in health courses for nurses and in schools of nursing (Holden & Littlewood, 1991), and, consequently, is being seen more and more as a tool to be used by nurses in their everyday working lives and not just as an academic subject.

Anthropological knowledge, the fruit of fieldwork by anthropologists in distant cultures, ensures that healthcare professionals in clinical practice gain sensitive insight into cultural practices of people from other societies.

■ THE APPLICATION OF FIELDWORK TO CLINICAL PRACTICE

The fieldwork method, or ethnography as it is sometimes called, can become a tool for learning (Dobson, 1986). Fieldwork is a participant-observer's method of research. How can healthcare professionals improve their practice by using ethnographic information? As Dobson pointed out, a wealth of texts, mostly in the field of social anthropology, can help healthcare professionals towards 'cultural discovery'. Clinical practitioners may develop a multicultural or transcultural awareness, and a positive insight into other people's practices, by undertaking small-scale projects based on ethnographic

research methods (Dobson, 1986). The application of the fieldwork method to develop better understanding of cultural differences can only enhance the quality of nursing care delivered. The relevance of research to nursing is not just a matter of attempts to fit ideas from other disciplines into nursing, but is essentially one of identifying and strengthening the professional foundations of nursing practice (Akinsanya, 1994). Ethnography is a research technique concerned with the direct observation of sociocultural groups (Abercrombie *et al.*, 1984), from which clinical nursing and medical staff can retrieve a wealth of information from the clients they encounter. Dobson (1986) suggested:

> While observation, participation and interviewing are skills which are central to nursing care, as ethnographic methods they take on a cultural emphasis. . . . Briefly ethnographic participation involves attending cultural functions and interacting with the people whose culture is under observation. Observational activities, however, focus both on the behaviour of the members of the cultural group chosen and the settings and circumstances in which such behaviours take place.

Interviewing and observing patients in their community settings are nursing activities usually undertaken by district nurses, community psychiatric nurses, and health visitors, for example. Dobson asserted that a small-scale ethnographic study is feasible in such circumstances. This will allow professionals to develop skills in data collection; they will also refine their cultural sensitivity and participate in offering guidance that is culturally acceptable. The knowledge obtained will also help professionals to work within a frame of reference that will serve them in planning and implementing holistic interventions by incorporating culturally sensitive care (Bushby, 1992).

Leininger (1983) strongly recommended the

application of her theory of diversity and universality of care, which comprises:

- The taking of deliberate cognitive steps to stimulate the expression of the clients' cultural beliefs, values, or practices.
- The concerted effort to preserve the integrity of a group's cultural values, beliefs, and practices.
- The use of creativity to restructure and reorganise different attributes of a culture, so that different or new patterns of care become evident.

Lipson and Meleis (1985), writing on immigrants in North America, explained how the effects of immigration can be traumatic for immigrants. They experience a sense of disorientation and disorganisation, a syndrome called 'cultural exhaustion'. Lipson and Meleis postulated that ethnographic studies, historical epidemiology, and observations in societies where a rapid increase of technology has occurred, show that people who are in a state of physical and cultural transition have a higher risk of illness— they develop high blood pressure compared with nonmigrants from the same society, and they are more prone to infection, chronic diseases, and other physical complaints. Any form of migration from one country to another is likely to affect an individual and cause stress, as well as predispose to mental illhealth (Helman, 1990). Revelations from ethnographic studies, as pointed out above, should be utilised by healthcare professionals to guide their clinical practice. In both hospital and community environments in Britain, the case of immigrants and their methods of adaptation should be assessed, and individual nursing care implemented.

Being admitted to hospital or being ill at home in an unfamiliar country can exacerbate the patient's condition. Consequently, care personnel should exercise tact, sensitivity, and understanding to minimise the negative effects of stress snd hence facilitate the patient's adaptation. To ease the transition of immigrants from their countries of origin to the host country, implementation of care should focus on the following guidelines:

- Develop a rapport with the client. This will contribute towards making the assessment procedure less traumatic.
- Aim at gaining an understanding of the social and cultural characteristics of the individual. (Specific information from relevant ethnographic studies may help.)
- Undertake a sensitive assessment to find out how the person is coping with difficulties regarding access to healthcare.
- Educate, as necessary, about practices, methods of treatment, and the importance of health education. Invite relevant specialist agencies to participate in the care: social care, dietetics, community agency, etc.
- Recruit interpreters if necessary.
- Invite appropriate religious leaders (who will explain usual religious practices).
- Identify the nonverbal and verbal communication style.
- Identify attitudes to health.

Dickinson and Bhatt (1994) conducted a fieldwork study between May and August 1991 on the attitudes of ethnic minorities in Britain to health. Their findings showed that most respondents perceived health to be an individual responsibility and not a 'matter of luck', albeit Chinese men and South-Asian women showed a slight tendency to believe the latter. The report concluded that generally there was an active and positive attitude to health, although the respondents wanted more health-related information. One general belief of the group was that too much thinking about health was itself detrimental to health. Some respondents expressed positive attitudes towards alternative medicine; others said that they would only see a doctor if they were 'really ill'. Chinese and Caribbean communities did not interpret serious illness to be the fault of the individual.

These findings have implications for the delivery of care. A failure to recognise and identify the health attitudes of the minorities means providing superficial care to a group who may have serious health needs. The group in question may not consider that they have any essential health needs if they believe that illness is not the fault of the individual or if they feel that a doctor must only be called in cases of serious illness.

The role of the care professional is to present a balanced perspective on health, its positive characteristics, and how it is interpreted in the western culture. It is an educational process for both the client and the therapist; one learns from the other. It is important for the clinician not to impose his or her westernised cultural beliefs. Active listening and appropriate psychological and cultural support should be provided.

According to McAllister and Farquhar (1992), there are several factors that may influence an individual's uptake of preventive health programmes:

- Cultural beliefs about health.
- Social background.
- Experience of health and illness.
- Exposure to health promotion.

An assessment of the client using the above framework will guide the practitioner towards a more realistic cultural-care intervention. Healthcare provision should reflect the individual needs of the person. As Watson (1993) put it, more understanding of commonly held notions about the social and cultural contexts of health, as a basis upon which to develop and implement health-promoting initiatives, should be seen in practice.

Healthcare knowledge pertinent to specific groups in a multicultural society can be gained from research findings. Socio-anthropological knowledge, assimilated from ethnographic studies of societies around the world, can facilitate the nursing process.

The contributions of ethnography to nursing research have been documented. Robertson and Boyle (1984), for example, reinforced the conceptual understanding of the relationships between health, illness, and culture. They affirmed that ethnographic methodology facilitates investigative processes in regard to the understanding of people's health beliefs and practices. They also asserted that improved understanding of the meaning of clients' behaviour will enhance nursing judgements and improve nursing care. The ethnographic perspective will enhance the richness of the investigations of nurse researchers, since it will bring them into closer contact with the circumstances in which peoples' health beliefs and practices evolve, and help them to identify cultural components of health and illness domains (Robertson & Boyle, 1984).

As pointed out already, the fieldworker or ethnographer, before undertaking fieldwork, needs to do some literature searches to gain an understanding of the customs and social patterns of the group to be investigated. Robertson and Boyle (1984) argued that a similar approach should be used by the nurse anthropologist:

> This means in effect that the ethnographer does not start out intellectually empty ended. Theoretical concepts are not created anew in each nursing ethnography, they are adopted from other studies, refined and applied to new interpretations of nursing problems. In this way, new insights into cultural

phenomena as they relate to health and nursing care are elaborated.

The contributions of ethnography to nursing knowledge are of prime significance. Their relevance and importance cannot be overemphasised. Robertson and Boyle (1984) argued that descriptive research, such as ethnography, contributes to a meaningful base of knowledge and theory, from which nursing practice can evolve. These authors point out that for nursing care to be culturally sensitive, a knowledge base with well-developed cultural elements related to health and illness issues would be useful; ethnographic nursing research could supply these needed data.

So far the relevance of ethnography to nursing has been emphasised from the angle of acquisition of knowledge about clients' health beliefs and practices. However, ethnography is just as relevant when the professional behaviour and practices of practitioners need investigating. As Field (1983) argued, if one accepts the premise that the core of any profession lies in its practice, then to understand that profession it is necessary to study practice within the contextual setting. Ethnography is invaluable because it paves the way for the fieldworker to penetrate nursing culture, to learn from other groups. In clinical practice, it permits access to other professional groups and observation of them at work. A thorough exploration of the context in which nursing is being practised (in hospital and community settings) may reveal an array of rituals, beliefs, good and bad practices, and the cultural climate in which patients are being nursed. Ethnographic findings may stimulate healthcare professionals to re-examine their own behaviour and cultural health beliefs.

Field (1983) described an ethnographic study, in Canada, into the various perspectives of public health and public-health nursing held by four nurses. The comparative framework of beliefs identified among the informants is shown in the list below:

(a) The goal of public health is health promotion and illness prevention.

(b) The goal of nursing is to help to achieve a healthier lifestyle.

(c) The role of the nurse is to:
- identify clients' needs and intervene to prevent potential problems;
- help the clients to identify problems;
- provide the clients with information;
- identify potential problems and provide education.

(d) The sources of the client's actual or potential problems are:
- social, psychological, and physical circumstances;
- insufficient knowledge to anticipate or cope with problems;
- multiproblem families with social, psychological and physical problems.

Although the above lists do not represent the full research findings, they are sufficient to give us a fairly accurate picture of the wide range of interpretations and nursing beliefs expressed by the informants during the fieldwork. These have implications for healthcare delivery. If beliefs about health are interpreted in a variety of ways, if the role of the care professional is interpreted differently and given alternative emphases, then nursing intervention is more likely to be influenced by the beliefs of the individuals and given different priorities.

To ensure uniformity and standardised approaches to healthcare delivery, an agreed and consistent framework for practice should be adopted by professionals. This should be based on a consensus of the role and functions of the nurse, as well as on their health beliefs.

The importance of ethnography as a tool for studying nursing culture was highlighted by Holland (1993). This author undertook an ethnographic study to explore ritualised practice in a ward setting. Holland noted that although rituals were found to exist in the working day of the nurses studied, there was no indication that ritualised behaviour was harmful to individualised patient care. Similar to studies undertaken by anthropologists in other cultures, she relied on informants within the cultural group being investigated. Her key informants were two student nurses and one qualified member of staff. Holland collected data by participant observations within the following contexts: social structures, systems of authority, economic system, communication, and socialisation. The task of the nurse ethnographer is to collect data in an objective fashion, ensuring that the clinical nursing image is represented as accurately as possible. Holland's study (1993) produced a wealth of information that reflected the ward climate at the time. The following is a summary of some aspects of the results:

- The social structures referred to in the study meant the physical environments, i.e. the wards or departments in which specialist intervention would take place: 'A cultural scene where patients came in with specifically diagnosed disordered body functions.'
- The economic activities were identified as the working day of the work force.
- The communication system focused on the nursing jargon used by the staff.
- Socialisation of the new members was observed, new members being student nurses, for example, considered a transient

workforce that only passed through the cultural setting.

■ CULTURAL NEEDS OF PATIENTS

The cultural needs of patients, both in the community and within hospital settings, should be considered just as important as the psychological, physical, and spiritual aspects of care by healthcare professionals. A 'transcultural' approach is therefore essential. Transcultural means going across and beyond the boundaries of cultures, including one's own culture, to meet the other person's cultural needs. Sometimes, the related terms 'crosscultural' and 'multicultural' are used. Transcultural care has been described as the interface between (DeSantis, 1994) or the blending of (Wilkins, 1993) anthropology and nursing. To achieve this transcultural approach, anthropological research findings should be utilised. Since social anthropologists study many cultures, their findings regarding norms and beliefs of groups are significant for effective care-planning by healthcare professionals. If the cultures of other people are of clinical significance, the application of anthropology can only predispose to culturally informed clinical practice.

Leininger (1983), a famous proponent of transcultural care and the founder of the field of transcultural nursing, emphasised:

Caring for people of diverse cultures and subcultures in the world is one of the greatest and most important challenges today for professional nurses. Cultural care means a conscious awareness and deliberate effort to use cultural values, beliefs and lifeways of an individual, family or group to provide meaningful assistance to those needing health care services. It means knowing and respecting the values and beliefs of different cultures or subcultures so that clients will receive care that is helpful to them. It is essentially a new and creative approach to client care.

Holden and Littlewood (1991) pointed out that nurses, who are predominantly white and middle-class, are increasingly encountering people from ethnic minorities, whose perceptions of the body and ideas of the self, of illness, and of social attitudes towards illness and disease can differ radically from their own. Gaining knowledge of such cultural diversity will help to bridge the gap between patients' needs and culturally sensitive care.

Nolde and Smillie (1987) asserted that culture comprises the learned ways of the acting and thinking of a group. These are transmitted from generation to generation, and provide guidelines for solutions to vital problems. In this way, inherent in the individual are his or her cultural norms. It is important, therefore, that an accurate cultural assessment is undertaken. As Dobson (1986) explained, it is essential for practitioners to use skills to discover and blend cultural knowledge with patient care.

Kitzinger (1982), referring to comparative studies of childbirth in Jamaica and Britain, noted that birth, like death, is not only a physiological act but also a social act. The social meanings of childbirth are perceived differently in Jamaica. Kitzinger described how for the Jamaican girl, as in many peasant societies, childbirth provides a ritual entry to the adult state; adulthood does not come so much with age or experience as with motherhood. The pregnant Jamaican woman follows the instructions of her 'nana' (midwife) as well as the traditional mythical beliefs; for example, no Jamaican woman who is pregnant must on any account look at a dead body. In contrast, in the British experience, Kitzinger (1982) argued, the highly formalised and circumscribed interaction of the hospital booking clinic, by which pregnancy is given public recognition, can all be seen as part of the rites-of-status transformation. Kitzinger stated that such comparative study suggests that all investigations of physiological states should focus on the dynamic interaction between meaning systems, social behaviour, and physiological functions. The author argued for a thorough understanding of the specific social context and a particular value system, an approach encompassing the needs of individuals and groups in 'defined relationships'.

Unless healthcare professionals become aware of such multicultural belief systems and meanings, patients' needs will remain unfulfilled. McGee (1994) emphasised the requisite for culturally sensitive care to consist of a sound knowledge base that incorporates an awareness of the nurses' own culture, preferences, and prejudices, alongside specific information about ethnic groups. Culture-specific care, Leininger (1983) explained, is becoming increasingly essential; when professionals fail to recognise cultural values, patients tend to become dissatisfied, withdraw, or may not have a favourable health outcome.

Manderson and Reid (1994) pointed out the complex interactions between culture and health. They explained how the interaction or influence of culture on health can be highly significant. For example, culture may influence food choice and cooking style; diet, for many people, plays a major protective factor against ischaemic heart disease. On the other hand, Manderson and Reid stated, the importance of culture can be overstated and, at times, it is equivocal whether the incidence of infection or development of disease, or the quality of treatment, is due to or determined by gender, class, race, ethnicity, or other factors. It is hence important for healthcare professionals to consider not only cultural factors during their assessment of patients, but also the biological, psychological, and spiritual dimensions.

To provide culturally sensitive care, healthcare professionals should recognise their own cultural beliefs and practices, as these influence their behaviour and perception: 'In terms of nursing care, it is the ability of nurses to temporarily step out of or suspend their own cultural traditions (values, beliefs, and practices) in order to perceive the situation as others do' (DeSantis, 1994). Healthcare professionals who do not 'step out of or suspend their own cultural traditions' are labelled as 'ethnocentric'. Ethnocentrism means centring on one's own cultural traditions and beliefs, and excluding other cultures. Professor Leininger (1983) reiterated the concept of ethnocentrism by linking it with the theory of cultural imposition. She argued that ethnocentrism refers to the belief that one's own values, beliefs, and practices are the best, most superior, and most desired. Cultural imposition, she expounded, is the tendency of a person to impose their values, beliefs, and practices upon another person, often without knowledge of the results of such actions. To prevent a superficial assessment of patients' needs, an objective approach is required, which involves the discarding of cultural stereotypes and ethnocentricity. The focus of care should be on the patient's personal and sociocultural realities. As Abdullah (1995) pointed out, nurses who adopt an ethnocentric attitude towards their clients may not be able to provide genuine unbiased care.

There is, however, another dimension to ethnocentrism: the patient's ethnocentricity. DeSantis (1994) used the term 'simultaneous dual ethnocentrism' to describe situations in which, for example, nurses are judging and reacting to patients according to their own perceptions of clinical reality and their expectation of patients; simultaneously, patients are judging nurses based on their beliefs about the healthcare encounter and their expectations of nurses.

Cultural care provides the 'bridge between sickness, illness and disease' (Germain, 1992). To provide culturally sensitive and appropriate healthcare, professionals in clinical practice must first identify the differences between 'illness' and 'disease' from a professional and a lay person's point of view. Manderson and Reid (1994) explained that illness is the human experience of symptoms and sufferings, including the physical dimensions (e.g. having a headache, feeling nauseous) and the social and behavioural consequences (e.g. taking drugs, not being able to work). Disease, on the other hand, refers to the pathological processes, the medical interpretation of biological changes.

A FRAMEWORK FOR CULTURALLY SENSITIVE CARE IN CLINICAL PRACTICE

(a) Identify and recognise the individuality of the patient, 'who may subscribe to the standards of his/her group to varying degrees and in varying situations' (Harwood, 1981). This implies responding to the fact that the client has ties with a social group from which he or she originates and to the powerful influences the group may exert on the individual.

(b) Acknowledge, as Mulholland (1995) advocated, that the central component of humanist approaches within nursing is to 'contextualise the interaction between the individual and his or her social context' in a rigorous manner.

(c) Provide nursing interventions that are tailored to meet the culturally diverse needs of patients by assessing their different social and family patterns, different religious and cultural beliefs, and different healthcare expectations and needs (Cortis, 1993).

Cultural sensitivity should be seen by the professionals to be a priority in the designing of a care plan and in the implementation of nursing care. Stevens *et al.* (1992) stressed how essential this approach is to the provision of holistic practice. These authors pointed out that the daily experiences of many cultural groups are unknown to health professionals. Their assessments tend to be founded on stereotypical ethnic and/or racial images. To prevent inefficient cultural care, they suggested, professionals should gain insight into the daily-living activities of the individual concerned.

The research Stevens *et al.* (1992) carried out focused on the everyday experiences of five ethnic and racial groups of female clerical workers in California, using narrative analysis. As the researchers explained: 'The interview study explored low income, urban women's experiences as workers, mothers and spouses. The stories participants told about integrating these roles provided insights into the totality of their everyday lives.' Stevens *et al.* (1992) concluded by saying that knowledge of the patient's cultural background may be gained by the use of narratives, 'because telling stories about one's life is a natural means of communicating personal and cultural information'. Such an approach will help professionals to learn about clients' everyday experiences, priorities, needs, and goals.

The impact of culture on pain was explored by Walker *et al.* (1995). Pain is a private and subjective sensation of hurt, acute discomfort, or damage. These authors described the individuality of patients' responses to pain based on their cultures. Culture influenced the way pain was experienced and the way pain relief was perceived and provided. Tolerance of pain was found to vary, both within the individual and between individuals.

Cultural aspects of care are just as relevant in psychological healthcare setting. The practitioner or the care-giver is also, in a variety of settings, the counsellor, ready to intervene in order to facilitate the healing process. Wright (1991), for example, claimed that traditional approaches to counselling have a 'disempowering' effect on the client, caused by an ineffectual assessment of the cultural context in which the client lives. Wright argued that psychiatric nurses 'have an opportunity to challenge some of the complexities and assumptions of traditional counselling models, and contribute towards the development of a helping approach, for those who are culturally 'different', which is both authentic and flexible'.

The role of the nurse manager is to integrate transcultural concepts into nursing practice. An awareness of the different beliefs and social practices of diversified groups of people in society requires developing. Harris and Tuck (1992) commented on the importance of the manager to be aware of the special needs of an ever-growing minority population, and the skills and knowledge needed by staff nurses to provide quality care.

■ KINSHIP

The admission of patients to hospitals and their care in the community always demand the filling in of relevant forms, whereby the patients are asked to name their next-of-kin. It is a routine, but nevertheless important, procedure. Very often the patients will respond by saying 'My wife' or 'My husband', sometimes 'My brother' or 'My sister', and so on.

One rationale given for the identification of the next-of-kin is to ensure that any future communication—which will consist of information giving, for example, details of surgery or the time of discharge home—is transmitted to the relatives. The importance, however, does not end here. Admission to hospital, or being ill at home, are stressful life-events for the patient. There is a severing of the moral obligations, duties, and social, spiritual, and economic activities that bind the individual with his or her kinship network. As Morrison (1994) wrote: 'Just like a child, the patient is relieved of responsibility while at the same time he/she loses the freedom to make decisions about their lives.' Identification of the wider kinship network is therefore essential. The patient's relations, and his or her perception of the relationships towards the kinship groups, are significant. The most common kinship pattern found worldwide is the multigenerational extended family (Helman, 1990). Helman explained the importance of the wider kinship groups in acting as miniature, self-contained communities, or self-help groups whose members have certain obligations to each other, by participating in many of the tasks and responsibilities of everyday life.

Patients whose norms, beliefs, and values revolve around the supportive networks of kinship groups are disadvantaged if appropriate and sensitive interventions do not match their needs. Significant others within the patient's circle may have a profound influence on the maintenance of a healthy psychological equilibrium. These wider kin, therefore, have a role in providing a sense of stability and continuity. Their participation in the care of their kin, upon agreement from the patient, should be considered during care planning.

Constraints in healthcare settings—such as the number of visitors allowed per patient, rules and regulations regarding visiting times and overnight stay—have implications for the patient who relies heavily on kinship support throughout his or her illness.

Morrison (1994) argued that an important aspect of the patient's personal concerns dealt with their families and friends. He stressed the buffering effects of these significant others in their interactions with the sick individual. The physical and psychological support that the kin network provides should not be underestimated. Their contribution towards patient care should be seen as a positive resource to be utilised by the care team. These family members, Morrison pointed out, may provide different forms of social support for patients.

However, not every patient will be fortunate to have such support, simply because they may themselves be the major supportive force in the lives of others outside the hospital. In this context, the patient's commitment to significant others is impaired. Concerns about the health of family members at home can be a very real source of anxiety and uncertainty for patients, and, consequently, will have detrimental effects on their psychological and physical wellbeing. Morrison (1994) noted how, in the busy hospital environment, these personal concerns for others outside hospital may often go unrecognised by nurses and doctors. The goal of healthcare professionals is to establish a rapport with the patient as soon as possible, to ensure a positive identification and assessment of the patient's needs. Acknowledging social-support groups as a communicative process (Kreps & Kunimoto, 1994) should be followed by care implementation, to relieve the anxieties and fears of patients with regard to the wellbeing of significant others.

Families may also have other negative influences on patients' health. The negative effects of kinship systems have been described by Helman (1990), who posited that myths regarding the natural and social world are created and transmitted from generation to generation. These myths prevail among some family systems—a form of 'family script' that guides behaviour. According to Helman, the script may also influence the clustering of certain symptoms within a particular family and how these symptoms are passed from parents to offspring. Family scripts, Helman (1990) noted, can be preserved by the family's own myths and folklore.

Mythical beliefs about health and illness in the family networks could easily affect the psychological and physical state of its members. Looking beyond the patient's clinical manifestations into the wider kin system is imperative, therefore, to ascertain that the aetiology of the illness is holistically investigated and understood.

Morgan *et al.* (1985) affirmed that the prevalent views seem to highlight the positive aspects of the family and kinship, whereas the negative features are overlooked. They postulated that what is considered 'normal' family life is very often a milieu full of 'disharmonies' with implications for the individual. The family, they asserted, may exert a constraining influence on the individual, preventing personal and social development. The authors cited case studies in which schizophrenic features could be perceived as meaningful in the context of the individual's family experiences, forming a natural response to an oppressive environment.

The positive and negative influences of kinship on care and treatment have also been documented. Morgan *et al.* (1985), for example, stated that studies of hospital patients have suggested that family members may exert either a positive or negative influence on compliance with treatment regimens, post-operative recovery, and adjustment to the psychological effects of surgery.

A kinship model of care could be designed to circumscribe salient features of patients' needs for social support during their periods of illhealth. This model could be based on the assessment of the following characteristics:

- The patient's kinship orientation.
- The patient's family's kinship orientation.
- The patient's subjective and objective view of the social world (including significant others).
- Individual health and illhealth beliefs.
- Kinship affinity (cohesiveness, bonds, obligations, duties).
- Lines of descent (patrilineal, matrilineal, etc.).
- Sociopsychological needs (anxiety, fears, depressive states due to social separation).
- Needs for therapeutic folk-medicine and combinations of medical-nursing interventions.
- Spiritual beliefs (ancestral spirits, mythical ceremonial beings, animal worship).
- Kinship power (family's physical proximity, healing touch—comfort, support).

▼ Review Questions

1   Describe the relationships between social anthropology and some other social sciences.

2   Examine and discuss the importance and relevance of fieldwork in anthropological studies.

3   Explain the importance and relevance of anthropology to clinical nursing practice.

4   Discuss how ethnographic research findings can facilitate the delivery of care in clinical practice.

5   Describe how ethnographic accounts may help in increasing cultural awareness and sensitivity.

6   Discuss the importance and relevance of culturally sensitive care in clinical practice.

7   Explore how a knowledge of kinship systems may help the healthcare professional to deliver appropriate care.

▼ References

Abdullah S. Towards an individualised client's care: implications for education. The transcultural approach. *J Adv Nurs* 1995, **22**:715–720.

Abercrombie N, Hill S, Turner B. *Dictionary of sociology.* London: Penguin; 1984:90.

Akinsanya J. Making research useful to the practising nurse. *J Adv Nurs* 1994, **19**:174-179.

Beals R. Fifty years in anthropology. *Ann Rev Anthropol* 1982, **11**:1–23.

Beattie J. *Other cultures: aims, methods and achievements in social anthropology.* London: Cohen & West; 1964.

Bell M. *Contemporary Africa.* Harmondsworth: Longman Scientific; 1986.

Burgess R. *Field research: a sourcebook and field manual.* London: Routledge; 1982.

Burgess R. *In the field. An introduction to field research.* London: Allen & Unwin; 1984.

Bushby A. Cultural considerations for primary health care: where do self care and folk medicine fit? *Holistic Nurse Pract* 1992, **6**:10–18.

Caplan P. Spirits and sex. A Swahili informant and his diary. In: Okely J, Callaway H, eds. *Anthropology and autobiography.* London: Routledge; 1992.

Carrithers M. *Why humans have cultures. Explaining anthropology and social diversity.* Oxford: Oxford University Press; 1992.

Cheater A. *Social anthropology, an alternative introduction.* London: Routledge; 1989.

Coleman S, Watson H. *An introduction to anthropology.* London: Apple Press; 1990.

Cortis J. Transcultural nursing: appropriateness for Britain. *J Adv Health Nurs Care* 1993, **2**:67–77.

Crick M. Anthropology of knowledge. *Ann Rev Anthropol* 1982, **11**:287–313.

Crick M. An essay in street-corner anthropology. Ali & me. In: Okely J, Callaway H, eds. *Anthropology and autobiography.* London: Routledge; 1992.

DeSantis L. Making anthropology clinically relevant to nursing care. *J Adv Nurs* 1994, **20**:707–715.

Dickinson R, Bhatt A. Ethnicity, health and control,

results from an exploratory study of ethnic minority communities' attitudes to health. *Health Educ J* 1994, **53**:421–429.

Dobson S. Ethnography: a tool for learning. *Nurse Education Today* 1986, **6**:76–79.

Field P. An ethnography: four public health nurses' perspectives of nursing. *J Adv Nurs* 1983, **8**:3–12.

Foote Whyte W. *Learning from the field. A guide from experience.* London: Sage; 1984.

Foster G, Kemper R. *Anthropologists in cities.* Boston: Little, Brown & Co; 1974.

Fox R. *Encounter with anthropology, 2nd ed.* London: Transaction Publishers; 1991.

Gannon M. *Understanding global cultures: metaphorical journeys through 17 countries.* London: Sage; 1994.

Gellner E. *The concept of kinship and other essays on anthropological method and explanation.* Oxford: Blackwell; 1987.

Germain C. Cultural care. A bridge between sickness, illness and disease. *Holistic Nurs Pract* 1992, **6**:1–9.

Hamnett C, McDowell L, Sarre P. *The changing social structure.* London: Sage; 1989.

Harris L, Tuck I. The role of the organisation and nurse manager in integrating transcultural concepts into nursing practice. *Holistic Nurs Pract* 1992, **6**:43–48.

Harwood A. Guidelines for culturally appropriate health care. In: Harwood A, ed. *Ethnicity and medical care.* Harvard: Harvard University Press; 1981.

Hastrup K, Hervik P. *Social experience and anthropological knowledge.* London: Routledge; 1994.

Helman C. *Culture, health and illness, 2nd ed.* Oxford: Butterworth Heinemann; 1990.

Hendry J. *Understanding Japanese society.* London: Routledge; 1987:110–113.

Holfstede G. *Culture's Consequences.* Beverly Hills: Sage; 1980.

Holden P, Littlewood J. *Anthropology and nursing.* London: Routledge; 1991.

Holland C. An ethnographic study of nursing culture as an exploration for determining the existence of a system of ritual. *J Adv Nurs* 1993, **18**:1461–1470.

Hunt R. *Personalities and cultures. Readings in psychological anthropology.* New York. Natural History Press; 1967.

International Encyclopaedia of the Social Sciences. Sills D. ed. London: Collier-MacMillan; 1968.

Keesing R. *Cultural anthropology. A contemporary perspective, 2nd ed.* New York: Holt Winston; 1981.

Kitzinger S. The social context of birth: some comparisons between childbirth in Jamaica and Britain. In: McCormack C, ed. *Ethnography of fertility and birth.* London: Academic Press; 1982.

Koentjaraningrat. Anthropology and non European–American anthropologists: the situation in Indonesia. In: Goodenough W, ed. *Explorations in cultural anthropology.* New York: McGraw Hill; 1964:293–308.

Kreps G, Kunimoto E. *Effective communication in multi-cultural health care settings.* London: Sage; 1994.

Kuper A. *The social anthropology of Radcliffe-Brown.* London: Routledge & Kegan Paul; 1977.

Kuper A. *Anthropology and anthropologists.* London: Routledge & Kegan Paul; 1983.

Leakey R, Lewin R. *People of the Lake Man; his origins, nature and future.* London: Collins; 1979.

Leininger M. Cultural care: An essential goal for nursing and healthcare. *AANNT JRNL*; 1983: 11–17.

Levine R. Witchcraft and sorcery in a Gusii community. In: Middleton J, Winter E, eds. *Witchcraft and sorcery in East Africa.* London: Routledge & Kegan Paul; 1963.

Lewis I. *Social anthropology in perspective. The relevance of social anthropology, 2nd ed.* Cambridge: Cambridge University Press; 1985.

Lewis J. *Anthropology made simple.* London: WH Allen; 1969.

Lipson J, Meleis A. Culturally appropriate care: the case of immigrants. *TCN* 1985, **7**:48–56.

Malinowski B. *Culture as a determinant of behaviour.* Cambridge: Harvard University Press; 1937.

Manderson L, Reid J. 'What's culture got to do with it?' In: Wadell C, Petersen A, eds. *'Just health'. Inequalities in illness, care and prevention.*

Edinburgh: Churchill Livingstone; 1994.

McAllister G, Farquhar M. Health beliefs: a cultural division? *J Adv Nurs* 1992, **17**:1447–1454.

McGee P. Culturally sensitive and culturally comprehensive care. *Br J Nurs* 1994, **3**:789–792.

Mitchell D. *A new dictionary of sociology.* London: Routledge & Kegan Paul; 1979.

Morgan M, Calnan M, Manning N. *Sociological approaches to health and medicine.* London: Croom Helm; 1985.

Morrison P. *Understanding patients.* London: Bailliere Tindall; 1994.

Mulholland J. Nursing humanism and transcultural theory: the 'bracketing out' of reality. *J Adv Nurs* 1995, **22**:442–449.

New Encyclopaedia Britannica Social Sciences. Chicago: University of Chicago; 1992: **27**:365–386.

Nolde T, Smillie C. Planning and evaluation of cross cultural health education activities. *J Adv Nurs* 1987, **12**:159–165.

Ohnuki-Tierney E. Structure, event and historical metaphor: rice and identities in Japanese society. *J R Anthropol Inst* 1995, **2**:227–254.

Pearson R. *Introduction to anthropology.* New York: Holt Rinehart & Winston; 1974:191–206.

Pelto G, Pelto P. *The human adventure. An introduction to anthropology.* New York: Macmillan; 1976.

Peoples J, Bailey G. *Humanity: an introduction to cultural anthropology, 3rd ed.* New York: West Publishing; 1994.

Powdermaker H. *International encyclopaedia of the social sciences, volume 5.* London: Macmillan; 1968:418–423.

Robertson M, Boyle J. Ethnography: contributions to nursing research. *J Adv Nurs* 1984, **9**:43–49.

Rodman W. Sorcery and the silencing of chiefs: 'words on the wind' in post independence Ambae. *J Anthropol Res* 1993, **49**:217–235.

Rogers A. *Guinness guide to peoples' cultures.* Enfield: Guinness Publishing; 1993:18–19.

Roth I. *Introduction to psychology.* Milton Keynes: Open University; 1990.

Rubel P, Rosman A. The past and future of anthropology. *J Anthropol Res* 1994, **50**:335–343.

Seymour–Smith C. *Macmillan dictionary of anthropology.* London: Macmillan; 1986.

Srinivas M. *Method in social anthropology.* Chicago: University of Chicago Press; 1958.

Stevens P, Hall J, Meleis A. Narratives as a basis for culturally relevant holistic care: ethnicity and everyday experiences of women clerical workers. *Holistic Nurs Pract* 1992, **6**:49–58.

Sutherland S. *Macmillan dictionary of psychology.* London: Macmillan; 1991.

Tambiah S. *Magic, science, religion and the scope of rationality.* Cambridge: Cambridge University Press; 1990.

Walker A, Tan L, George S. Impact of culture on pain management: an Australian nursing perspective. *Holistic Nurs Pract* 1995, **9**:48–57.

Watson J. Male body image and health beliefs: a qualitative study and implications for health promotion. *Health Educ J* 1993, **52**:246–252.

Wilkins H. Transcultural nursing: a selective review of the literature, 1985–1991. *J Adv Nurs* 1993, **18**:602–612.

Wood C. *Human sickness and health, a biocultural view.* California: Mayfield Co; 1979.

Wright J. Counselling at the cultural interface: is getting back to roots enough? *J Adv Nurs* 1991, **16**:92–100.

▼ Further Reading

Bignold S, Cribb A, Ball S. Befriending the family: an exploration of a nurse–client relationship. *Health Social Care Commun* 1995, **13**:173–180.

Bond J, Bond S. *Sociology and health care.* London: Churchill Livingstone; 1986:115–117.

Burrows A. Patient-centred nursing care in a multi-racial society: the relevance of ethnographic perspectives in nursing curricula. *J Adv Nurs* 1983, **8**:477–485.

Cohen P. Young carers: looking after Mum. *Community Care* 1995, **16**:18–19.

Cuff E, Sharrock W, Francis D. *Perspective in sociology, 3rd ed.* London: Unwin Hyman; 1990:71–73.

Dobson S. The concept of culture now that they are caring for the health needs of various ethnic groups in Britain. *Nursing Times* 1983 Feb **9**:53–57.

Dobson S. Under the Punjabi sky. *Nursing Times* 1985 Feb **13**:45–46.

Dobson S. Conceptualizing for transcultural health visiting: the concept of transcultural reciprocity. *J Adv Nurs* 1989, **14**:97–102.

Ellis P. European ethnic identity research and its relevance to community care. *Health and Social Care* 1993, **1**:55–58.

Foote Whyte W. Intervening in field research. In: Burgess R, ed. *Field research: a sourcebook and field manual.* London: Routledge; 1982.

Fuller J, Toon P. *Medical practice in the multi-cultural society.* Oxford: Heinemann; 1988.

Gans H. The participant observer as a human being: observations on the personal aspects of fieldwork. In: Burgess R, ed. *Field research: a sourcebook and field manual.* London: Routledge; 1982.

Giddens A. *Sociology.* Cambridge: Polity Press; 1989:384–386.

Hammond P. *An introduction to cultural and social anthropology, 2nd ed.* New York: Macmillan; 1978.

Hastrup K. Writing ethnography: state of the art. In: Okely J, Callaway H, eds. *Anthropology and autobiography.* London: Routledge; 1992.

Logan B, Dawkins C. *Family-centred nursing in the community.* California: Addison-Wesley; 1986:110–117, 708–709.

Malinowski B. The diary of an anthropologist. In: Burgess R, ed. *Field research: a sourcebook and field manual.* London: Routledge; 1982.

Mares P, *et al. Health care in multi-racial Britain.* Cambridge: NET; 1985.

McGee P. Educational issues in transcultural nursing. *Br J Nurs* 1994, **3**:1113–1116.

Outhwaite W, *et al. Blackwell dictionary of 20th century social thought.* London: Blackwell; 1994.

Papadoulos I, Alleyne J, Tilki M. Promoting transcultural care in a college of health care studies. *Br J Nurs* 1994, **3**:1116–1118.

Papadopoulos I, Alleyne J, Tilki M. Learning from colleagues of different cultures. *Br J Nurs* 1994, **3**:1118–1124.

Payer L. *Medicine & culture. Notions of health and sickness.* London: Victor Gollanz; 1988.

Rajan M. Transcultural nursing: a perspective derived from Jean-Paul Sartre. *J Adv Nurs* 1995, **22**:450–455.

Robertson L. The giving of information is the key to family employment. *Br J Nurs* 1995, **4**:692.

Sorby M. Kalymnos: island of care. *Elderly Care* 1994, **6**:35.

Stanhope M, Lancaster J. *Community health nursing. Process and practice for promoting health.* St Louis: Mosby; 1988:357–359.

Torkington N. *Black health—a political issue. The health and race project.* London: Catholic Association for Raenal Justice; 1991.

Young A. The anthropologies of illness and sickness. *Ann Rev Anthropol* 1982, **11**:257–285.

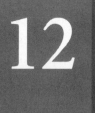

12

Social Econom
Health, Ill-health, and
Care Provision

▼An Explanation of Social Economics

The word 'economics' is in common usage in advanced eastern and western societies. Economics is the science of the methods employed in the production and distribution of resources (wealth); one may, for example, make reference to the 'economics of publishing'

(*Oxford Concise Dictionary*, 1991). An econo-mist is a person who manages financial or eco-nomic affairs. When politicians, social scientists, and economists make allusion to the 'economy', they mean the wealth and resources of a community; the production processes; the consumption of goods; and the services avail-able. The economy, therefore, is related to the allocation of resources by an economic system. This system can be broadly defined as 'the net-work of institutions and arrangements direct-ed towards using scarce resources of a certain organisation' (Eidem & Viotti, 1978). According to Bendavid-Val (1977), pure eco-nomics quantifies everything, including the 'non-quantifiable', in terms of money (pro-duction gained or foregone) and benefits (pro-duction gained).

Social economics, on the other hand, is (Rohrlich, 1974):

- The application of economics principles to social problems.
- A branch of applied statistics: the numerical measurement of the extent and constitution of social problems.
- The study of the social causes of economic behaviour ('economic ecology').
- The study of social consequences of economic behaviour ('welfare economics').

Hence, compared with the principles of pure or conventional economics, social economics is concerned with the relationships between market goods and services, and how human satisfaction may be achieved and social prob-lems more effectively and economically tack-led. Social economics recognises the human factor in the process (Bendavid-Val, 1977).

According to Stanfield (1990), formal eco-nomics is based on rationalistic psychology,

taking the individuals as a datum, whereas social economics is more behaviouristic in its psychological reach, and centres on the *forma-tion* of individuals. As Lutz (1990) reaffirmed when discussing the evolution of American social economics, the main concern of this dis-cipline is to do with the social welfare of the people and the framework within which it operates: the sociocultural environment, with all its conditions and laws.

Social economics, therefore, may be inter-preted to reflect 'welfare economics'. Bohm (1987) postulated that welfare economics is the branch of economics that among other things attempts to explain how to identify and reach socially efficient solutions to the resource-allocation problems of the national (or local) economy.

Welfare, Lai (1994) explained, is 'struct-urally and contextually built in the public domain', and has both a fiscal and social dimension. The fiscal dimension (banking net-work systems) deals with economics; the social dimension is represented by the intervention of the consumers (the citizens), whose role is to make use of the resources made available to them through the market mechanism. The inter-relationships of these two dimensions are best observed in the processes at play with wel-fare-state benefits (e.g. unemployment allowance and social insurance), which are almost without exception bound with labour market status (Lai, 1994). These mechanisms, Lai stated, are in motion to enhance an indi-vidual's performance in the production sector.

The ethos of social economics is encom-passed in its focus on socio-economic problems and how resources are employed for the benefit of the individual. Hill (1990) gave this definition:

> Social economics may be defined as the socio-economic analysis of human behaviour within a broad social and

political context for the purpose of improving the quality of life and enhancing human welfare. Social economists have always expressed and demonstrated a very special concern for the economically deprived people, the have-nots of our society.

Hill affirmed the features of social economics to consist of measures to meet the needs of the disadvantaged in society; for example, the poor, the homeless, the elderly who live in poor housing conditions, the ethnic minorities and their uptake of health facilities, single-parent families, vagrants, the unemployed, the disabled, people with learning difficulties, and any subjects who are entitled to healthcare or benefits from the welfare state but are unable to claim, either through a lack of access (transport, distance, etc.) or simply through ignorance about what they are entitled to. Hill also pointed out that social economics aims towards social improvement rather than the preservation of the status quo. Social economists are believed to be agents of change within the boundaries of the social context. Social economists consider both the sociocultural context and the ecological dimension in which the individual lives. As far back as 1974, Rohrlich expressed personal concern that our understanding of, and concern for, our social habitat (in contrast with our natural surroundings), and the aetiology of its state of jeopardy (what Rohrlich called social ecology) is limited.

When social economists examine the economic activities of society, their analysis will be aided by an understanding of any social problems that may result from the said activities. As Hill (1990) argued, the aim of social economists is to help the economically deprived in society by 'using normative value judgements as intellectual tools for the solving of socio-economic and political problems'.

Stanfield (1990) expounded on the concept by arguing that social economics is the study of the interaction of economy and society; in other words, social economics is concerned with factors that influence economic institutions and behaviour in the 'social, political and cultural realms'.

The economics of social problems—with the human factor being the central figure in the equation—focuses on the achievement of *efficiency* and *equity* (Le Grand *et al.*, 1992). 'Efficiency' refers to the provision of the number of homes, hospitals, schools, residential institutions, and so on that yield the greatest level of aggregate (net) benefit to the community. 'Equity' is about fairness and justice, and implies, for example, that everyone should have an opportunity to attain their full potential for health (Calman, 1995) and that entitlement to benefits from available resources should be accessible to the community as a whole. Calman explained that 'equity' is sometimes used interchangeably with *equality*, despite important distinctions between the two. He pointed out that 'equality' is about comparisons between the level of health or the ability to obtain access for care, and is a principle that may be applied to other aspects of social economics.

Another area of interest for the social economist, which may be used to explain further the concept of this discipline, is unemployment. Some effects of unemployment are both economic and social (Sharp *et al.*, 1994). As Sharp and colleagues pointed out, although the social effects of unemployment are more difficult to pinpoint and measure, they are just as real as the economic effects.

The application of economics to social areas is an important measure for humankind. It is the social areas that form the core components of social economics; considering and examining problems of for example, social security, healthcare, education, poverty and housing.

The mobilisation of available resources—such as technological devices, information technology—and computer technology, can help to empower clients who have disabilities. Information technology, for instance, is useful for social-security claimants (Cahill, 1994), as it makes the identification of claims more efficient: an example of the consumer/citizen reaping the socio economic benefits at his or her disposal.

▼ The Concept of Health

Health is the most valuable resource for both animals and humans; without it, any living organism will malfunction and die. Health is a broad concept. It means different things to different people. The meanings and definitions of health may alter, for example, depending on the age of the individual (Smith and Jacobson, 1991), or the context in which the term is used. It is a relative concept (Baggott, 1994). As Smith and Jacobson (1991) explained: 'If health is defined in terms of the state of fitness of our leading athletes then most of the rest of us would have to be considered seriously disabled.' Hence, the sociocultural framework, as well as the expectations of the individual, should be remembered whenever one is discussing the subject.

A common point of reference is to apply the definition provided by the World Health Organization (WHO) in 1946, which stipulates that health encompasses not only the absence of bodily changes due to pathology, but also the psychological and social wellbeing of the person. However, it is argued that this definition, although giving us an idea, a model, or framework to work on, only provides an abstraction, an ideal, or utopian view (Baggott, 1994).

Seedhouse (1986) asserted that there is a state of confusion created by the multitude of writings on health, which leads to a lack of clarity concerning 'what is being talked about when health is discussed'.

> The word 'health' is used to mean different things. For a medic health might mean physical fitness, absence of disease, or the harmonious functioning of the organs of the body. For an administrator in a hospital health might mean the state of a person when that person is discharged; for a member of the World Health Organization health might mean complete physical, social and mental wellbeing; for a health educator health might be essentially a freedom to make choices about personal habits and activities, and for a social scientist health might mean a person's ability to function according to social customs and norms or it might mean the opposite of this if the scientist does not think these norms desirable (Seedhouse, 1986).

The relative nature of health and its interpretations are made more evident when one considers the following definitions of health (Seedhouse, 1986):

● A 'commodity' to be given and possessed.
● A particular ideal state.
● A variable state that enables a person to function normally.
● A reserve of strength.
● An ability to adapt to changing circumstances.
● A resilient spirit.

The dimensions of health are wide, not easily defined, sometimes unclear, and sometimes confusing, especially when one makes allusions to what is normal and not normal, negative or positive. These features give the concept its abstraction or, as Jones (1993) explained, a mythical quality. When health is defined along a 'continuum between illness and complete wellness', people tend to interpret the absence of health as a 'socially unacceptable state, and at worst, as deviant from normal' (Jones, 1993).

Health and illness, Jones argued, are two dimensions belonging to the same process: the life process. Thus, a person who is able to use inner potential continually in order to meet the demands of everyday life will attain a high-level of health (Murray & Zentner, 1989). Using the continuum of physical, psychological, emotional, cognitive, developmental, spiritual, and social components of the health concept, one finds that health and illhealth (or disease or illness) become a 'complex dynamic' set of processes (Murray & Zentner, 1989).

How the public consider health will embody some of the dimensions mentioned above. Ewles and Simnett (1992), for instance, explained that some people argue that health has something to do with being 'robust' and 'resistant' to infection; whereas others contend that it is associated with moods and feelings, a sense of balance and equilibrium.

O'Donnell and Gray (1993) proposed that notions of health from an individual's context should be examined by looking at the whole person and to such aspects of their overall pattern of life as feeling confident to cope, enjoying life, and being able to adapt to change. This holistic approach accepts the individual as the central point of reference: how he or she feels; their ability to develop and maintain social relationships and interactions with others; their experience of, and ability to cope with, a range of emotions; their inner strength and resilience in adversity.

To be resilient and have strength of the inner-self form part of the health-belief model of some groups in society. Webb (1994) described this interpretation of health as 'something internal and individual, closely linked with temperament and heredity'. The person who holds such beliefs, she argued, regards what is within to be easily controllable, whereas external factors (e.g. pollution, infection) are beyond individual control.

The many dimensions of the health concept are perhaps best reflected in the *Health of the Nation*, a consultative document published by HMSO in 1992. This document was aimed to stimulate a period of widespread public and professional debate on health and how it might be improved. It covered areas such as biological (physical) health, social health, public health, sexual health, occupational health, socio-economic health, and environmental health.

Health theorists have circumscribed in their analysis some of the topics listed above. For example, according to Cavanagh (1991), Orem (1980) defined health in terms of 'structural and functional soundness and wellness', relying heavily on a medical model based on the absence of signs and symptoms. Health is also conceptualised in relation to an inability to look after oneself. It is also understood in terms of the individual and his or her relationship with the environment. The environmental aspect of health, however, is not made explicit in Orem's model of health, Cavanagh (1991) pointed out.

Neuman's theory of health (1982) is founded on the interactions of the individual with 'stressors' in the environment (e.g. occupational hazards, overcrowding). Reed (1993) commented: 'In the Neuman model, health status is reflected by the level of client wellness. Health and wellness are considered to be the same. When system needs are fully met a state of optimal wellness exists and the client is healthy.' The environmental and sociocultural context of the person provide the framework of the interrelationship, including the biological dimension too. As Akinsanya (1994) affirmed when describing Roy's theory of adaptation(1984): 'Health and illness occur in a continuum. . . . There is a constant interaction between the individual and the environment which calls for adaptive responses.'

Health–human–environment are therefore important interconnected variables in theorising about the health concept. Humans are seen to be in a state of constant co-existence with their environment; humans, as organisms, maintain their health equilibrium within an environmental framework. Kikuchi and Simmons (1994) labelled this line of thinking 'the man–living– health theory'.

The existence of humankind cannot be segregated from the broad view of health. Health, as pointed out already, is a dynamic process containing all perspectives of human life (Herberts & Erikson, 1995). There is no doubt that feeling well physically, emotionally, socially, and spiritually are features associated with being healthy. This multidimensional nature of health is well illustrated by the views on health held by nursing leaders and caring staff, as reported by Herberts and Erikson (1995):

- 'Health' is more than just being 'healthy'.
- A multitude of perspectives on aspects of life are contained within the concept.
- It is an experience of wellbeing based on individuals' interpretations and perception.
- Health is related to the inter-relationships of the individual with social networks: a state of balance and harmony, as well as of communion, within the family, among friends, and at work.
- 'Health' correlates with physical health and strength.
- It is associated with a positive attitude and harmony of existence.

The many levels of health also include the positive effects of religious faith and belief, which may beneficially influence the emotional and psychological wellbeing of the individual.

However, there is a school of thought that postulates that our definition of health may be influenced by sociological writings, which emphasise the social and cultural aspects, rather than the biological, medical, or pathological ones (Mitchell, 1996). However, this is more likely to have an effect on professionals, who have a penchant for the social and cultural dimensions; the lay person is likely to define health in a different way. Pridmore and Bendelow (1995) found that primary school children in England perceived being healthy as related to diet (healthy food: fruit, vegetables), exercise, sport, hygiene, not smoking, and sleep. Primary school children in Botswana, on the other hand, perceived food to be the main category associated with health; whereas the Bushmen children in Ghanzi district, Botswana reported food, exercise, medicine, and hygiene to be essential categories.

These health interpretations from children are probably the results of primary and secondary socialisation. In their interactions with parents, peers, and others in their social network, children acquire their beliefs about health and health-related matters (Chevannes, 1995). One should not overlook family and outside-family influences in shaping and structuring these views.

Images of health held by older people contrast sharply with those held by children. In a replication study in Seattle, USA, on older women's (70–91 years) definition of health, Perry and Woods (1995) revealed:
- At least 100 images of health.
- A common theme of health definition based on beliefs in the following: energy, independence, realistic optimism, taking care of oneself, functioning effectively by

participating in daily-life activities.

- Older women retain positive images of health into very advanced years.
- Health to women aged 18–45 years means exuberant wellbeing, healthy lifestyle, positive self-concept and self-body images, flexible adjustment to the environment, ability to interact, stamina, and strength.

For most people, health still is the presence or absence of illnesses, with all the signs and symptoms that accompany them. They perceive health to be 'what people have when they are not sick or dying' (Edlin & Golanty, 1992).

It is interesting to note that care professionals' perceptions of health may differ, depending on the type of work they do. For example, Davis (1995) found that nurses working in a neuro-rehabilitation unit equated physical independence with wellness, and, therefore, physical dependence with illness. Positive wellness, Edlin and Golanty explained, is made up of the freedom from symptoms of disease and pain; the freedom to be active, and to be in good spirits.

To conclude, health is not static (Webb, 1994); it is a dynamic process; it is a relative concept (Baggott, 1994); and it is multidimensional in nature.

▼ Chronic Illness, Carers, and Care Provision

The onset of illness, whether acute or chronic, and health disfunction are very likely to affect the person in a multidimensional way. Chronically ill individuals require adjustments in their life styles: physiologically, there is decreased general functioning; psychologically,

they may experience mood changes and depression; socially, their interpersonal relationships with their families may be undermined, due to, for example, the socio-economic effects of a decrease in their working hours or of unemployment (Hwu, 1995).

The impact of chronic illhealth is also felt by significant others in the individual's immediate social environment. These are the carers: relatives, friends, and neighbours who are responsible for caring for the sick. Taylor *et al.* (1995) argued that carers have been identified as 'a risk group'. These authors referred to the 'burgeoning research literature' showing that caring involves considerable sacrifices, ranging from the loss of career prospects and income, to detrimental effects on the carers' health. Illhealth not only disrupts the life style and socio-economic status of the sufferer, but has impact on the carers too. Carers, therefore, may find themselves sociopsychologically, physically, and socio-economically affected. As Taylor *et al.* (1995) described: 'It has been frequently argued that the combination of unemployment and caring causes a "pile up" of demands which interact to increase the likelihood of stress, breakdown and illhealth.' The critical issue, Taylor *et al.* affirmed, especially at a time of resource constraint, is what proportion of carers are in need of health and/or social care? A similar question should, nevertheless, be asked simultaneously in relation to the chronically ill patient.

Carers often cope unaided. Social support, Baggott (1994) posited, is lacking, and respite care is inadequate. The burden of delivering care to the chronically sick causes excessive fatigue, a loss of social opportunities, financial problems, and an increased stress level. The community-care philosophy, Baggott argued, which aims at economising resources by shifting the burden of responsibility for care from the state to the individual, has not considered the health and socio-economic implications for the carers. The literature suggests that the problems experienced by informal carers have not altered. For example, Smith and Jacobson (1991) highlighted the plight of carers as follows:

> The mainstay of support for old people continues to come from self-care and unpaid female relatives. Despite changes in the social roles of women, they continue to shoulder this responsibility willingly often with very little outside support and at great personal cost, including restrictions in personal freedom and high levels of anxiety and depression.

The quality of life of carers should become a priority in the prevention of illhealth and in the allocation of scarce resources by health and social services. Carers should be made aware of services available to them. Sheffield Health Authority's Community Nursing Service, for example, offers respite care for overstressed carers by caring for older dependants for regular two-week stays in Coleridge House Respite Unit (Halliday, 1991).

The provision of such facilities is essential. The NHS and Community Care Act 1990, Mandelstam and Schwehr (1995) highlighted, does not make reference to carers, their needs, or the conditions they work under. These authors argued that policy guidance states that 'carers can request assessments'. Local authorities have a role to play in 'assessing the ability of that other person to continue to provide such care on a regular basis'.

Conflict sometimes occurs between carers and the chronically sick patient. It is thus important to assess the needs of carers individually.

> In evidence to the Health Committee (1993, vol 1, p22), the Institute of Health Services Management made the point that there were no 'widely disseminated protocols for managing conflicts between a user and a carer'. For example, the need for separate carer assessments to resolve conflicts may arise because 'in a climate of tight resources the needs of carers might be subordinated to those of users; for example, a programme of closure of long stay institutions might continue in spite of little account being taken of the resulting additional pressure on carers' (Mandelstam & Schwehr, 1995).

The financial implications of neglecting carers will have an impact on scarce health resources. Although the act of caring in the community is a philosophy to be aimed for, if the people doing the caring are not cared for themselves, the socio-economic burden will most likely remain unaltered. Unless support is at hand, the chronically sick will receive substandard care and the carer will show signs of stress and 'burnout'.

Philp *et al.* (1995) undertook a comparison study of the financial burden, use of services, and perceived unmet needs in family supporters of elderly people with and without dementia in community care in the city of Dundee. The investigation revealed the following facts:

- In spite of regular commitment, supporters of people with dementia did not report a high level of perceived financial impact; some household expenses were incurred, however.
- Supporters who were more closely involved in caring for those with dementia made use of formal services (home help, day care, district nursing).
- There was a low level of perceived need for secondary care and private services.

The findings from the study further reinforce the fact that both the care-consumer and the care-giver are prone to socio-economic problems. The researchers felt that the low uptake of private services by carers might have suggested a lack of knowledge about these services. The low financial impact on both carers and the elderly could be due to differences in local authorities' financial arrangements, under which local authorities in parts of Britain charge for day care and home help (Philp *et al.*, 1995). The study concluded that carers are in need of more support because of the intensity of the care expected in cases of dementia.

▼ Psychological Disfunction and Care Provision

Individuals with psychological illhealth or disfunction (mental illness or learning disabilities) may have a major impact on healthcare resources. These individuals need special healthcare provision because of their vulnerability. They may, in exceptional circumstances, become key consumers of specialised healthcare provision: for example, the client with challenging behaviour who is in need of intensive psychiatric care; the very depressed, suicidal individual; the person with altered perception caused by, for example, drug addiction; the client with cognitive impairment, whose ability to learn is disabled.

To meet the needs of such groups, an effective mobilisation of resources is needed. At government level, it is believed that the relocation of psychiatric services from large institutions to a community-based pattern would achieve the objective of meeting clients' needs (Gill, 1988). However, Gill argued that the move from institutions to the community was precipitated by a motivation to reduce costs: 'The capital cost of maintaining old Victorian buildings with no growth in existing revenue makes closure attractive, especially so if sites are commercially valuable.'

The move from institutions to community-based care provision has been severely criticised. Community care for the mentally ill has been described as the consequence of policy shambles

(Robin, 1995). Robin reported that the client and individuals (like Jayne Zito) who are caught up in the client's mental illness are equally victims of the community. Zito's husband was killed in an unprovoked attack by a diagnosed schizophrenic patient. Her experience exposes the failures of community services, and their lack of comprehensiveness regarding care provision. Hendra (1994) in an interview with Zito reported the latter saying, 'that community care is under-resourced, 'that it is failing thousands in distress and leaving many people at risk in the community'.

It is evident that concerns and apprehension about present community-care facilities for the individual with psychological illhealth are feelings shared by the public (Lucas, 1994). The public, it is argued, favours community-based services in principle, 'but is overwhelmingly critical of the practice' (*Anonymous*, 1994). According to a report by MIND, based on a national survey conducted in January 1994, the public's priority is 'a properly funded *community* service'. Although community care is a sound and popular idea (Gill, 1988; Emery, 1994), the system is failing simply and mainly due to inadequate allocation of funding and resources.

The above criticisms of community-care intervention in meeting the needs of a population with psychological disfunction, however, should not be accepted as a complete failure. For instance, Williams and Wilkinson (1995), in the introduction to their article 'Patient satisfaction in mental health care' wrote: '. . . the results of a survey by MIND of users' views of psychiatric care . . . revealed a level of dissatisfaction. In response, a letter appeared questioning the findings and pointing to higher levels of satisfaction in a patient sample.'

This comment indicates that community care is not altogether failing to meet clients' needs. In an evaluation of community-based psychiatric care for people with treated, long-term mental illness, Wilkinson *et al.* (1995) concluded: 'Integrated, multidisciplinary, community-based psychiatric care for people with treated long-term mental illness is feasible in a semi-rural setting: patients receiving pharmacotherapy, and regular psychosocial treatments remain relatively stable on clinical and social measures over two years.'

However, analysis of research projects and review of the literature are likely to produce differing viewpoints. For instance, Kingdon and Sumners (1995) reported that a recent survey of general practitioners by the British Medical Association had found that, of the third who returned their questionnaires, almost half thought that community-care services had deteriorated and only a quarter felt that they had improved.

These findings, among others, suggest that all is not well in the provision of community services. Shortfalls in funding and resources (human and capital) are the factors that impinge on the effectiveness of healthcare delivery. The management of healthcare resources is reliant on a realistic assessment of the care needs of special groups; for example, the mentally ill and those with chronic illnesses. However, socio-economic forces (social status, social deprivation, financial constraints, incompetent allocation of health-focused resources) exercise a widespread influence throughout the structures of society, to include other groups too. For instance, the elderly, the homeless, women with cervical cancer, the unemployed, children, ethnic minorities (and their uptake of healthcare provision), and the terminally ill are some of the groups classified as consumers of healthcare resources.

▼ Summary

Social economics comprises the application of conventional economic principles to social issues, such as poverty, unemployment, the elderly, healthcare, housing, and other aspects that have impact on the citizens of a society. Since the basic premise of pure economics is the mobilisation and distribution of available scarce resources, social economics is concerned with the consequences of 'economic behaviour' on people in society. The impacts that unemployment or a lack of healthcare facilities have on a particular community are examples of topics for analysis by the social economist. Because the focus of social economists is on how humans are affected by decisions made regarding the distributive forces of economic-resource allocation, they tend also to refer to their discipline as 'welfare economics'. There is a humanistic component associated with social economics, whereas conventional economics deals only with quantifiable data, market mechanism, supply and demand, and the statistics associated with these concepts.

The traditional view of health given by the World Health Organization is now regarded as static, non-dynamic, and utopian. Although initially it had the desired impact, it is rather a restrictive definition. Case studies and other related research have pointed to the multidimensional nature of the concept. Health should be defined in terms of the quality of life of the person; it should also be interpreted as the individual's total existence—the holistic view of health. The notions of health are varied and complex. To some people, health is to do with resilience and robustness, with being resistant to infection or disease; to others, health means physical fitness, and an ability to cope with adversity and to interact with others in a meaningful way. Independence, energy, and feeling well emotionally, physically, and spiritually are other attributes believed to be linked with the health concept. A state of positive wellness, forming freedom from disease and pain, is another image held by some.

Children's views of health are influenced by parental socialisation, and focus mainly on the biological aspects. Older women, on the other hand, believe that health is related to 'energy to participate in life's daily activities' and 'being able to look after oneself and not be dependent on other people'.

Health theorists have examined health as one of the variables in the conceptual framework of humans and their environment. The interactions involved in the dynamic process of living and adapting to the environment, and the coping strategies utilised to deal with life stressors, are formulae contained in their theories.

Illhealth has an impact on the wellbeing of people. Chronic illness affects not only the sufferer, but also the relatives, neighbours, and friends whose responsibility it is to care for the sick. These individuals are known as the informal carers. It is thought that caring has been identified as a new social problem. During caring, carers may experience frustrations due to conflict with the sick person; they may experience mood changes; they may feel depressed; some may experience financial constraints caused by the increased expenditure. Interpersonal relationships suffer in cases of decreased working hours and unemployment. The life style of both the sufferer and the carer is likely to be modified as a result. It is believed that carers and the chronically sick could become socio-economically disadvantaged. This may be a consequence of not being informed about services available to meet their needs and to minimise their social problems. The inadequacies in social support and respite care lead to increased stress. The provision of facilities becomes a priority for local authorities, whose role is to assess and identify social needs.

It is argued that the move from institutional care to community care for mentally ill clients has not been successful; that these individuals are not receiving the best resources because of cutbacks, and motivation by the government to reduce costs.

▼ Application to Clinical Practice

The effects of economics on health practices, nursing interventions, and medical practices have been documented. For example, according to the NHS Centre for Review and Dissemination, expensive specialist beds are not effective in the prevention of pressure sores (*Anonymous*, 1995). The article highlighted that although the prevention and treatment of pressure sores is a multibillion-pound industry, available research has shown an 'unacceptably high' proportion of hospital patients continue to develop them. If care intervention is to be economically effective, it is suggested, 'a rigorous evaluation' of the equipment to be used—whether expensive or not—should be done by hospitals before purchasing.

If patient-centred care is to be achieved effectively, with the prevention of wastage in scarce resources, 'the structure and processes involved in delivering care should be shaped by the need to develop a decentralised organisational structure with resources allocated based on the needs of patients' (Buchan, 1995). Patients' needs are more realistically assessed using the skills of the care professionals.

The clinical nurse specialists, Sturdy and Carpenter (1995) argued, have the closest continuing contact with patients during their stay in hospital, and are more likely to know more about them than any other group of healthcare professionals; hence, they are in the best position to provide the necessary information regarding the patient's needs. Sturdy and Carpenter asserted that nurses must be involved in providing high-quality, cost-effective care, based on an assessment of 'individual need' with participation from relevant multi-disciplinary teams.

The impact of socio-economics, however, does not affect solely the nursing practice. Bunker (1995) referred to 'the increased substantial gains in life expectancy and quality of life' that can be achieved by medical care intervention and productivity. He argued for an efficient management and investment of resources that are available but incompetently allocated. Allocation of scarce resources is therefore a priority in medical and nursing practice. This becomes more imperative as the population ages. It is estimated, for example, that future trends will show evidence of major resource implications regarding the cost of treating hip fractures in the twenty-first century, as the population of England ages (Hollingworth *et al.*, 1995). As the elderly become older, their frailty increases and they are more prone to accidents. The authors recommend a programme of preventive measures to include:

- A more complete understanding of the epidemiology of falls.
- Attempts to increase the consumer's awareness of the benefits of positive health practices, aimed at modifying behaviour.
- An exercise programme to increase physical fitness and agility, although the implications of increased activity (associated with the increased risks of falls) should be borne in mind.
- Alterations to the environment (home alterations, for example).

Opportunities to participate in health-education and health-promotion programmes should be grasped by care professionals in all settings, to ensure that the client's proneness to illhealth is minimised or prevented.

Although advances in technology and science have made major contributions towards the alleviation of suffering—such as improving communication and so on, as pointed out above—Hawthorne and Yurkovich (1995) explained that these advances can sometimes impede the delivery of care:

> ... a surfeit of information tends to be overwhelming and immobilising, clouding the clarity of thought required for reflecting on our experiences thus hampering us from finding meaning and purpose in our lives. When we are hampered from finding meaning and purpose, caring for and about each other is diminished.

Hawthorne and Yurkovich (1995) commented that the technological care settings in which the professionals are operating impede their ability to find this meaning and express themselves in their caring role. The humanistic aspect of nursing and care should take priority over scientific and technological intrusion. As Goose (1995) wrote, clinical leaders and managers are the key resources for good patient care. Patient care consists of the interactions between the care professionals and the client; technology, however, if used sensibly, can contribute to the process.

Dawson (1995) argued that care can be enhanced and improved if clinical practitioners make more effective use of research technology and findings. She also stressed the importance of cost–benefit analysis. This entails a systematic exploration and study of the effectiveness of expenses on resources, and whether they are of benefit to the consumers by attaining the desired goals. A systematic uptake of bio-medical research findings and 'development through implementation in everyday clinical practice', Dawson argued, would ensure the attainment of these objectives. She explained that, at present, professional relationships between communities of clinical practitioners and scientific researchers are 'usually distant', which does not help in bridging the gap between them:

> Clinicians are preoccupied with doing their clinical work in 'tried and tested' 'good enough' ways, which reflect the principles of their own education and training and the norms of practice for many of their respected colleagues. Practitioners are frequently unaware of the results of research and development and even if they are aware they are often sceptical about the feasibility of general application (Dawson, 1995).

Dawson affirmed the potential that is inherent in the utilisation of available research in technology, and how 'its transfer could usefully be taken as a basis for determining fruitful avenues for developing the relation between research and practice in the health sector'.

The transfer of appropriate research findings to clinical practice becomes the responsibility of the care practitioner. If research improves the health status of the client in practice, it is also likely to improve his or her economic and social status (return to work, improved social contact, etc.). Hence, knowledge of the basic principles of social economics is necessary in clinical practice; the broader framework of the client will be better appreciated.

Dawson (1995) argued, however, that the transfer of technology research findings to clinical practice may not be an easily achievable goal:

> Changes indicated by research may lead to a

reluctance to change either because fewer resources are required and therefore empires may be threatened or because more resources are required and therefore already overstretched budgets for purchasing health care may be stretched beyond their limits. Conditions previously untreatable may become treatable, new investment in equipment may be required, and the drugs bill may escalate.

As described above, a critical evaluation of resources to be used must be done by clinical managers in healthcare settings, based on patients' needs. The evaluation should also include the outcome of health intervention, to determine the effectiveness of care delivered. Expensive resources (human and material) may be used that may not be positively beneficial to the patient.

On the assessment of the benefits of health-care, Ryan and Shackley (1995) expressed these views:

> The application of the techniques of economic evaluation to health care is becoming increasingly commonplace. This is shown by the increasing number of published evaluations and is to be welcomed. Despite this progress, however, we believe that current economic evaluations of health care interventions may fail to take into account potentially important sources of benefit and disbenefit to individual patients.

They expressed concern that the evaluation of healthcare technologies may sometimes be incomplete, 'while interventions that are thought to be efficient may in fact be inefficient and vice versa'. Economic evaluation should start by accepting the patient as a valuable participant in the care process. The clinician may be a facilitator; it is at the bedside that 'the sources of health care benefits can be determined by the consumers, as only they can make the link between the consumption or availability of health care or both, and the effects that has on their utility' (Ryan & Shackley, 1995).

Health is the most important resource in society; without it, the socio-economic systems and other interconnected systems (legal, educational, etc.) would not exist. It is for this reason that society makes provision to ensure that the health of the nation maintains its integrity. Healthcare professionals form one of the major groups of individuals whose role it is to educate the public and to promote the beneficial effects of health. Since health is defined in a way that takes account of the whole person, the promotion of health includes any activity that enhances positive health and wellbeing (O'Donnell & Gray, 1993).

The education of parents in their homes becomes the responsibility of community services. Health visitors who have regular contact with families aim towards increasing public awareness of health practices that enhance health status. Knowledge about the multidimensional nature of health, gained in the interactions with professionals, can only help the development of increased individual responsibility about health maintenance. To educate patients regarding health matters—with the involvement of the primary-care team—is to carry out a preventive approach to the occurrence of illhealth.

As many sociologists have explained, the most basic—and one of the most important—unit in the social system is the family. It is at this micro-level of society that primary socialisation is nurtured, developed, and influenced. Therefore, it makes sense for any community healthcare professionals to focus their health-education and health-promotion activities within the heart of the family system networks. As pointed out already by Chevannes (1995), the family is influential in developing children's

knowledge of health and health matters. Children learn by imitation and examples (social learning theory). Smith and Jacobson (1991) pointed out: 'The health of children and their parents is inextricably linked. The impact of parents' health and behaviour on that of their children is well documented in some respects, and we know that parents who smoke or drink heavily are more likely to produce children who do likewise.' Hence, the authors concluded, childhood is a time when opportunities for maximising health potential are likely to be great.

The prevention of illhealth should begin, therefore, by educating parents in the community, with the support and professional help of the primary-care team. Establishing a professional rapport with parents and their children is a priority to be aimed for and achieved at a very early stage. An assessment of parents' definition of health is also important, as this will allow a better understanding of their attitudes and knowledge. Care should be taken to avoid what Seedhouse (1986) called 'indoctrination', because 'the long term effect of its continued use is the undermining of some of the essential conditions which make up individual health'.

The implementation of preventive medicine in the community could be realised by using the framework of beliefs detailed in the HMSO's *Health of the Nation* document of 1992. For example, section A of the document states that it is generally accepted that the main risk factors for coronary heart disease (CHD) and stroke are cigarette smoking, raised plasma cholesterol, raised blood pressure, and a lack of physical activity. This information could be used in the assessment of the client's smoking habits by the care professional, who could:

- Invite discussions regarding the client's knowledge of the dangers of smoking.
- Identify extraneous factors that may

precipitate the motivation to smoke (e.g. peer pressure, occupational stress).

- With the participation and consent of the client and significant others, explain the links that exist in the causation of CHD and stroke, as listed in the document.

As the *Health of the Nation* document states, individuals should be made aware of the risk factors associated with CHD and stroke, and how to make the life style changes necessary to avoid them. The nurse, the physician, and allied personnel have the expertise to impart appropriate knowledge and information on matters related to health and illhealth; their role in prevention, early detection, treatment, and rehabilitation cannot be overemphasised.

On diet and nutrition, the document emphasises the importance of a balanced intake of nutrients 'for the repair and maintenance of every part of the body throughout life'. To achieve this target, healthcare professionals must first increase their own knowledge of dietetics by making use of research findings. They should display positive health beliefs by acting as role models, and disseminate information about healthy eating, so encouraging and enabling changes in the population's diet. The transmission of information can take place in a variety of settings: the domestic environment, nursing homes, hospitals, day centres, health farms, gymnasiums, health centres, general practitioners' surgeries, and so on.

Although the *Health of the Nation* document specifies key target areas and objectives on the psychosocial and biological aspects of health, spiritual health is not mentioned.

The following extract comes from Ross (1995), following an encounter with a terminally ill patient:

Having been asked if she would like a passage read to her from the Bible lying on her locker, the change in this woman's expression was remarkable. Instead of lying sleeping, or staring blankly into space, her eyes widened, she strained to raise her head, smiled and attempted to speak for the first time in several months. Later, just before she died, she expressed how much this, together with prayer, had meant to her. She had a spiritual need which she wanted to be met.

Health, living, and dying all form part of the life process. The spiritual dimension is important for the attainment of an overall sense of health and wellbeing, and quality of life (Ross, 1995). In any settings, and at any stage of the life process, care personnel should assess and identify the client's needs for spiritual support. It is a vital— but complex—part of good nursing practice (Gill, 1995) and medical intervention too.

The special problems that face people in other groups, such as unpaid part-time or full-time carers, must also be considered (HMSO, 1992). Chronic illness has a debilitating effect on both the sufferer and the carer. The progressive nature of some diseases (e.g. metastatic carcinoma, multiple sclerosis, presenile dementia) entails a long-term commitment by many carers. For the healthcare professional, this means the implementation of long-term monitoring (Hwu, 1995). The aims of care are to develop strategies that may help both the carer and the sufferer cope with the situation in a more effective way. Another aim is for the professional to assess the impact of the condition on the individuals; to observe and report the responses to chronic conditions, so that individual care can be delivered.

Chronic illness exerts 'psychological, social and activities of daily living changes' (Hwu, 1995); therefore, it is essential to intervene in a holistic way to ensure all needs are being considered. Lassitude, social deprivation, and emotional outbursts are some of the ill-effects that the patient and carer may experience. Carers with dependants may also have feelings of anxiety and fear (Phair, 1995); for example, they may worry about having an accident while being away from their chronically sick relative. Phair suggested using a card system to 'give carers more peace of mind'. The card would contain details of the dependants and a phone number to contact.

If the disease develops (for example, in a person who is terminally ill), every available resource should be utilised. Many patients prefer to be in the comfort of their own homes during the last stages of the life cycle. Nash (1995) suggested the effective employment of Macmillan carers, who operate flexibly in response to the needs of families—sometimes working very few hours in a week, sometimes many more. Other attributes of the Macmillan carers consist of the ability to recognise the individual needs of family carers and the sick, being prepared to accept beliefs and attitudes other than their own, and good communication skills (Nash, 1995).

During home visits, the community-health practitioner should exercise tact and professional judgement in the assessment of the families that are in need of support. Dearden et al. (1995) highlighted the concern regarding the large number of children who are providing primary care for family members in the community. Children are caring for relatives suffering from a variety of pathological conditions (e.g. Parkinson's disease, Huntington's disease). Dearden et al. (1995) referred to the complex consequences that caring can have on children:

- Poverty caused by the loss of parental earning, long-term illness, and the fact that young carers do not receive benefits from the welfare system.
- Health problems, such as back injury caused by poor lifting technique.
- Impairment of psychosocial health development.
- Loss of social contact with their peer group.

Therefore, it is imperative for professionals to recognise, identify, and support these children. It is a social issue, as well as a health one.

The role of nursing and medical personnel, Dearden and colleagues explained, is to use sensitivity and tact to obtain the trust of young carers. They recommended:

- Active listening of the young carer's viewpoint.
- Adopting a nonjudgemental approach.
- Setting up additional support, with the carer's consent.
- Showing respect for the carer, who feels the need to care.
- Imparting relevant educational information that will help them to cope.

The authors also emphasised the anticipation of children's needs when admitting and caring for adults with a chronic illness or disability, or a condition that is likely to require care following discharge. It is essential during discharge procedures, therefore, to investigate the patient's social background to identify the possible existence of young carers at home, so that they may receive professional help.

The NHS and Community Care Act has recognised the important role of carers in the community (George, 1995). George explained that a new act is now being implemented that will give carers the right to have their needs assessed. This can be seen as the carrying out of the 'collaborative caring' principle, which involves the collaboration of professionals from various health settings. Assessment of needs will ease access to support services by carers who have health problems, often a mixture of mental health difficulties, stress-related conditions, and especially musculoskeletal problems (George, 1995).

■ CLIENTS WITH PSYCHOLOGICAL DISFUNCTION

In England, as in all other westernised countries, there are variations in health status between different socio-economic groups within the population.

There will need to be improved supervision of patients' care in the community. . . . Most, if not all, seriously mentally ill people who commit suicide are in contact with specialist services (HMSO, 1992).

Correlations between socio-economic factors and mental illhealth (HMSO, 1992), and between mental illhealth (suicide, parasuicide) psychiatric admissions and socio-economic deprivation (Gunnell *et al.*, 1995), have been documented.

In a study of social deprivation and psychiatric admission rates among different diagnostic groups, Harrison *et al.* (1995) found that patients with schizophrenia or delusional disorder had higher rates of admission than those in other groups (organic brain syndromes, mania, depression, personality disorder, and substance abuse). The researchers concluded: 'The association between psychiatric admission rates and measures of deprivation varies considerably with diagnosis. Measures of social deprivation may indicate need for services for patients with psychotic disorders; admission rates for non-psychotic illnesses may reflect the availability of beds rather than need.'

A 17-year, retrospective, follow-up study to assess the relationship between socio-economic status and mental illness in Finland found that patients with schizophrenia showed a constant downward drift, commonly to unemployment, and had a high risk of social dropout (Aro *et al.*, 1995).

The research described above gives a clear idea about the effects of socio-economic factors on mental illhealth morbidity. These findings should help care professionals in clinical practice to implement more effective sociopsychological assessment of the clients, and to intervene with more insight, depending on the individual needs of the client.

Social deprivation (unemployment, financial impotence, social isolation, homelessness, inaccessibility to health care provision, etc.) affects individuals in a multitude of ways. It is evident from research findings that the mentally ill require support in the community and in other settings, to help them cope with the psychosocial pressures impinging on their wellbeing.

If mental illhealth results from social deprivation, an assessment of the social background of the client is necessary to identify key factors that may have precipitated the psychological disturbance. Nevertheless, caution should be exercised: mental disfunction may not necessarily be the consequence of socio-economic factors. Many clients are admitted to mental health units because of pathological changes in brain functioning or systemic physiological alterations (renal failure, brain failure, intoxication from alcohol abuse, or medication overdose).

The role of professionals is to accept the client as an individual with problems of living, and to discuss aspects of social life that impinge on his or her social adaptation or functioning. As much as possible, the nurse or medical practitioner should attempt to reinstate the client's full awareness of 'the factors which can affect their basic foundations for achievement' (Seedhouse, 1986). Seedhouse explained that these foundations are impaired by 'racial discrimination, grossly unequal distribution of income and power, inadequate housing, a poor education and service, and low levels of fulfilling employment'. These may all play a very significant role in the client's present state of illhealth.

▼ Review Questions

1 Discuss how resource allocation may have an impact on consumers in society.

2 Explain by giving examples the humanistic approach of social economics in comparison with conventional economics.

3 Give an account of the measures healthcare professionals may take to ensure patients' needs are met effectively and socio-economically.

4 'It is believed that scientific and technological resources can impede the act of caring.' Discuss this statement.

5 'Health is a dynamic and multidimensional concept.' Discuss this statement with reference to the traditional definition of health provided by the World Health Organization.

6 Describe the role of healthcare professionals in health education and health promotion.

7 Explain how primary healthcare personnel may develop the client's knowledge of health practices.

8 Discuss the measures that may be taken to prevent stress-related illness among carers of the chronically sick.

9 Examine the factors that influence care delivery in the community.

References

Akinsanya J. Introduction to Roy Adaptation Model. In: Akinsanya J, et al. The Roy Adaptation Model in action. Basingstoke: Macmillan; 1994.

Anonymous. 'News'. 'We'll pay more tax to help people with mental health problems.' Open Mind 1994 67:6.

Anonymous. 'News' Expensive special beds may be useless. Nurs Manage 1995, Vol 2: 7:4.

Aro S, Aro H, Keskimaki I. Socio-economic mobility among patients with schizophrenia or major affective disorder. Br J Psychiatry 1995, 166:759–767.

Baggott R. Health & health care in Britain. New York: St Martin's Press; 1994.

Bendavid-Val A. Social economics. 'An innovative practical approach'. In: Pettman Barrie O, ed. Social economics—Concepts and perspectives. Bradford: MCB Books; 1977.

Bohm P. Social efficiency: a concise introduction to welfare economics. London: Macmillan; 1987.

Buchan J. 'Patient-focus pocus?' Nurs Manage 1995, 2:6–7.

Bunker J. Impact of economics on medical practice. J R Soc Med 1995, 88:667–668.

Cahill M. The new social policy. Oxford: Blackwell; 1994.

Calman C. On the state of public health. Health Trends 1995, 27:71–75.

Cavanagh S. Orem's model in action. Basingstoke: Macmillan; 1991.

Chevannes M. Children's views about health: assessing the implications for nurses. Br J Nurs 1995, 4:1073–1080.

Davis S. An investigation into nurses' understanding of health education and health promotion within a neuro-rehabilitation setting. J Adv Nurs 1995, 21:951–959.

Dawson S. Never mind solutions: what are the issues? Lessons of industrial technology transfer for quality in health care Quality Health Care 1995, 4:197–203.

Dearden C, Becker S, Aldridge J. Children who care: a case for nursing intervention? *Br J Nurs* 1995, **4**:698–701.

Edlin G, Golanty E. *Health & wellness. A holistic approach, 4th ed.* London: Jones & Bartlett; 1992.

Eidem R, Viotti S. *Economic systems. How resources are allocated.* Oxford: Martin Robertson; 1978.

Emery R. Building support for MIND's community care campaign. *Open Mind* 1994, **68**:6.

Ewles L, Simnett I. *Promoting health: a practical guide, 2nd ed.* London: Scutari Press; 1992.

George M. 'Collaborative caring'. *Nurs Stand* 1995, **9**:22–23.

Gill J. Managing contracting psychiatric institutions. *Health Care Manage* 1988, **3**:21–27.

Gill. J. Spiritual care of the terminally ill. *Community Nurse* 1995, **1**(2):23–24.

Goose M. Human resource issues in the NHS. *Br J Hosp Med* 1995, **54**:587–590.

Gunnell D, Kammerling R. Relation between parasuicide, suicide, psychiatric admissions and socio–economic deprivation. *Br Med J* 1995, **311**:226–229.

Halliday M. *Our city, our health.* Sheffield: Healthy Sheffield Planning Team; 1991.

Harrison J, Barrow S, Greed F. Social deprivation and psychiatric admission rates among different diagnostic groups. *Br J Psychiatry* 1995, **167**:456–462.

Hawthorne D, Yurkovich N. Science, technology caring and the professions: are they compatible? *J Adv Nurs* 1995, **21**:1087–1091.

Hendra A. 'Jayne Zito joins Mind campaign' *Open Mind;* 67: Feb/Mar 1994.

Herberts S, Erikson K. Nursing leaders' and nurses' view of health. *J Adv Nurs* 1995, **22**:868–878.

Hill L. The institutionalist approach to social economics. In: Lutz M, ed. *Social economics: retrospect and prospect.* London: Kluwer Academic; 1990.

HMSO. *Health of the nation. A strategy for health in England.* London: HMSO; 1992.

Hollingworth W, Todd C, Parker M. The cost of treating hip fractures in the twenty-first century. *J Public Health Med* 1995, **17**:269–276.

Hwu Y. The impact of chronic illness on patients. *Rehabil Nurs* 1995, **20**:221–225.

Jones S. Personal unity in dying: alternative conceptions of the meaning of health. *J Adv Nurs* 1993, **18**:89–94.

Kikuchi J, Simmons H. *Developing a philosophy of nursing.* London: Sage; 1994.

Kingdon D, Sumners S. Community care and general practice. *Br Med J* 1995, **311**:823–824.

Lai O. Farewell to welfare statism! More happiness in welfare market? Putting consumption in (post) modern context. *Int J Soc Economics* 1994, **21**:43–54.

Le Grand J, Propper C, Robinson R. *The economics of social problems, 3rd ed.* London: Macmillan; 1992.

Lucas J. Community care campaign. *Open Mind* 1994, **67**:4.

Lutz M. *Social economics: retrospect and prospect.* London: Kluwer Academic; 1990.

Mandelstam M, Schwehr B. *Community care practice and the law.* London: Jessica Kingsley; 1995.

Mitchell D. Post modernism, health and illness. *J Adv Nurs* 1996, **23**:201–205.

Murray R, Zentner J. *Nursing concepts for health promotion.* New York: Prentice Hall; 1989.

Nash A. Macmillan carers: a practical approach to home care. *Int J Palliative Nurs* 1995, **1**:148–154.

Neuman B. *The Neuman's systems model: application to nursing education and practice.* Appleton-Century Crofts East Norwalk (1982).

O'Donnell T, Gray G. *The health promoting college.* London: Health Education Authority; 1993.

Orem D. *Nursing: concepts of practice.* New York: McGraw-Hill (1980).

Perry J, Woods N. Older women and their images of health: a replication study. *Adv Nurs Sci* 1995, **18**:51–61.

Phair L. A card to give carers more peace of mind. *Nurs Stand* 1995, **9**:44.

Philp I, McKee K, Meldrum P. Community care for demented and non-demented elderly people: a comparison study of financial burden, service use, and unmet needs in family supporters. *Br Med J* 1995, **310**:1503–1506.

Pridmore P, Bendelow G. Images of health: Exploring beliefs of children using the 'draw and write' technique. *Health Educ J* 1995, **54**:473–488.

Reed K. Betty Neuman. *The Neuman system model.* London: Sage; 1993.

Robin N. Victims of community care. *Mental Health Nurs* 1995, **15**:26–27.

Rohrlich G. *Social economics: concepts and perspectives.* Patrington: Emmasglen; 1974.

Ross. The spiritual dimension: its importance to patient's health, well being and quality of life and its implications for nursing practice. *Int J Nurs Stud* 1995,**32**:457–468.

Ryan M, Shackley P. Assessing the benefits of health care: how far should we go? *Quality Health Care* 1995, **4**:207–213.

Seedhouse D. *Health—the foundations of achievements.* Chichester: Wiley & Sons; 1986.

Sharp A, Register C, Leftwich R. *Economics of social issues, 11th ed.* Sydney: Irwin; 1994.

Smith A, Jacobson B, Whitehead M, *The nation's health. 'A strategy for the 1990s'.* London; King Edwards Fund: 1988.

Stanfield J. Understanding the welfare state: the significance of social economics. In: Lutz M, ed. *Social economics: retrospect and prospect.* London: Kluwer Academic; 1990.

Sturdy D, Carpenter I. 'Right plan for elderly care' *Nurs Stand* 1995: **2**(7):16–8.

Taylor R, Ford G, Dunbar M. The effects of caring on health. A community-based longitudinal study. *Soc Sci Med* 1995, **40**:1407–1415.

Webb P. *Health promotion and patient education. A professional's guide.* London: Chapman & Hall; 1994.

Wilkinson G, *et al.* An evaluation of community-based psychiatric care for people with treated long-term mental illness. *Br J Psychiatry* 1995, **167**:26–37.

Williams B, Wilkinson G. Patient satisfaction in mental health care. Evaluating an evaluative method. *Br J Psychiatry* 1995, **116**:559–562.

World Health Organization. *Constitution: basic documents.* Geneva: World Health Organization; 1946.

▼ Further Reading

Aldridge J, Becker S. Excluding children who care. *Benefits* 1993b, **7**:22–24.

Ashton J. *Healthy cities.* Milton Keynes: Open University Press; 1992.

Bruyn S. Social economy: a note on its theoretical foundations. *Rev Social Economy* 1981, **34**:81–84.

Cairns J. The cost of prevention. *Br Med J* 1995, **311**:1520.

Clark N, McLeroy K. Creating capacity through health education: what we know and what we don't. *Health Educ Q* 1995, **22**:273–289.

Clarke R. Ageing populations. In: Eatwell J, Milgate M, Newman P, eds. *Social economics.* Basingstoke: Macmillan; 1989:1–3.

Clarke R, Spengler J. *Economics of individual and population ageing.* Cambridge: Cambridge University Press; 1980.

Dockrell J, Gaskell G, Normand C. An economic analysis of the resettlement of people with mild learning disabilities and challenging behaviour. *Soc Sci Med* 1995, **40**:895–901.

Donaldson R, Donaldson L. *Essential public health medicine.* Lancaster: Kluwer Publishers; 1993.

Eatwell J, Milgate M, Newman P. *Social economics.* Basingstoke: Macmillan; 1989.

George M. Social benefits: phased changes. *Nurs Stand* 1994, **8**:22–23.

Guadagnoli E, Cleary P, McNeil B. The influence of socio-economic status on change in health status after hospitalisation. *Soc Sci Med* 1995, **40**:1399–1406.

Hellzen O, Norberg A, Sandman P. Schizophrenic patients' image of their carers and the carers' image of their patients: an interview study. *J Psychiatr Mental Health Nurs* 1995, **2**:279–285.

Labonte R. Population health and health promotion: what do they have to say to each other? *Can J Public Health* 1995, **86**:165–168.

Meredith H. Supporting the young carer. *Community Outlook* 1992, **2**:15–18.

Minkler M, Wallace S, McDonald M. The political economy of health: a useful theoretical tool for health education practice. *Int Q Commun Health Educ* 1995, **15**:111–125.

Peterson J. Michigan's elderly hope for a brigher future. *Michigan Med* 1994, **93**:34–36.

Petrou S, *et al.* Cost and utilisation of community services for people with HIV infection in London. *Health Trends* 1995, **27**:62–67.

Poulson K, *et al.* Estimated costs of post-operative wound infections. A case control study of marginal hospital and social security costs. *Epidemiol Infect* 1994, **113**(2):283–295.

Reijneveld S, Gunning Schepers L. Age, health and the measurement of the socio-economics status of individuals. *Eur J Public Health* 1995, **5**(3):187–192.

Smith A, Baghurst K, Owen N. Socio-economic status and personal characteristics as predictors of dietary change. *J Nutr Educ* 1995, **27**:173–181.

Smith K, Shah A, Wright K. The prevalence and costs of psychiatric disorders and learning disabilities. *Br J Psychiatry* 1995, **166**:9–18.

Whittick J. *Carers of the dementing elderly: coping technique and expressed emotion,* PhD Thesis. Glasgow: University of Glasgow; 1993.

13

Socio-Economic Problems:
Poverty, Homelessness and Unemployment

▼ Poverty

■ DEFINITION OF POVERTY

Poverty is an emotive word. In societies throughout the world there are people who live in conditions that we would consider deprived: lack of sanitation; food shortages; financial insecurities caused by unemployment; slum areas or ghettoes; homelessness and exposure to the environment. The media frequently portray the extremes of poverty: children half naked, gasping for food and drink, with flies hovering over them; parents too feeble to hold them, starving, and dehydrated. And then one sees their harsh, barren, living environment: a scarcity of houses, but evidence of many shed-type shelters. In comparison, our standard of living is remarkably different: modern housing in the suburbs with cars in the drives; supermarkets with an abundance of food; schools; leisure complexes; airports teeming with holidaymakers; the housewife experimenting with her new dishwasher or computerised vacuum cleaner; school children with computers and video games. These stark differences in material possessions make us realise the socio-economic contrast that demarcates what one considers wealth from what one considers deprivation or poverty.

What is poverty? Sociologists, economists, social policy-makers, social economists, and others have grappled with the concept for many years. Townsend (1979) commented that the term could be defined objectively and applied consistently only in terms of the idea of relative deprivation. Objectivity—rather than subjectivity—is essential, he argued, to gain an understanding of its nature. Thus, he posited, families and groups are seen to be existing in poverty when they lack the resources to obtain the type of diet, participate in the activities, and have the living conditions and amenities that are customary (or at least encouraged or approved) in the societies to which they belong.

Although this approach provides a framework towards an understanding of the meaning of poverty, it is limited because the term is being used in different senses (Atkinson, 1989). To clarify the underlying concept, Atkinson argued, it is crucial to determine the poverty standard.

■ ABSOLUTE AND RELATIVE POVERTY

'Absolute' concepts of food and material requirements, and those poverty scales that are 'relative', need to be considered. Absolute poverty means living in conditions under which a person is unable to obtain the basic necessities of life (Brown & Payne, 1990; Byrne & Padfield, 1990a). Le Grand et al. (1992) argued that absolute poverty is a term that can be applied at all times in all societies, and includes, for instance, the level of income necessary for bare subsistence. Similarly, Spicker (1990) interpreted poverty in its 'absolute' form to be founded on subsistence and the minimum standard needed to live. Sharp et al. (1994) explained that poverty problems in the United States are defined in terms of 'absolute income levels', and are caused by defective income distribution.

These theories of absolute poverty were formulated by two eminent figures in the history of social thought: Charles Booth (1840–1916) and Seebohm Rowntree (1871–1954). Their research was used by the State (in line with the Beveridge recommendations in the early 1940s) to calculate the level at which benefits should be paid, a traditional approach that the State still tends to follow.

It is argued that Charles Booth's method of

investigating poverty became a starting point for others interested in the subject (Holman, 1978). Booth concentrated his research on the population of London. He undertook a detailed house-to-house investigation using the interview technique. His understanding of absolute poverty was related to people described as 'living under a struggle to obtain the necessaries of life and make both ends meet'.

Rowntree's analysis of poverty was centred in the city of York. He was particularly interested in 'physical efficiency' as the main criterion in his differentiation between poverty and non-poverty (Holman, 1978). As Holman explained, he then expanded by attempting to assess exactly how much money was required to ensure physical efficiency. To do this, he had to know how much food was required, for which he turned to the work of two nutritionists.

However, the approaches of Booth and Rowntree do have limitations: the physiological assessment of needs in relation to physical efficiency provides a rather inflexible definition of poverty (Holman, 1978) and their 'stringent standards' in defining poverty 'are hardly adequate for a society whose average standard of living is well above mere subsistence level' (Brown & Payne, 1990).

The concept of absolute poverty has been widely criticised. Its definition assumes a narrow perspective of the realities of a social problem. Using nutrition, shelter, and clothing as criteria does not give a thorough interpretation of other variables, such as basic cultural needs. Lack of nutrition, shelter, or clothing in one society may not necessarily mean poverty: 'Within the same society, nutritional needs may vary widely, between for example, the bank clerk sitting at his desk all day and the labourer on a building site' (Haralambos, 1985).

Brown and Madge (1982), too, discussed the limitations of using the concept of absoluteness for deprivation. While acknowledging the widespread deprived states of some families with multiple problems—'who are undeniably badly off regarding income, housing, diet, employment and other respects'—they affirmed that there are too many variables at work to legitimise an absolute deprivation line that is unaltered over time and transferable from person to person.

There is no agreement as to what a poverty line is, although it is argued that the idea of a *relative* standard of measurement is the one most frequently employed (Holman, 1978; Townsend, 1979; Brown & Madge, 1982; Haralambos, 1985; Young, 1989). Although there is no official set 'poverty line' in Britain, the level of income at which Income Support allowances are payable is usually, in practice, treated as a measure of poverty. The accepted European level appears to be households with half-average income.

The utilisation of relative concepts takes into account the fluidity of society: the fact that the standards, needs, and demands of society are in a continual state of motion and change. It is a dynamic process caused by social and technological changes, as well changes in interpretations of measurements and standards.

Relative poverty is a term that is applied to individuals whose living conditions are considered far below those of the rest of the society in which they live. Such measurement contains a comparative approach. One group is compared to another in terms of, for example, their income level, their potential in accessing social amenities, and their ability to afford certain items of food or clothing. For instance, one person may be a regular customer at an exclusive department store, whereas another may be able to afford clothing only from a charity shop.

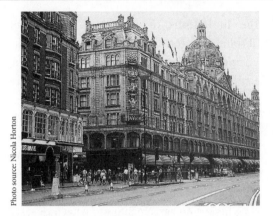

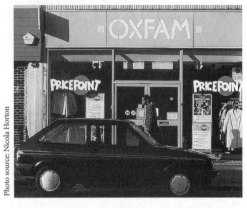

▲ *A difference in income levels: do you shop in expensive department, or make more purchases*
from charity shops?

The relative concept examines individuals in their social context, and their relationships with other groups in society regarding 'the gap or distance between the lowest and the average or normal standards' (Holman, 1978). The absolute poverty level, as pointed out previously, is focused on subsistence criteria and physical efficiency.

Inclusion of the social dimension gives a comparative framework for us to understand poverty, and shows the degree of inequality in existence among various groups.

However, at the same time as one must emphasise the relative nature of poverty, Brown and Madge (1982) argued, it must be effectively disentangled from a general observation of differences and inequalities. These authors explained the need to recognise the depth of inequalities and differences by examining groups who are *in* poverty. For example, Philo (1995), writing about the social geography of poverty in the UK, commented as follows:

> Social inequality increased in numerous ways: between the employed and the unemployed; between those in high-earning managerial and financial professions and those in low-wage, low skill, unstable and

often marginal jobs; between an expanding home-owning majority and a residualised minority of homeless; between those living in deprived inner-city areas and those in the more prosperous suburbs and shires.

The relative poverty illustrated in this extract should be seen in a realistic social context, bearing in mind that within the groups identified there are many individuals who live *in* poverty.

■ OTHER THEORIES OF POVERTY

SUBJECTIVE POVERTY

Subjective poverty is a different dimension to the concepts outlined above. This perspective looks at persons as individuals: how they think and feel about their existing living standards or status, and how they feel they are affected by them. For example, an Australian aborigine living in the remote deserts may argue that he has everything a human needs in life: food (in the form of lizards or snakes), water from cacti plants, rocky caves to shelter from the elements, clothing made from the skins of animals he has killed, and freedom. On the other hand, a city dweller who works in a factory and drives a budget-class car may argue that he is in poverty.

PRIMARY AND SECONDARY POVERTY

These theories originated from Rowntree, based on his research on poverty among the people in York. Primary poverty refers to a person's inability to maintain an adequate standard of physical efficiency due to insufficient income. Secondary poverty, on the other hand, applies to those people who, although having sufficient resources to avoid absolute (or primary) poverty, nevertheless fall into that condition because they mis-spend their incomes on items that are not essential, such as cosmetics (Byrne & Padfield, 1990a).

THE CULTURE OF POVERTY

This theory originated from the anthropological studies of Oscar Lewis (Townsend, 1979). The main features of this perspective are:

● The social context in which the poor find themselves shows a varying degree of reactive behaviour to their poverty problems (e.g. alcoholism, wife beating).

● Overcrowded quarters, absence of savings, lack of concern for the future, child labour, and unemployment are some of the social problems associated with poverty.

● The poor believe that their social state cannot be improved and that they are merely existing in a highly stratified and unequal society.

THE CYCLE OF DEPRIVATION

This theory found its origin from one politician: Sir Keith Joseph, Secretary of State for Social Services in 1972. The concept is defined as the reproduction of deprivation and poverty perse. Individuals who are born into poor families are said to be inescapably caught up in this cycle. This theory is associated with the culture of poverty, and stems from inadequate chil-

drearing practices. There is a failure to prepare children for effective participation in the prevailing culture. Thus, working-class families will encourage their children to obtain employment as early as possible, instead of undertaking further education studies as their middle-class counterparts do. There is a tendency for immediate gratification, probably due to a shortage of money. Gaining employment in factories will counteract the financial problems. Cultural influences have a role to play in the process too. If grandparents and parents have always earned a living doing menial tasks in factories, this belief may be transmitted to the children, who grow up accepting their social living as the accepted and respected norm for that particular family. After that, the cycle is set in motion, with cultural values transmitted from one generation to the next.

However, theories about the culture of poverty and the cycle of deprivation can be challenged. Oppenheim (1993), for example, argued that there is poverty in employment: 'The poverty of low wages and poor working conditions is often still a hidden factor in the poverty debate.' She also asserted that low-paid people do not receive benefits as a whole; people with disabilities live on very low incomes, often with very little chance of participating fully in society.

Oppenheim (1993) exposed the causes of poverty by emphasising that the social structure is the main predisposing factor: 'access to the labour market; inadequate governmental policy framework; discrimination based on "class, gender, and race"; disability and sickness as well as old age'. She concluded by blaming the system: 'In each of these cases social security benefits have failed to pull people out of poverty, often leaving them to manage on the most meagre incomes.'

On the increasing level of poverty in Britain, Oppenheim (1993) argued that the main factors are economic recession, the increasing level of unemployment, and the inadequacy of the social security system to deal with today's problems: 'Designed for a full time male workforce, it [the social-security system] discriminates against those who have been low paid, or unemployed, against those who have worked part time and people who have come to this country from abroad.'

▼ Homelessness and Housing Provision

■ A BRIEF HISTORY OF HOUSING

Shelter, in the form of houses, is an essential resource in society. No house to live in means no home for the person faced with this predicament. The social history of housing reveals the struggles of the poor: accompanying poverty one finds either homelessness or accommodation of poor quality, which impinge adversely on the health status of the individual. Social concerns about the plight of the poor and their housing needs have been reflected in the multitude of policies aimed at counteracting the harmful consequences of either housing shortages or substandard dwellings. The poor are not the only group who experience housing problems; there are also the disabled, the elderly and the mentally ill, for example. The problems for these special groups may be compounded if, as well as physically, psychologically, or socially disabled, they are also poor and there is a lack of housing provision for their specific needs.

Social history depicts contrasting modes of housing between the rich and the poor. Hibbert (1987), in his survey of social history from 1066 to 1945, reported the splendour and lavishness of the houses owned by the wealthy during the ages

of Shakespeare and Milton:

> The great chamber, the principal room in the house, was now often known as the dining chamber; but it was also used for games, dancing, plays, for the lying-in-state of deceased owners, and distinguished members of their families, and where there was no chapel, for household prayers. Plays were also performed and games sometimes played in the hall.

In contrast, social historians described housing conditions for the poor as pathetically below standard. This feature has not changed much from the Victorian era to modern times. Hibbert (1987), drawing from the social research of Charles Booth, illustrated the plight of the poor in some London dwellings:

> Fifteen rooms out of twenty were filthy to the last degree, and the furniture in none of these would be worth twenty shillings, in some cases not five shillings. Not a room would be free from vermin, and in many life at night was unbearable. . . . The houses looked ready to fall, many of them being out of the perpendicular.

Despite the Housing Act of 1924 that encouraged house building by granting subsidies—only the relatively better-off could afford houses of a comfortable standard (Hibbert, 1987):

> For the poor . . . housing conditions were still pitiably inadequate; and despite the large number of new council houses, two thirds of all householders continued to pay rent to private landlords, a large proportion of them having to part with as much as a third of their incomes for inadequate accommodation, in many cases without a piped water supply.

Burnett (1986), in his social history of housing between 1815 and 1985, explained how cellar dwellings represented one type of housing for many urban working-class workers in the early nineteenth century: 'To the contemporary mind the cellar dwelling seemed to represent the lowest general category of accommodation that was available for human or subhuman existence.' Living conditions, according to his account, were atrocious, with the high risk of illhealth due to unhygienic situations. A similar picture would be found, he noted, in the lodging houses—another category of housing—in Leeds, London, Birmingham, and so on.

Burnett (1986) also referred to another category of accommodation: tenement houses. He defined 'tenementing' as the subdivision of existing houses into separately occupied floors or single rooms. These, he explained, were for longer tenancy than the lodging houses, although the occupants did not adhere faithfully to the rules. The standards of conditions in tenement houses varied, but mostly were no better than those in the other housing categories. Burnett described how tenement houses were specially subject to such deficiencies as lack of water supplies; inadequate number of privies; no proper arrangements for cooking, sanitation, sewerage, and removal of refuse; and how, all too often, they lacked supervision from absentee landlords.

Another type of housing—the 'back-to-back'—was designed by builders of the time to meet the emergency needs of the population. Burnett (1986) postulated that this category of housing was considered to provide an improvement in living standards: 'In this sense, the back to back did not represent a deterioration of previous standards so much as an improvement in the slow continuum of vernacular housing.'

Terraced houses were developed in the first half of the nineteenth century. These were seen as a major improvement on the other types of houses described already. However, as Burnett

(1986) pointed out, only a minority of the urban working class would have been able to afford them: 'The terraced house in a respectable part of town or in one of the new inner suburbs, involving a weekly rent of 5s to 7s-6d, and more in London, represented the upper limit of working class housing in mid century.'

Other types of housing facilities occupied by the working classes at that time were known as 'workshop houses' and 'employer houses'. Workshop houses were those buildings modified to suit the needs of craftsmen (e.g. handloom weavers, silk and ribbon weavers), who lived and worked in them. Employer houses, as the term implies, were the houses provided by the employers to workers in the factories or mines; some of these houses were considered of good standard, others were not so good.

The middle-class housing in the suburbs, however, was of a different character. Spaciousness, private, and well located near the places of business, the homes of the middle classes stood out in their higher profile.

The above description gives an overview of the housing situation from 1815 to 1850. From 1850 to 1914, although houses were being built, the 'horrors of slums and overcrowding' were still in existence (Burnett, 1986). Some acts of parliament—the Public Health Act of 1858, for example, which passed regulations regarding the building of back-to-back houses, and the Local Government Act of 1858 for the control of buildings—came into force due to concern about unsafe and overcrowded dwellings being a source of danger to public health. For most of the working classes, however, housing problems remained very common features of their lives. Meanwhile, the suburban middle classes continued to prosper.

From 1918 to 1939, housing problems still existed. There was the realisation that private enterprises would not be able to supply houses to meet the demand. State intervention came in the form of acts of parliament: for example, the Housing and Town Planning Act of 1919, which allowed local authorities to assess housing needs in their areas. Houses built during this period were of a good standard, and became known as 'council houses'. Many slums were cleared, too. However, 'housing problems and housing issues were far from resolved in 1939' (Burnett, 1986).

From 1945 to 1985, houses were being built at a greater rate. The feeling of prosperity after the war years was evident in the provision of better housing amenities, local authorities being more involved in the implementation of safety regulations for buildings, and by increases in the availability of private houses. The working classes, Burnett (1986) pointed out, began to enjoy a higher standard of housing.

However, the policies of the succession of Conservative governments since 1979 have had an effect on the housing situation. For example, the 1980 Housing Act brought in the right for council tenants to buy their own homes. Encouraging home ownership has led to difficulties for people to obtain a council house or flat, so reducing the availability of cheaper housing for rental. The statutory involvement in building more council houses from the proceeds of sales has not been satisfactory. According to Burnett (1986), the ominous presence of deprivation, poverty, and homelessness still prevailed in 1985:

> Now in 1985, public concern over housing problems has again led to a major Inquiry into British Housing. . . . The Inquiry stresses the very real housing problems of those with low or limited incomes. . . . It catalogues . . . the growth of homelessness . . . the deterioration in the condition of housing . . . the 'totally unsatisfactory environment' around many council estates

and the particular shortages of accommodation in London and the southeast.

■ HOMELESSNESS

Hills and Mullings (1991) stated that the number of people living in bed-and-breakfast accommodation at the end of 1988 was 11,011; 6523 were in hostels, including women's refuges, and 13,200 were in short-life tenancies. The same authors quoted a study in London in April 1989 in which an estimated 75,000 were found to be 'overtly' homeless. According to Jones (1991), there were an estimated 400,000 homeless people at the end of 1989. Some key findings from Oppenheim (1993) revealed that in the early 1990s about 420,000 adults and children were accepted as homeless by local authorities in England; the number of 'unofficial homeless' was estimated to be approximately 1.7 million. London and other urban areas show an acute condition of homelessness. Oppenheim (1993) also pointed out that since 1978 to the early 90s, the number of homeless had nearly tripled. In spite of knowledge gained from social history concerning the problems of housing shortages, the effects on those unable to afford accommodation, and the perennial problems of homelessness, one finds similar dissatisfaction being expressed from many quarters in the 1990s.

Homelessness in the 1990s is the concern of many: from the politicians to the ethnic minorities, women, the elderly, the disabled, and migrants. It has become a major social and political issue (Denscombe, 1992).

Ginsburg and Watson (1992) expressed their views regarding the inadequacy of the Housing Act of 1985 (formerly known as the Homeless Persons Act). They argued that ethnic black minorities are becoming an official growing group of homeless people, 'while their rights and their treatment under the Act have been inferior'. The reluctance to carry out the Act is perhaps illustrated by what Ball *et al.* (1988) called the 'unwillingness' of social housing organisations to house an increasing proportion of lower income households, including groups such as the ethnic minorities and one-parent families. These authors also referred to the 'restrictive lending policies' of financial institutions, applied in areas where there are high concentrations of low-income households and ethnic minorities. Building societies and estate agents have shown discriminatory practices against black people (Young, 1989).

The whole social structure, however, shows an increase in homelessness. It is important to emphasise that the meaning of homelessness should include any person whose housing stan-dards consist of inadequate protection from the elements, a lack of access to safe water and sani-tation, and a lack of safety (Fallis & Murray, 1990).

Denscombe (1992) argued that homelessness should also include people living in 'temporary accommodation'; that is, those who have been given shelter by local authorities, according to their statutory duties, but who cannot be consid-ered as living in a 'place of their own'.

When one considers Denscombe's (1992) argument, it is realistic to propose that 'not hav-ing a roof over one's head' is a very restrictive definition of homelessness. Thus, people who live in bed-and-breakfast accommodation around London and other parts of the country, in unhygienic conditions in overcrowded rooms, with an unreliable supply of hot water and heat-ing, are classified as homeless (Conway, 1988).

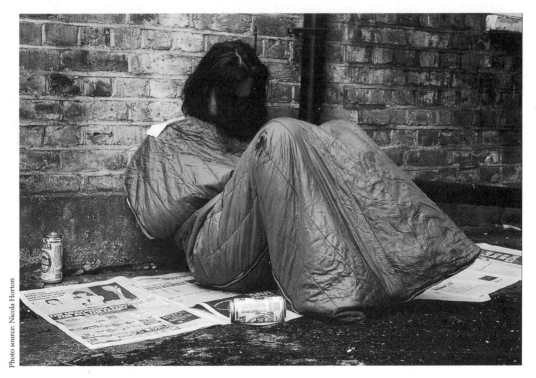

Photo source: Nicola Horton

▲ *One of London's many homeless people*

HOMELESS WOMEN

The scale of homelessness among women and black people is well documented (Hutson & Liddiard, 1994; Douglas & Gilroy, 1994; Dhillon-Kashyap, 1994; Ginsburg & Watson, 1992).

There is a Code of Guidance (1991) that local authorities are expected to use to help them to carry out the Housing Act of 1985 regarding homeless persons' needs (Douglas & Gilroy, 1994). According to the legislation, women who are in need of housing must either be pregnant or have dependent children, who are expected to reside with them, to receive priorities in terms of housing allocation.

Douglas and Gilroy (1994) made particular reference to the growing number of young homeless women who are experiencing problems in securing accommodation. They argued that the Children Act of 1989 specified the duty of social services to provide 'accommodation to any child in need—this covers any person up to and including those aged 17 who fall within certain categories'.

The housing system is, however, not fully meeting the housing needs of young homeless women: 'In some local authorities there are still no clear policies between Housing and Social Services as to which young people are to be accommodated, and who will accommodate them' (Douglas & Gilroy, 1994).

There are many homeless women in society who are not included in the statistics. As Hutson and Liddiard (1994) argued: 'The key to understanding the relative invisibility of young women and young black people in such homelessness statistics is to understand more about the nature of their homelessness.' Women are more, and feel more, vulnerable; it is understandable why not many are visible on the streets. They are prone to sexual harassment; they are discriminated against if they are of ethnic origins and black (Hutson & Liddiard, 1994).

There are other vulnerable groups in society who are homeless and in need of support services: the mentally ill and the elderly are two examples.

HOMELESSNESS AND THE MENTALLY ILL

The de-institutionalisation of mental healthcare to the community destabilised the secure hospital environment that many psychiatric patients were used to. Care in the community meant the re-allocation of the mentally ill from hospital to facilities that were, according to Watson and Austerberry (1986), largely nonexistent. Consequently, these authors argued, discharged patients found themselves homeless, without any neighbourhood networks to support them. In the 1980s, as the move from hospitals to community-care services gathered pace, mental healthcare workers and other community-care professionals realised the housing implications for clients with mental illhealth. Community services could not meet the demands. Patients were therefore housed in bed-and-breakfast or other accommodation (Young, 1989).

The discharge of such patients to community care makes them candidates for homelessness, Fallis and Murray (1990) argued. A failure to maintain stable relationships with others in the community, and the stress experienced in resettling in new types of accommodation, are factors that may not only cause a recurrence of mental symptoms but also create tension in relationships. Many psychiatric patients are found in this category. Many become homeless and sleep rough because of low incomes and the refusal by some members of the community to offer them dwellings.

THE HOMELESS ELDERLY

The physical and psychological impairments that accompany old age, not omitting the social and financial implications of retirement, contribute to the causation of homelessness in this group. The housing conditions for the elderly are poor (Sykes, 1994). Similarly to the other groups outlined above, the elderly are disadvantaged. Although not all elderly people experience housing problems or homelessness, a high percentage (1.3 million according to Sykes) are living in substandard conditions.

Many elderly people live in isolation and poverty; they need support if they are to remain in their own homes (Tossell & Webb, 1994). Tossell and Webb argued that local authorities are not directing resources to meet the needs of the elderly. A lack of resources for the elderly could lead to their inability to afford the rent and fuel bills. The purpose of the Housing Act of 1985 (part 3, Homeless Person Act) was to empower 'local authorities to work in a preventive way and to make arrangement for families and individuals before they become homeless in order to lessen the trauma' (Tossell & Webb, 1994). To become homeless is a traumatic experience for any individual. The elderly are a vulnerable group; their housing needs must be anticipated and prioritised.

■ CAUSES OF HOMELESSNESS

There are many causes of homelessness, for example:

- A shortage of housing available for rent at a reasonable price (Oppenheim, 1993).
- Poverty (Hutson & Liddiard, 1994): a low income means the inability to afford to rent or buy a house.
- Marital breakdown; spousal abuse; wife battering (Fallis & Murray, 1990).
- Problems of unemployment and inequality (Hutson & Liddiard, 1994).
- House repossession: failing to pay the mortgage.

- Mental illhealth and disabilities.
- Violence and racial harassment (Cooper & Qureshi, 1993), which can discourage tenants from seeking accommodation.
- Relatives or friends telling them to leave accomodation (Denscombe 1992).

Homelessness is not a new feature in British society, as pointed out in the historical account at the beginning of this section. However, it is necessary to re-emphasise that, in spite of past experiences, this social problem has not been eradicated. Concerns about its nature, its effects, and its implications as a socio-economic problem have been expressed repeatedly.

Murray (1995a), for example, wrote about the £100 million cut in grants for new building schemes and the reduction in housing benefits for those under 25 years, thought 'certain to put an added strain on cheap private rented accommodation which is widely exploited by unscrupulous landlords'. Murray also referred to the freeze in council rents, which, he felt, would lead to a fall in the amount of money available to maintain these properties and a decline in services.

In a different article, Murray (1995b) argued that a new Housing Bill—to be introduced by the government to create a further 1.5 million home owners over the next decade—was 'attacked' by Labour, local authorities, and housing charities 'as a recipe for homelessness', as very few would be able to afford to buy.

The debate on housing and homelessness will remain a perpetual one, although different kinds of legislation are in existence.

▼ Unemployment

■ THE UNEMPLOYED

The transition from full-time education to full-time or part-time employment is a major step for many individuals in society. To be employed, to have a job, creates a sense of fulfilment, achievement, satisfaction, and self-actualisation to many people. Employment also gives a sense of responsibility; the person who is employed is participating in the maintenance of society's economy and its functions. There is also the personal economic role or function of the person who is employed: the breadwinner of the family, the wage earner, a financial resource for the family.

However, employment is a major social issue too. If employment opportunities are not available, tension is created in society. The individuals who become unemployed feel the most affected. The absence of work is dispiriting (Bilton *et al.*, 1987); it creates psychological as well as material hardship (Giddens, 1989). Families and friends express compassion; politicians and the media constantly express their views on the subject; the topic becomes the focus of lively debates.

Unemployment—or 'worklessness' (Hayes & Nutman, 1981)—relates to one's perception of being a potential member of the workforce and being seen as having this aptitude by others, but being unable to gain employment. It means being out of paid work or work in a recognised occupation (Giddens, 1989), for example doing housework.

There are many individuals in society who want to work but are unable to find suitable employment. These include both men and women, young and old. Unemployment is higher among men than women; although there are many unemployed women, the statistics seem to disguise the unemployment figures among this group (Hayes & Nutman, 1981; Bilton *et al.*, 1987). Other groups that experience higher levels of unemployment are the ethnic minorities (Giddens, 1989; Beharrell, 1992; *Central Statistics Office*, 1995).

Unemployment—a social problem that affects so many groups of individuals in society–has shown an insidious trend since 1948. The Central Statistics Office (1995), for example, outlined the developing trends by pointing out that the long-term unemployed accounted for about 45% of all ILO* unemployed in Spring 1994, up from 28% in 1991, but lower than the 48% recorded in 1984.

Other statistics show the unemployment rates by gender and age as follows (*Social Trends*, 1995):

- In 1991, males aged 16–19 years had a higher rate (16.5%) of unemployment than age-matched females (13.2%). In 1994, the numbers had increased to 21% and 16%, respectively.
- In 1991, 12.3% of men and 9.4% of women aged 20–29 years were unemployed. In 1994, the number for men had increased to 14.8%, whereas the women showed a slight decrease at 9.3%.

The level of unemployment is also analysed and compared in different parts of the country. The ILO* unemployment rates (*Central Statistics Office*, 1995) showed that in 1986 the North had an unemployment rate of 14.6%; in 1994, 11.7%. In comparison, figures for the Southeast were 8.5% and 9.6%, respectively.

From looking at such trends, we can see that there has been a gradual rise in the number of unemployed people in Britain. O'Donnell (1993) argued that the number of unemployed people went above 10% in September 1992, and was rapidly rising. However, Macintyre (1995) asserted that in September 1995, compared with the French—who had shown a rise in unemployment for the second consecutive month, from 11.4% to 11.5%—Britain's unemployment rate in September had 'dropped for the 25th month in a row, to 8.1%, the lowest level since 1991'.

■ CAUSES OF UNEMPLOYMENT

The following have been put forward as possible causes of unemployment:

- The fact that the long-term unemployed are 'demotivated', 'lack skills', and a have a tendency towards being 'labour inflexible' (McDonnell, 1993). Labour inflexibility means an attitude of not being prepared to lower wage expectations sufficiently to get a new job.
- Lack of skills or qualifications, and discrimination (e.g. the person with a disability, the mentally ill, newly released prisoners) (Young, 1989).
- Lack of purchasing power (Giddens, 1989).
- Lack of demand or a lull in economic activity; decreased consumer spending (Beharrell, 1992).
- Mechanisation and technological advancement, such as microchip engineering.
- Too many people and not enough jobs (Beharrell, 1992).
- The economic recession and inflation. This puts the blame on the sociopolitical structures of society rather than the individual; the idea that in society there are many well-motivated workers who are simply not able to obtain a job that will match their expertise and experience.

■ THE EFFECTS OF UNEMPLOYMENT

It is a fairly common theme when the subject of unemployment is brought to our attention by the media and politicians to underline the statistical aspect of this topic. We are told about the *number* of unemployed in a particular region; we are made aware of the *number* of redundancies for a set period; thereafter the discussion develops along the line of the industries and corporations that are affected. Further statements and debates may look at what the other political parties are proposing to do about unemployment, the weaknesses of their proposals, or their failings in tackling this social problem. The feelings of the unemployed person—who is struggling socially and financially to survive the hardship of unemployment—do not receive a similar focus of heated debates and attention.

Losing one's job after many years of application and hard work creates in anyone a deep sense of loss that is similar to the grief process. It is a state of deprivation—financially, socially, and psychologically. The person is overwhelmed, denies anything has happened, and becomes depressed (Hayes & Nutman, 1981). Unemployment is said to be linked to mental illhealth and physical suffering, too (Balloch *et al.*, 1985).

The social impact is traumatic. The unemployed person is unable to afford the usual luxuries of treating friends to a meal or drinks, because of financial constraints. There is an implicit separation of relationships. Friends do not make invitations for parties; the unemployed person may lack the financial confidence to organise family activities and to participate fully in social life. There is evidence that a deterioration in social wellbeing is a possible consequence (Balloch *et al.*, 1985). The unemployed find that they have to rely more heavily on the

Welfare State for unemployment benefits.

Social consequences of unemployment include other problems, such as increased crime and the predisposition to alcohol abuse and drug addiction. Financial problems lead to an inadequate uptake of a well-balanced diet; hence, it is not surprising to find unemployed people showing signs of weight loss. The whole person is affected. This perspective becomes more evident in the 'Application to Clinical Practice' section, where other features of the effects of unemployment are considered.

▼ Summary

Poverty is a term used in the identification of a person's socio-economic status. Sociologists, social economists, policy-makers, and academicians have analysed the concept from a variety of perspectives. Most writers on poverty will refer to the works of two well-known figures in social history: Charles Booth and Seebohm Rowntree. Booth investigated the extent of poverty in London, whereas Rowntree concentrated his studies in York. Their findings helped them to reach a conclusion in relation to a definition and measurement of poverty. To Booth, poverty is when a person is unable to acquire the 'bare necessaries of life'; to Rowntree, poverty is when someone's physical efficiency is impaired due to an inability to meet the expected nutritional status.

Both Booth's and Rowntree's definitions are focused on the concept of absolute poverty. This has been described as being too inflexible, since there are other variables to consider. Consequently, the term 'relative poverty' is used. Relative poverty has a social orientation; it examines and compares the socio-economic status of one social group to another; the poor are identified in relation to, or relative to, other groups in society.

There are several theories of poverty. For example, there is primary poverty, when someone's income is so low that he or she cannot afford the basic necessities of life; secondary poverty occurs when incomes are adequate but mismanaged, so causing deprivation. Poverty is also examined from a personal perspective. This refers to the subjective experience of the person, who may or may not consider that he or she is poor. The culture of poverty is another theory. According to one anthropologist, Oscar Lewis—Townsend (1979) argued—this consists of the transmission, from generation to generation, of patterns of childrearing and socialisation that implant values and forms of behaviour. The attitude that poverty should be accepted as a way of life is passed on by parents; the children are not thereafter psychologically equipped to remove themselves from the deprived culture. The cycle of deprivation is a related theory. It was Sir Keith Joseph who explained this theory by arguing that families are caught up in a cycle of deprivation because of the culture of poverty they live in. This culture is transmitted and repeats itself. Although these latter perspectives are of some relevance, they lead to a tendency to blame the individual rather than the social system, which, it has been argued, is inadequate in its implementation of benefits' policies, showing a failure in commitment to a wide-ranging strategy.

Historical accounts have shown us that housing has been an ongoing major social problem. A survey of the literature shows that the group of people in society who are most likely to be affected by housing problems are the low-income groups: the working classes and those living in poverty; ethnic minorities; the elderly; the mentally ill. White women and black women also fall into a high-risk category, although it has been posited that the latter are more likely to be disadvantaged than the former.

There are many homeless persons in society, despite legislation such as the Housing Act of 1985. Homelessness does not necessarily mean rooflessness or no home to live in; other conditions—such as substandard housing, a lack of basic amenities, overcrowding, or an unhygienic living environment—are also be included in this definition.

Several causes of homelessness have been identified. Poverty is one factor; marital breakdown, abuse in the family, unemployment, violence, and racial harassment are some other reasons given for homelessness.

Unemployment, another social problem, is often the focus of lively debates in parliament and in the media. It is defined as a state of worklessness; the ability to do a job but the inability to find one. The level of unemployment has been rising since 1948, and has continued to increase throughout the 1990s. The level of unemployment was higher among males aged 16–19 years in 1991. There are regional differences, with the North showing a higher level of unemployment than the Southeast.

Several causes of unemployment have been outlined: demotivation, lack of skills, mental illhealth, and physical disability. Other possible causes are technology and mechanisation.

Unemployment is said to affect the person in many ways: psychosocially, financially and/or economically, and physically.

▼ Application to Clinical Practice

■ POVERTY

Current literature largely shows that poverty and social deprivation—which are common features among the low-status socio-economic groups—are associated with poor clinical outcomes. This finding is reinforced by the Child Poverty Action Group in their account of poverty in the UK (Dyer, 1995). They reported that disease processes such as prostate, lung, and breast carcinomas are higher among the underprivileged.

There is evidence too, according to research carried out by Bindman *et al.* (1995) in California, that race and poverty act as barriers to outpatient care. The researchers postulated that: 'Preventable hospitalization rates may be greater in poor or minority areas because these areas have more individuals who experience a clinical deterioration in their health.' Homer *et al.* (1995) found that the rate of paediatric hospitalisation in the United States was higher among poor children compared with 'non-poor' children.

The incidence of tuberculosis in England and Wales is associated with deprivation (Catchpole, 1995). However, Smith (1995) argued that an assessment of the high rate of tuberculosis among 'economically disadvantaged people' should consider their propensity for 'a higher risk of infection or a higher rate of progression from infection to disease or both'. Other authors, for example Doherty *et al.* (1995), although acknowledging the importance of poverty and overcrowding in the incidence rate of tuberculosis, have argued that the analysis to some extent show that ethnicity is more important than social deprivation in explaining variation in the rate. The association between poverty and tuberculosis in England is, nevertheless, accepted as a strong link (Mangtani *et al.*, 1995).

Low socio-economic status may also be linked with other conditions, such as diabetes (Crow *et al.*, 1991; Connolly & Kelly, 1995). HIV and/or AIDS, Small (1995) argued, should be seen from a *poverty* perspective rather than the 'general heading of behavioural explanation under which we understand the pandemic'. Small stated: 'The prevalence of HIV in sub-Saharan Africa, India and some other south-east Asian countries, can be closely identified with both the poverty of the populations most affected and also the poverty of the preventive and treatment facilities available to combat the virus.'

At a societal level, the gap between the poor and the rich is widening. The rise in poverty is affecting families who are feeling the detrimental effects of low incomes (Health News, 1995). From a health perspective, the inequality shown in relative wealth—rather than absolute poverty—is significant (Morris, 1995). The low income of some groups should make care professionals aware of the possible health implications. However, Judge (1995) pointed that although income distribution has an effect on life expectancy (the poor are more likely to die earlier and have the worse health), one should recognise that there may be other factors at play; dietary and sociocultural influences, for example.

The specific socio-economic problems faced by the severely disabled have been documented. Phillips (1995) identified the variations in community care among severely disabled people on low incomes. The data, he argued, showed inefficient healthcare support for this group. The vulnerability of the impoverished disabled is further reinforced by the inevitable trappings of debt and illness (Grant, 1995). Their social status and physical condition contribute to make their lives difficult, 'because of the way they are marginalised, degraded and devalued by society' (Grant, 1995).

Low-income single mothers make up another vulnerable group. In a study to assess the coping behaviours of such individuals in a city in the mid United States, Sachs *et al.* (1995) reported that poverty was the great stressor faced by single mothers and their families. Poverty is a stressful life-event that produces anxieties, destabilises the family, affects self-worth, and leads to depression.

To live in poverty in any society is a daunting experience. Frequently, the literature does not use the word 'poverty', but instead refers to low socio-economic status, deprivation, or being disadvantaged. These terminologies may sometimes mask the true nature of a growing social problem. To the poor person, poverty is a harsh reality.

Although poverty usually means a lack of material resources to cope with the demands of daily living, it is nevertheless good practice to extend the concept to include the 'emotional' and 'social' dimensions. Emotional poverty can be the consequence of unemployment (Barnes, 1987), or failed marriages and relationships (Sachs *et al.*, 1995).

Mental health workers have a role in assessing the coping strategies used by the clients. These may include, for example, social isolation, if the individual feels unwanted and threatened. Sachs *et al.* (1995) described the coping strategies used by low-income single mothers in their study for economic, physical, and emotional survival. Sensitivity to the mothers' repertoires of coping strategies and behaviours is important.

The focus of care should include the children of the mothers, too. It is argued that the social inequalities in health are related to increased child adult morbidity (Hobbs *et al.*, 1993). If one takes the theories of the 'culture of poverty' and the 'cycle of deprivation' into consideration, one finds 'the continuum of poor socioeconomic circumstances in childhood leading into disease developing in later life' (Hobbs *et al.*, 1993). Poverty is therefore a predisposing factor in the aetiology of pathological changes in later life.

When basic needs for a well-balanced diet are not met, growth and health status are affected. Food expenses are the main priorities for anyone; the poor find 'unhealthy' food to be cheaper. The intake of poor-quality nutrients has implications for health.

Poverty is also associated with problems of living in substandard housing. Hobbs *et al.* (1993) pointed out: 'Thus not only are children living in cramped unsuitable housing, it is also damp, cold, unhygienic and unsafe. High rise flats are unsuitable for children, young and older, who need safe supervised playing areas.'

The prevention of the consequences of deprivation, disadvantage, and poverty should be aimed for; or, as Polnay and Hull (1993) emphasised, the effects should at least be minimised. Preventive measures can be implemented by the mobilisation of resources from the primary healthcare team. Their role in the alleviation and reduction of the impact of poverty on the disadvantaged should not be underestimated. Baly *et al.* (1987) outlined the aims of primary healthcare as:

- The promotion of health in its broadest terms through education, support, and the encouragement of self-care.
- The prevention of illhealth by prophylaxis, early diagnosis, education, and advice on the value of early contact with primary healthcare services.
- The caring, treating, and rehabilitating of those who are acutely or chronically ill.
- The referral of patients to specialist services, where necessary, and the provision of continuing care following specialist treatment.

There are some community programmes designed to meet the needs of the poor or disadvantaged groups (Polnay & Hull, 1993). The programmes are tailored to provide preschool education for the children; and, for the parents, support and an important element of 'parenting the parents'. A multidisciplinary team approach is used by these family centres. Activities are aimed to empower, through education, families who are socially disadvantaged. This is achieved by: individual reviews and counselling; group work and practical activities; education regarding health, budgeting, and literacy; and guidance on childcare, play, family life, bereavement, and working.

Inequality remains a persistent and significant health problem in the UK (Morris, 1995) and throughout the world. In spite of available evidence showing that poverty is linked to the aetiology of illnesses and illhealth, government documents such as *Working for Patients* (HMSO, 1989a) and *Caring for People—Community Care in the Next Decade and Beyond* (HMSO, 1989b) do not make reference to poverty and its impact on the health of the population. Poverty, Oppenheim (1993) posited, leads to the risk of a shorter lifespan and a predisposition to illhealth and disability.

Blackburn (1991), on the other hand, discussed the relationship between health and poverty by stressing the need to use a micro-perspective, looking at the life style of the individual. She argued that the processes that influence the causation of illhealth are intertwined with the concept of poverty. For example, poverty, which constrains an individual's access to material resources and increases his or her vulnerability to health hazards, will affect the person physiologically by reducing their ability to combat infection.

Financial deprivation also takes its toll on both mental wellbeing (Blackburn, 1991) and social wellbeing. Recognising the dimensions of poverty, and its interconnectedness with other social factors (such as housing and unemployment), is essential.

■ HOMELESSNESS

Homelessness is another social problem that has implications for health and healthcare provision. For example, it is currently argued that homeless people are susceptible to tuberculosis (Mangtani *et al.*, 1995). Higher notification rates have been seen among these groups and the poorer section of the community.

When a homeless person encounters the care professional in clinical practice, it is important to bear in mind that he or she may have endured traumatic experiences on the streets, such as harassment of a sexual or racial nature, or both. There is also the likelihood of physical and psychological abuse. Physical abuse results from personal neglect, alcoholism, poor nutritional status, and surviving in an unhygienic environment. Psychological abuse is the consequence of the continuing impact of social isolation, the feeling of being discarded by relatives and friends, the depression that follows, and the anxieties and fears generated by a life of uncertainties.

There are homeless individuals living in cities throughout Britain, young and old, who are classified as 'missing' (Payne, 1995). This group of homeless 'are vulnerable to exploitation and at risk of committing crime and suffering from other social difficulties'. Payne

asserted that this group leave behind families with practical and emotional difficulties. The nurse and medical practitioner should undertake an assessment of the person's own emotional and practical difficulties. This should give an insight into the individual's mode of thinking and reasoning about his or her behaviour.

Once a thorough assessment has been made, an investigation of the wider kin network of the homeless should be carried out, assuming the client agrees. The rationale behind this approach is to consider the needs of families left behind. If the client is a child, the possibility that he or she may have left home because of domestic violence and abuse should be borne in mind. As Payne (1995) explained, there is a tendency to ignore this possible association. Although 'going missing' and homelessness are two different issues, Payne pointed out that it is nevertheless the task of the professional to realise that there may be a connection between them.

Following assessment, a decision has to be made regarding the involvement of other agencies, such as the social services, to gain specialist advice. The vulnerability of children who are homeless—for whatever reasons—must not be underestimated. 'Children who are homeless face unique challenges in their day to day lives. The task of providing basic necessities while they are homeless frequently leaves parents overwhelmed, preoccupied, and distracted' (Percy, 1995).

The impact of homelessness on any child is very severe, but particularly so among children who are not only homeless but do not have relatives or friends to support them. Children with families may be experiencing 'the same crises as their parents without the life experience or cognitive ability to understand the situation fully' (Percy, 1995). It is therefore advisable for the clinician to anticipate the psychosocial and biological needs of these children. Since homelessness is associated with poverty, their nutritional status will probably be substandard. The possibility of dehydration, electrolyte imbalance, respiratory tract infection, weight loss, mouth ulcers, and vitamin deficiency should be borne in mind during assessment procedures. From a psychological perspective, 'manifestation of severe anxiety and depression once their families become homeless' may be observed (Payne, 1995). A psychotherapeutic approach is recommended, with the parents being included in the counselling process. The aim is to enable the homeless families to identify their problems, and to assess the methods or coping strategies at their disposal to help them cope with their situations. The clinician—as a facilitator of this process—helps to guide them in a sensitive way towards expressing their care needs and finding solutions for their problems.

Payne emphasised how a holistic perspective of nursing is vital to understanding the complexities of childhood. A holistic view of the child, she argued, will help us to understand the multiple needs and fears inherent in homelessness.

The educational needs of homeless children are important issues to be considered, too. For homeless families living in temporary accommodation, the setting up of a professional link with the school nurse and the health visitor in the area will enhance team support in identifying and meeting the educational needs of these children and their families (Clarke, 1995). Clarke explained that the aim of this link is to establish communication to achieve the following objectives:

- To offer school health-service support to families and their children.
- To encourage and support children back

into schooling, hence maintaining their education.
- To minimise stress and insecurity.
- Health education.
- Liaison with other agencies: social services, city housing, and education, for example.

A multidisciplinary team approach is recommended, since children's needs are many. Some children may exhibit behaviour that is not easy to define; they may be labelled as having 'behavioural problems'. In a cross-sectional study of homeless primary school children and permanently housed control children in an outer London borough, Amery *et al.* (1995) concluded that there is evidence of 'behavioural problems' among the disadvantaged homeless groups. The authors did not explain fully, however, the meaning of what they considered to be 'behavioural problems'. This study, they argued, showed 'concerns about the mental health of a disadvantaged group'. Healthcare professionals need to examine any research findings that may help therapeutic interventions and guide them in targeting this vulnerable group.

Homelessness and child health are issues that become the healthcare professionals' main priorities in the delivery of care to this group. As pointed out already, the effects of homelessness are wide ranging. Jenkins (1993) emphasised other health issues of concern to the clinician: high rates of infectious illness and hospital admissions; risks of accidents to children; and the low uptake of developmental checks and immunisation. She reported that the conditions in which children live (overcrowded bed-and-breakfast accommodation, no play-area facilities) predispose them to stress and illness; cause behavioural and emotional problems; and increase the risk of accidents such as burns and scalds. Jenkins (1993) also reiterated that behavioural and development problems are common in childhood, and are associated with maternal stress and depression.

Primary healthcare teams have a responsibility to investigate and identify the healthcare needs of children and their families and to prevent further deterioration in health-status standards. To meet homeless families' healthcare needs, an integrated strategy must be implemented (Lee & Goodburn, 1993). These families, Lee and Goodburn pointed out, need support and understanding to overcome the initial shock of being homeless. Other health-promoting measures consist of the role of health visitors and allied professionals in:

- Raising awareness of child safety.
- Highlighting the dangers of overcrowding and unhygienic living.
- Developing a closer relationship of trust and communication with the client.
- Involving parents at the primary-care level.
- Liaising with centres for homeless families.
- Participating in drop-in centres for families.
- Advising, as required, on housing benefits and any other social entitlements.
- Recognising that there is a higher rate of depression among adults in temporary accommodation (Seymour, 1994).
- Identifying existing links between health agencies, housing departments, and homeless persons' units (Firth, 1995).
- Making a health assessment of the individuals and responding to their immediate needs, before referral to more specialist services (Haigh & Elliott, 1994).
- Raising the awareness of the homeless to specialist-interest groups.
- Locating and contacting homeless families, and facilitating access to and uptake of primary services (Hutchinson & Gutteridge, 1995).
- Recognising that environmental factors

influence client-use of the healthcare system: for example, clients whose housing is marginal or who experience daily dangers from abusive partners or drug dealers may have little interest in keeping healthcare appointments (Kinsey, 1995).

Other vulnerable groups, such as the elderly and the mentally ill, must have their needs met, too. The elderly tend to be frail and prone to illhealth. There are older homeless people with mental problems who live in isolation (Smith, 1992). The elderly are in need of continuing care and supervision from the primary care services. Discharge planning from the hospital and emergency department, Smith argued, is often poorly arranged. Discharge planning should form a joint effort based on 'an interdisciplinary perspective involving doctors, environmental health officers, health visitors and housing managers' (Ormandy, 1993).

Similar approaches to the ones outlined above can be used in the case of clients with mental illhealth. It is estimated that between 25 and 40% of the homeless population are likely to have serious psychiatric problems (Community File, 1993). The resettlement of homeless mentally ill people into the community needs preparation, as suggested by Sone (1995) reporting on the Lambeth High Street project in London. This project was aimed at resettling street-living homeless people into newly built flats and a hostel. Clients who have been used to a life of misery on the streets may need time to adapt to conventional settings. Their psychological disfunction (cognitive impairment, hallucinatory experiences, emotional and motivational disablement) hinders their social skills. It is for these reasons that they need—as Sone put it—*time, space, and stability.* The community health worker should ease this process.

Resettlement also means helping the homeless client to forge links with neighbours, as a component of relationship building and socialising skills. The benefits for clients in building positive relationships with their neighbours, Dunn (1995) argued, will extend into the wider community, as hopefully their neighbours can advocate for them in other arenas.

Caring for any category of homeless people in society is a demanding task for all healthcare professionals. It is an immense endeavour, requiring the mobilisation of effective healthcare resources through interdisciplinary teamwork. Several points must be noted:

- Strategic healthcare intervention should be based 'on the real experiences of individuals, families and communities; particularly the most deprived' (Rayner, 1996).
- Housing is a key instrument of healthcare (Conway, 1995).
- The extension of community nursing 'to the public health perspective will enhance its impact and that of health visiting on individual areas of clinical and management practice, widening future health priorities' (Nicholas, 1996).
- A holistic view of the homeless is imperative in care delivery.
- Poverty, unemployment and homelessness are all related.

■ UNEMPLOYED

In caring for the unemployed client in healthcare settings—in hospitals or in the community—several points must be noted:

- The unemployed client with either a mental or physical ailment may be poor and homeless too.
- The impact of unemployment has psychological, physical, and socio-economic implications.
- To be unemployed, poor, homeless, and sick, augments the stress factor; it is an added strain on the person's coping strategies.
- Hospitalisation and its effects on individuals may impede recovery if care is not tailored to meet the individual needs of this group.
- Increased vulnerability, heightened by admission to hospital, is worsened by exposure to clinical procedures such as tests, investigations, and treatment.
- The psychological impact is as traumatic as the physical and/or biological conditions that caused the client to be admitted; the risk of suicide or attempted suicide is a reality.

In the assessment of health and illness, the social and psychological factors are as important as the physical assessment of the disease (Rowden, 1993). For example, irritable bowel syndrome, peptic ulceration, or palpitations may originate from the stresses caused by unemployment. Rowden argued that any physical illness has a psychological component. Similarly, concerning the social component, unemployment, for example, could be the precipitating factor in the aetiology of psychological or physical illhealth. Brooking *et al.* (1992), however, believe that the link between unemployment and poor physical health is weak. The evidence, they asserted, shows a stronger link with poor mental health, which worsens as the duration of unemployment increases: the unemployed show increasing signs of depression, neurotic behaviour, dissatisfaction, have lower self-esteem and confidence, and are unhappy. Thus, unemployment is not only correlated to mental illhealth, but to mental wellbeing too.

In a review of the literature, Owen and Watson (1995) pointed to several studies showing the relationships between unemployment and mental health. They noted that poor mental health peaks three months after redundancy, and tails off to a plateau at 9–12 months after redundancy. The authors argued for governmental policies to consider the implications of this finding. Courses, workshops for training skills, and education for the unemployed, Owen and Watson (1995) explained, should aim to prevent individuals from adopting a fatalistic attitude to unemployment, which could exacerbate their mental health difficulties.

In health settings, the professionals (mental health workers, general nurses, physicians, psychiatrists, and others) should create an environment for the client that is conducive to the achievement of not only physical care but also social and psychological care. Thus it may be necessary to employ the skills of an experienced counsellor, as well as the counselling skills of nurses, physicians, and allied personnel. The role and functions of relatives in this process should be considered too, since these individuals may possess valuable information regarding the client's sociopsychological state.

The psychological impact of unemployment on the patient can be so traumatic that the individual becomes predisposed to self-inflicted injuries. The literature gives a series of discussions and arguments concerning the correlation between unemployment and suicidal behaviour:

- Crombie (1989) pointed to studies that showed increasing unemployment and evidence of an association between suicide and unemployment in the late 1970s: 'This study found a remarkable correlation between the trends of unemployment and suicide rate in men. . . . A simplistic interpretation would be that an increase in unemployment brings about an increase in suicide.'

- Similarly, Homer (1994) reported that recent studies in the UK have confirmed the association between suicide, parasuicide, and unemployment: 'The evidence relating to unemployment and parasuicide has been consistent over time with the parasuicide rate among unemployed people reported to be up to 30 times greater than the rate among employed.'

- Owen and Watson (1995) found similar relationships to those detailed above, but explained that suicide is a fatal act that is caused deliberately to self, whereas parasuicide—termed 'attempted suicide'—is a non-fatal act intended to cause injury.

Although studies tend to show the link between mental illhealth and unemployment to be stronger than that between physical illhealth and unemployment, the latter correlation should nevertheless not be ignored. Price (1995), for example, writing on youth unemployment, asserted: 'The first belief is that to be unemployed occasions illhealth, both *physical* and *mental*'. Increases in mortality due to coronary heart disease, accidents, and increased blood pressure—as well as suicide—have been found to be associated with unemployment (Hammarstrom, 1995). Cooper (1995), on unemployment and health, stated: 'Deterioration in physical health has been linked to a combination of poverty, diet, increased smoking, drug and alcohol abuse, psychological problems and stress, which are all associated with unemployment.'

In view of reported findings on the effects of unemployment on the individual, the multidisciplinary teams, in both community and hospital settings, have a major responsibility to consider not only the mental health effects on the person, but also the physical and social perspectives.

It is essential to realise in the day-to-day delivery of care to the client that admission to a general ward (e.g. for surgery) does not preclude the risk of suicide or parasuicide. Inattention and a lack of adequate discrete supervision give the depressed and psychologically distressed unemployed client ample opportunities to attempt suicide.

Writing about the 'Confidential inquiry into homicides and suicides by mentally ill people', set up by the Department of Health in 1992, Morris (1996) concluded that failures in communication between professionals, lack of clarity about care plans, and lack of time for face-to-face patient contact, increase patients' vulnerability to self-harm. Clear, concise, specific communication regarding the behaviour (psychological, mental, and social) of the client in any healthcare settings is a priority. This may be achieved by increasing face-to face contact time with the client and by a comprehensive care-planning programme, followed by effective implementation measures from a multidisciplinary team.

Community support is an invaluable asset to some groups of unemployed clients. Based on their findings from a study of mental health among unemployed men in England and Wales, Jackson and Warr (1987) suggested that community support in areas of long-term unemployment may help to protect unemployed men psychologically. This aspect should be borne in mind in the implementation and delivery of care. For example, involving friends, neighbours, and nearby relatives could reduce the impact of the stress caused not only by unemployment but by hospitalisation as well. Whelan (1993) emphasised that social support can act as a buffer against the negative consequences of stress: 'Social support means access to and use of individuals, groups or organisations in dealing with life's vicissitudes.'

This philosophy is reflected in 'community solution' strategies, which are aimed at enhancing the general wellbeing of mentally ill people who are unemployed. Local Exchange Trading (LET) systems provide both genuine employment opportunities and therapeutic benefit to mentally ill people (Wray, 1995). As Wray explained:

> The system is essentially an organised way of exchanging favours, and therefore has a considerable potential to create a sense of community among its participants. Having your clothes made by someone or doing gardening work for someone is an effective way of building and extending social networks within a community.

Hence, the LET system is a community initiative that allows people with mental health problems easy access to community resources. Consequently, the mentally ill have an opportunity to use their skills to the benefit of themselves and their community.

Other projects that aim at enhancing the life style of people recovering from mental health problems by helping them find employment are based on training and understanding, which can lead to rehabilitation (McCrone & Young, 1995). The main objectives of the Pecan project, the authors explained, are to increase confidence, overcome obstacles, develop interests and skills, and explore issues about work.

In face-to-face interactions, professionals such as health visitors can help unemployed people by disseminating information (Robertson, 1988). Social workers, mental health workers, and general nurses could supplement the client's knowledge regarding education and training. For example, there are opportunities available in 'youth training', introduced in May 1990; 'modern apprenticeships' and 'accelerated modern apprenticeships' are new choices for young people. These schemes offer the opportunity to acquire the skills and qualifications needed to become technicians or managers in the future (Slade, 1995). Training and work experience, Slade postulated, help people to obtain jobs.

It must be pointed out, however, that unemployment does not affect only the individual, but family and friends in the individual's immediate environment too. As discussed above, financial constraints impair social activities. Consequently, families are unable to participate fully in leisure activities, for example. There is a need to budget carefully, because unemployment benefits do not match the previous financial status of the person. The needs of families are therefore as important as the individual's needs.

▼ Review Questions

1 Explain how social economists have attempted to define poverty.

2 'Disadvantaged and deprived families in society have healthcare needs.' Discuss.

3 Describe the effects of substandard housing among homeless people.

4 'A holistic view of the homeless is necessary to understand the true nature of homelessness.' Discuss this statement with reference to the role of healthcare professionals.

5 Explain the importance of a thorough assessment of homeless people's social, psychological, and biological status.

6 The impact of unemployment on the individual is considerable. Examine and discuss the following:
(i) its socio-economic consequences;
(ii) its psychological and physical effects.

7 Unemployed clients in healthcare settings are prone to self-harm. Discuss how the multidisciplinary team may help clients to cope with the stress of being unemployed.

▼ References

Amery J, Tomkins A, Victor C. The prevalence of behavioural problems amongst homeless primary school children in an outer London borough: a feasibility study. *Public Health* 1995, **109**:421–424.

Atkinson A. Poverty. In: Eatwell J, Milgate M, Newman P, eds. *Social economics.* London: Macmillan; 1989.

Ball M, Harloe M, Martens M. *Housing and social change in Europe and the USA.* London: Routledge; 1988.

Balloch S, *et al. Caring for the unemployed people.* London: Bedford Square Press; 1985.

Baly M, Robottom B, Clark J. *District nursing, 2nd ed.* Oxford: Heinemann Nursing; 1987.

Barnes A. *Personal and community health. 'Disadvantaged families'.* London: Bailliere Tindall; 1987.

Beharrell A. *Unemployment and job creation.* London: Macmillan; 1992.

Bilton T, *et al. Introductory sociology, 2nd ed.* Basingstoke: Macmillan; 1987:395–403.

Bindman A, *et al.* Preventable hospitalisations and access to health care. *J Am Med Assoc* 1995, **274**:305–311.

Blackburn C. Poverty and Health: Working with Families. Buckingham: Open University Press; 1991.

Brooking J, Ritters S, Thomas B. *A textbook of psychiatric and mental health nursing.* London: Churchill Livingstone; 1992.

Brown M, Madge N. *Despite the Welfare State. A report on the SSRC/DHSS programme of research into transmitted deprivation.* London: Heinemann; 1982.

Brown M, Payne S. *Introduction to social administration in Britain, 7th ed.* London: Unwin Hyman; 1990.

Burnett J. *A social history of housing 1815–1985, 2nd ed.* London: Routledge; 1986.

Byrne T, Padfield C. *Social Services, 4th ed.* Butterworth: Heinemann; 1990a:35.

Byrne T, Padfield C. *Social Services.* Oxford: Butterworth Heinemann; 1990b:343–359.

Catchpole M. Tuberculosis in England & Wales. *Br Med J* 1995, **311**:187.

Central Statistics Office. *Regional Statistics.* London: Central Statistical Office; 1995.

Central Statistics Office. *Social Trends.* London: Central Statistical Office; 1995.

Clarke L. Special report improving school nursing care for homeless children. *Community Nurse* 1995, **1**(9):37.

Community File. Mental illness and homelessness. *Professional Nurse* 1993, **8**(10):674.

Connolly V, Kelly W. Risk factors for diabetes in men. *Br Med J* 1995, **311**:188.

Conway J. *Prescription for poor health. The crisis for homeless families.* Rochdale: LFC, SHAC; 1988.

Conway J. Housing as an instrument of health care. *Health Social Care Community* 1995, **3**:141–150.

Cooper J, Qureshi T. Violence, racial harassment and council tenants. *Housing Studies* 1993, **8**:241–255.

Cooper S. Unemployment and health. *Br J Nurs* 1995, **4**:566–569.

Crow Y, Alberti K, Parkin J, Insulin dependent diabetes in childhood and material deprivation in Northern England, 1977–86. *Br Med J* 1991, **303**:158–160.

Crombie I. Trends in suicide and unemployment in Scotland, 1976–1986. *Br Med J* 1989, **298**:782–784.

Denscombe M. *Sociology update.* Leicester: Olympus Book UK; 1992.

Dhillon-Kashyap P. Black women and housing. In: Gilroy R, Woods R, eds. *Housing women.* London: Routledge; 1994.

Doherty M, *et al.* Ethnic origin is more important than social deprivation. *Br Med J* 1995, **311**:187.

Douglas A, Gilroy R. Young women and homelessness. In: Gilroy R, Woods R, eds. *Housing women.* London: Routledge; 1994.

Dunn S. Helping clients build links with the neighbours. *Br J Nurs* 1995, **4**:94–96.

Dyer O. North–South divide does not explain British poverty. *Br Med J* 1995, **311**:82.

Fallis G, Murray A. *Housing the homeless and poor. New partnerships among private, public and third sectors.* Toronto: University of Toronto Press; 1990.

Firth K. Opening the door to homeless households. *Health Visitor* 1995, **68**:97.

Giddens A. *Sociology*. Cambridge: Polity Press; 1989:502–507.

Ginsburg N, Watson S. Issues of race and gender. In: Birchall J, ed. *Housing policy in the 1990s*. London: Routledge; 1992.

Grant L. Poverty: disabled people 'head above water'. *Community Care* 1995, **1095**:26–27.

Haigh J, Elliott P. The Hanover Project. *Health Visitor* 1994, **67**:274–275.

Hammarström A. Health consequences of youth unemployment. *Public Health* 1994, **108**:403–412.

Haralambos M. *Sociology: themes and perspectives*. London: Unwin Hyman; 1985:140–144.

Hayes J, Nutman P. *Understanding the unemployed. The psychological effects of unemployment*. London: Tavistock Publications; 1981.

Health News. Families worst affected by rise in poverty. *Health Visitor* 1995, **67**:216.

Hibbert C. *The English. A social history 1066–1945. 'The ages of Shakespeare and Milton'. 'Country houses and country people'*. London: Guild Publishing; 1987.

Hills J, Mullings B. Housing: A decent home for all at a price within their means? In: Barr N, Coulter F, Evandrou M, *et al*. eds. *The state of welfare. The welfare state in Britain since 1974*. New York: Oxford University Press; 1991: 135–203.

HMSO. *Caring for people—community care in the next decade and beyond*. London: HMSO; 1989a.

HMSO. *Working for patients. The Health Service*. London: HMSO; 1989b.

Hobbs C, Hanks H, Wynne J. *Child abuse and neglect. A clinician's handbook*. Edinburgh: Churchill Livingstone; 1993.

Holman R. *Poverty explanations of social deprivation*. London: Martin Robertson; 1978.

Homer C, *et al*. Effect of socio–economic status on variation in paediatric hospitalisation. *Ambulatory Child Health* 1995, **1**:33–43.

Homer M. Links between unemployment and mental health problems. *Nursing Times* 1994, **90**:42–44.

Hutchinson K, Gutteridge B. Health visiting homeless families: the role of the specialist health visitor. *Health Visitor* 1995, **68**:373–374.

Hutson S, Liddiard M. *Youth homelessness. The construction of a social issue*. London: Macmillan; 1994.

Jackson P, Warr P. Mental health of unemployed men in different parts of England & Wales. *Br Med J* 1987, **295**:525.

Jenkins S. Homeless and child health. *Maternal Child Health* 1993, **18**(7):198–202.

Jones K. The making of social policy in Britain 1830–1990. London: Athlone; 1991.

Judge K. Income distribution and life expectancy: a critical appraisal. *Br Med J* 1995, **311**:1282–1285.

Kinsey K. Risky business: managing the health care of urban low-income families. *Holist Nurs Pract* 1995, **9**:41–53.

Lee H, Goodburn A. Developing an integrated strategy to meet homeless families' health needs. *Health Visitor* 1993, **66**:51–53.

Le Grand J, Propper C, Robinson R. *The economics of social problems, 3rd ed*. Basingstoke: Macmillan; 1992:184–187.

Macintyre B. Rising jobless toll has France eyeing Britain with envy. *The Times* 1995 Nov 2:13.

Mangtani P, *et al*. Socio-economic deprivation and notification rates for tuberculosis in London during 1982–1991. *Br Med J* 1995, **310**:963–966.

McCrone P, Young M. Pecan choose. *Health Service J* 1995, **105**:33.

McDonnell B. Unemployment and economic policy. In: O'Donnell M, ed. *New introductory reader in sociology*. Walton-on Thames: Nelson & Sons; 1993, 254–259.

Morris M. Inequality: a health problem resistant to intervention. *Br J Nurs* 1995, **4**:553–554.

Morris M. Homicides and suicides by mentally ill people: resources highlighted. *Br J Nurs* 1996, **5**:2.

Murray I. Help and incentives for new buyers. *The Times* 1995a Nov 16:11.

Murray I. Public sector hit by £160m cut. *The Times* 1995b Nov 29:14.

Nicholas A. Making it happen: community nurses' public health role. *Health Visitor* 1996, **69**:28–30.

O'Donnell M. *New introductory reader in sociology, 3rd ed.* Walton-on-Thames: Nelson; 1993:254 .

Oppenheim C. Poverty the fact. London: CPAG; 1993.

Ormandy D. Homes above all. *Health Visitor* 1993, **66**:62.

Owen K, Watson N. Unemployment and mental health. *J Psychiatr Mental Health Nurs* 1995, **2**:63–71.

Payne M. Understanding 'going missing'. Issues for social work and Social Services. *Br J Social Work* 1995, **25**:333–348.

Percy M. Children from homeless families describe what is special in their lives. *Holist Nurs Pract* 1995, **9**:24–33.

Phillips V. Community care for severely disabled people on low incomes. *Br Med J* 1995, **311**:1121–1123.

Philo C. *Off the map. The social geography of poverty in the UK.* London: CPAG; 1995.

Polnay L, Hull D. *Community paediatrics, 2nd ed.* Edinburgh: Churchill Livingstone; 1993.

Price B. Youth unemployment: effects on health and happiness. *Br J Nurs* 1995, **4**:892–895.

Rayner G. Public health, health alliances and primary care. *Health Visitor* 1996, **69**:26–27.

Robertson C. *Health visiting in practice.* London: Churchill Livingstone; 1988.

Rowden L. Mind and body—the emotions and physical illness. In: Wright H, Giddey M, eds. *Mental health nursing from first principles to professional practice.* London: Chapman Hall; 1993.

Sachs B, Hall L, Pietrukwicz M. Moving beyond survival: coping behaviours of low-income single mothers. *J Psychiatr Mental Health Nurs* 1995, **2**:207–215.

Seymour J. Homeless families face closing doors. *Health Visitor* 1994, **67**:151.

Sharp A, Register C, Leftwich R. *Economics of social issues.* Burr Ridge–Illinois: Irwin; 1994:265–266.

Slade E. *Employment handbook, 9th ed.* Croydon: Tolley; 1995.

Small N. Don't die of poverty. *Health Matters* 1995, **23**:12–13.

Smith I. Define high risk behaviours, not high risk groups. *Br Med J* 1995, **311**:187.

Smith J. Are the needs of older homeless people being ignored? [Editorial]. *J Adv Nurs* 1992, **17**:763.

Sone K. Mental health practice: lessons in responsibility. *Community Care* 1995, 29 June–5 July: **1074**; 21.

Spicker P. *Social housing and the Social Services.* Harlow: Longman Group; 1989.

Sykes R. Older women and housing—prospects for the 1990s. In: Gilroy R, Woods R, eds. *Housing women.* London: Routledge; 1994.

Tossell D, Webb R. *Inside the caring services.* London: Edward Arnold; 1994.

Townsend P. *Poverty in the United Kingdom. A survey of household resources and standards of living.* Harmondsworth: Penguin Books; 1979.

Watson S, Austerberry H. *Housing and homelessness. A feminist perspective. Homeless women and the labour market.* London: Routledge & Kegan Paul; 1986:129–148.

Whelan C. The role of social support in mediating the psychological consequences of economic stress. *Social Health and Illness* 1993, **15**:87–100.

Wray S. A community solution to unemployment for mentally ill people. *Mental Health Nurs* 1995, **15**:6–8.

Young P. *Mastering social welfare, 2nd ed.* London: Macmillan; 1989.

▼ Further Reading

Anderson I. Housing policy and street homelessness in Britain. *Housing Studies* 1993, **8**:17–28.

[Anonymous]. Further work for colleges. *The Times Higher Education Supplement* 1995 Nov 17.

Bassett P. W H Smith makes job centre deal on recruitment. *The Times* 1995 Nov 8:26.

Blom-Cooper L, Hally H, Murphy E. *The falling shadow*. London: Duckworth; 1995.

Brindle C, Brown K. *Community health care*. London: Macmillan; 1991.

DasGupta P. *An enquiry into wellbeing and destitution*. Oxford: Oxford University Press; 1993.

DasGupta P. Population, poverty and the local environment. *Sci Am* 1995, **272**:40–45.

Davis K, Schoen C. *Health and the war on poverty. A ten year appraisal*. Washington DC: Brookings Institution; 1978.

Duggan J, Roper H. The benefits of simplicity and the scourge of poverty. *Br J Midwifery* 1996, **4**:14–17.

Dwelly T. New deal for young homeless. *Roof* 1995, March/April:18–19.

Ferrie J, *et al*. Health effects of anticipation of job change and non-employment: longitudinal data from the Whitehall Study. *Br Med J* 1995, **311**:1264–1269.

Garrett G. But does it feel like home? Accommodation needs in later life. *Professional Nurse* 1992, Jan:254–257.

Gershuny J, Pahl R, Nabarro R, et al. Unemployment and the black economy. A New Society. *Social Studies Reader*. London: New Society Schools; 1980.

Griffiths S. Housing: discouraging independence. *Community Care* 1995, June 29-July 5.

Hammarstrom A. Health consequences of youth unemployment—review from a gender perspective. *Soc Sci Med* 1994, **38**:699–709.

Lahelda E. Unemployment and mental well being. *Int J Health Services* 1992, **22**:261–274.

Lahelma E, Mandebacka K, Rakikonen O, Karisto A. Comparisons of inequalities in health: evidence from national surveys in Finland, Norway and Sweden. *Soc Sci Med* 1994, **38**:517–524.

Monsuez J, *et al*. Cutaneous diptheria in a homeless man. *Lancet* 1995, **346**:649–650.

Norman I, Parker F. Psychiatric patients' views of their lives before and after moving to a hostel: a qualitative study. *J Adv Nurs* 1990, **15**:1036–1044.

RCP. *Report of the confidential inquiry into homicides and suicides by mentally ill people*. London: Royal College of Psychiatrists; 1996.

Redelmeier D, *et al*. A randomised trial of compassionate care for the homeless in an emergency department. *Lancet* 1995, **345**:1131–1134.

Sherman J. Brown forced to tread carefully after policy row. *The Times* 1995a Nov 24:12.

Sherman J. Now Labour tells young jobless 'get on your bike'. *The Times* 1995b Nov 9:1.

Thompson A. Policy: housing. No place like home. *Community Care* 1992, Oct 26–Nov 1 **940**:14–15.

Townsend P, Davidson N. *Inequalities in health: the Black Report*. Harmondsworth: Penguin Books; 1982.

Turok I. Tackling poverty through housing investment: an evaluation of a community self-build project in Glasgow. *Housing Studies* 1993, **8**:47–59.

14

Social Policy

▼ What is social policy?

The character of social policy is not easy to define because the whole concept comprises an amalgamation of attributes. Social policy is understood to be related to social welfare and its development. It is an interdisciplinary subject: it has links with social provision and sociology, and action-oriented activities by the government; it has a peripheral link with public policy; and it is concerned too with non-public matters such as community care (Bulmer *et al.*, 1989).

It is said that social policy is concerned with public expenditure, which contributes to public welfare (Hill, 1993b). However, Hill stated that this interpretation raises 'a most misleading and widespread false assumption' about its character; to argue that social policy is mainly centred on welfare provision, gives a restrictive definition of its true nature.

There is an undeniable relationship between social policy and the governmental action-oriented programmes that aim at improving the welfare of citizens; for example, policies on poverty, unemployment, housing, the aged, and the disabled. However, this notion of social policy, Hill (1993b) postulated, has also been challenged from many quarters: 'Several recent discussions of social policy have suggested that welfare policies are promulgated not from humanitarian concerns to meet needs but as responses to social unrest.'

Hill (1993) referred to other arguments which point towards a Marxist interpretation of social policy: the view that the purpose or objective of policy is to maintain the ideology of a capitalist society, 'which requires an infrastructure of welfare policies to help maintain order, buy off working class protest and secure a workforce with acceptable standards of health and education'. This perspective may be said to contain a sociological interpretation, which again shows the interdisciplinary nature of the topic. Other perspectives on the subject, Hill (1993) argued, show social policy 'as sustaining not only class-based patterns of domination but also patriarchy and racial inequality'.

The origin of social policy must nevertheless be located within the governmental political framework. Therefore, the making and implementation of social policies should be objectively assessed and evaluated in regard to their outcome or consequences on the welfare needs of the citizens.

It is important to adopt a more open and balanced view of social policy to include not only humanitarian objectives but non-humanitarian ones too. The possibility of altruistic motives in the evolution of policy, as well as manipulative and social-control-motivated actions (Hill, 1993), should be considered.

The domain of social policy is vast. There are aspects of social life, such as expenditure on defence, that are not conventionally perceived to be social policy, but play a major role in its contribution to welfare (Hill, 1993). Monetary management, expenditure, and redistribution of benefits, as in social-security provision, may all be encompassed within the realm of social policy, but with the emphasis on the economic nature that it reflects. Hence,

social policy is linked with economic policy.

Thus, from the above discussions, a common theme may be identified:

● Social policy does not occur in a vacuum: there are social and political forces, as well as economic pressures, involved.
● Social policy is the consequence of government action; policies are formulated at government level.
● Social policies are interlinked with broader policies, e.g. defence policies.

The Welfare State is an umbrella term that covers a multitude of services–social and occupational —aimed at ascertaining the provision of social measures to meet the needs of citizens. Sullivan (1994) explained that the Welfare State is an aspect of social policy development. In particular he argued that the growth of 'institutionalised state welfare services is understood as stemming from increasing awareness of social problems and an accompanying moral conviction that they should be resolved'.

The Welfare State, many writers on the subject would agree, found its origin from the framework provided by the Beveridge Report of 1942 (Rimmer, 1981). Fraser (1984) claimed that the report was an immediate best-seller and was 'the culmination of a lifetime's influence upon social administration which had begun with Beveridge's advocacy of labour exchanges and insurances in 1909'. The ethos of the report is perhaps better defined by what Abel-Smith (1983) described as the spirit of consensus in society following the Second World War; consensus regarding the imperative need to combat poverty, squalor, homelessness, unemployment, and illhealth. The aims of Beveridge's social programmes were to tackle the five giants: Want, Disease, Ignorance, Squalor, and Idleness. Beveridge had provided the means to dispose of want: poverty could be abolished by flat-rate social-insurance benefits provided to those legitimately off work, and family allowances for all, starting from the second child (Abel-Smith, 1983). The landslide victory of the Labour Party in 1945 allowed the government to implement forcefully the recommendations of Beveridge. The success of the plan, Fraser (1984) pointed out, was based on three assumptions: the time was ripe for revolutionary changes; social insurance was to be an important part of social policy; there was to be the provision of social security with state intervention and individual participation.

The report gave undivided attention to the health of the nation, inspiring the provision of the NHS, the purpose of which was to prevent and cure disease and disability (Pope *et al.*, 1986).

Midwinter (1994) saw the whole process leading to the implementation of the Beveridge Report as a 'silent revolution of the 1940s'. The report, he argued, demonstrated the Labour Government's dedication to 'construct something closer to a programmed welfare state'. 'The salient features', Midwinter (1994) pointed out, 'were the National Health Service, the attendant social insurance schemes of Beveridge Report, the continuation of new town and municipal housing, and a determination to offer all children access to secondary education.'

▼ Approaches to the Study of Social Policy

To study social policy is to study one of the many facets of social life. Social life is governed by social structures. The structures of society (the legal, educational, community, health, and social-services frameworks, to mention but a few) only become operational after the formulation and implementation of policies.

Policy formulation and implementation require the support and authorisation of groups situated at the higher level of social organisation: the central government. Therefore, the study of social policy requires students to be sensitive to the political realities that form one of the forces impinging on and influencing the policy-making mechanisms.

Hill (1993) believed that social policy may be studied in a number of ways. This is true, since social policy—its formulation, implementation and, not least, its evaluation—demands a multidimensional approach. For instance, policies concerning healthcare provision can be examined, assessed, and debated in regard to their effectiveness within a very broad social framework: how the health needs of citizens are being catered for—occupationally, socially (family health), psychologically, from a social services and a community perspective, as well as legally and economically in response to demands and resource availability. On the other hand, as Hill (1993) suggested:

> We may merely set out to determine the main policies in the areas in which we are interested. What is our system of social security? What benefits does our health service provide? How has government intervened in the housing market? These and similar questions need to be answered by those who want to understand social policy.

Therefore, one may approach the study of social policy by an examination of the broad interrelated institutional structures of society, within which provisions of services are located. If, for example, one is studying housing market policies, their relationship with health and safety cannot be ignored; consequently, a look at health policies would be advisable. The provision of community services for the mentally ill cannot be implemented without due consideration of the role of health providers, hospital trusts, and general practitioners.

In the implementation of policies for the unemployed and homeless people, one has to ask:

- Will the benefits provided be sufficient to raise the standard of living of these groups and meet their health needs?
- To what extent are social policies creating inequalities or reducing their impact?
- Do welfare policies reduce individual initiative and enterprise?
- To what extent do policy initiatives from central government fail to realistically counteract existing social problems?

These are some of the questions and alternative approaches that may be used in the study of social policy.

Other basic approaches can be used; for example, the belief that citizenship entitles a person to a set of rights—and this includes economic and welfare rights, such as rights to health services, a certain level of education, and so on (Ware & Goodin, 1990). This principle may be studied in relation to the debates on whether it is the duty of the state to supply resources and services to every citizen, commensurate with those rights being respected (Ware & Goodin, 1990).

The socio-economic and political dimensions of social policy are just as important; so is the sociological perspective. In attempting to assess and understand how the Welfare State 'deals' with women, it may be relevant to consider the feminist perspective or interpretation. The following extract should make this point clearer: 'What we should have at the end of such an investigation of social policy is a new understanding, not only of the way the welfare state deals with women, but also of social policy itself' (Pascall, 1986).

Another approach would be to gain insight into some wide-ranging theories on the Welfare State; this would lead to an understanding of the effects of social policy. For instance, under the heading of 'demand theories' the student of social policy could investigate the formulation of welfare policies that are dependent on class structures or the economic development and size of ascriptive groups such as the aged (Pampel & Williamson, 1989). The redistributive process (benefits for the disadvantaged groups) classified under demand theories could be evaluated by looking at evidence of fairness and equality: Are political institutions independent in their decision-making mechanisms and free from external influences (e.g. pressure groups and economic pressures)? Are social policy changes the consequence of technification?

Although the above approaches are relevant to the study of social policy, an even more important stance is to scrutinise the progress of social policy implementation by assessing objectively and in an unbiased fashion 'the actual impact of any policy upon the public' (Hill, 1993). As Hill (1993) explained: 'The implementation process throws light on the strengths and weaknesses of a policy, and experience at the implementation end (by junior officials and by the public), gets fed back into the policy process to influence future policy changes.'

How the reader or student of social policy approaches the subject is a matter of individual choice. Awareness that social policy cannot be isolated from the other social sciences will enrich the student's repertoire. For example, can it be argued that social anthropology, sociology, and social economics are relevant to the study of social policy Adoption of such beliefs would cause the implementation of policies of a rudimentary nature. Social policy decisions must be studied from within and without a global framework: for example, if social anthropology informs us on other cultures' ways of life, social policy should be tailored with minority groups in mind.

A sociological insight will pave the way to understanding the social factors (class structure, gender, education, politics, and economics, for example) that energise the creation and implementation of social policies.

There are other relevant areas of interest too: the inter-relationships of local authorities (in their various forms), the institutions of the NHS, quasi-governmental bodies, and the central government, which are seen to be major executants of welfare policy.

Butcher (1995) argued that there are two public faces of welfare government in Britain:

> One face is made up of a small number of central government social service departments who are not normally delivery agencies of welfare . . . but are primarily concerned with the functions of policy making, resource allocation and supervision. The other public face of welfare consists of a range of non-departmental organisations, notably local authorities and health authorities.

Hence, the study of social policy should not be concerned simply with the identification of policies for citizens' welfare; it should include approaches aimed at scrutinising the processes, the mechanisms, the relationships of government bodies, and their methods of delivery as well.

▼ Policy-Making

Policy-making, or the formulation of policies, needs to be understood in terms of the complexity of processes that contribute to its development: from the point of an idea concerning the improvement of social welfare conditions and problems, to its acceptance and further development into principles to be embodied in legislation, and finally to its acceptance as policy. These factors refer to the complex network of the 'legislative process and of intricacies of local administration, its financial management and the balance between central departments and local authorities in the working of decisions regarding services' (Brown & Payne, 1990).

Policy-making is a process; it is to do with development; it is seen as an 'activity of many different types of public institution: not just governments but also aid agencies, non-governmental organisations, community groups, collectives and political movements' (Mackintosh, 1992). To think of policy as a social process, Mackintosh pointed out, is to realise that the nature of the policy-making institutions matters a great deal.

■ THE ROLE OF GOVERNMENT IN POLICY-MAKING

What is the role of government in this social process? What measures should government take to counteract social problems? These are some of the questions asked when a society is facing problems that cause hardship to its citizens. To obtain an awareness of this policy-making mechanism, an insight into the structures of government is needed.

Government is sometimes referred to as the British Constitution. Norton (1991) defined a constitution as the 'collectivity of laws, customs and conventions that define the composition and powers of organs of the state and regulate the relations of those organs to one another and to the individual citizen'.

A macroscopic view of the state shows the Crown (Monarchy) at the top, followed by the House of Commons and House of Lords adjacent to each other. The House of Commons is made up of ministers and other Members of Parliament (MPs)—representing the majority party and other parties—who won a seat at the most recent general election or by-election. The House of Lords consists of hereditary members of the peerage and life peers. Central government comprises of; the Prime minister and cabinet, ministers and their departments, and the civil service.

Cocker (1993) described the concept of parliament as a body made up of three elements—the House of Commons, the House of Lords, and the Crown, collectively termed the legislative assembly. Hill (1993) pointed out that the Crown (Monarchy) and the House of Lords formally do not have much influence in the policy-making process. The House of Commons is believed to be the most dominant element.

The House of Commons has many facets and functions. One facet to consider is the many different kinds of structures enmeshed in its framework: Government, the governing party, the opposition front bench, the opposition party, the other parties.

The functions of the Commons may be summarised as its representative functions: the electorate is represented in the House; this feature is perceived to be the foundation of the other roles of the Commons. Cocker (1993) explained: 'In a democracy the representative principle underpins the right of the representatives to act on behalf of the voters, and endorse or reject the legislation of the government itself drawn from parliament'. This feature is important for policy-making. Citizens in the various constituencies will express their welfare needs and concerns to their appropriate MPs. MPs are therefore the voices of the people (in the constituencies), as well the voices of pressure groups and, of course, the voices of the

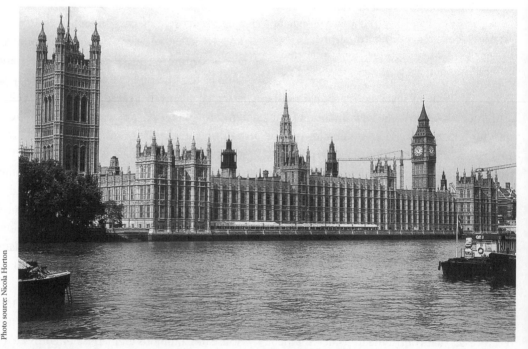

Photo source: Nicola Horton

▲ *The British Houses of Parliament*

political parties they represent. The transmission of information by MPs in the Commons concerning citizens' dissatisfaction with policies in force exerts a powerful pressure on government ministers to review existing legislation and social policies.

Although the power of the Commons has been criticised in regard to its effectiveness in legislation and legitimisation, the goverment—which the House of Commons represents—is still the fount of legislation and policy, with Parliament playing a supportive if critical role (Cocker, 1993).

The Commons has vital scrutinising functions. The behaviour of governmental legislation is critically assessed, evaluated, and sometimes rejected; this particular feature may be seen on the television screen, with opposition parties, and even members of the majority government, forcefully opposing certain policies, and then accepting or rejecting them according to an assessment of their particular value or appropriateness. The Commons, however, still has the ultimate sanction on government policy and legislation. The House of Commons, hence, is an extremely important arena in government structures.

The 'Cabinet' is another such structure. This term is sometimes used to mean the Government, although, it is argued, this can lead to a misinterpretation of its true nature in the political framework:

> The 'Government' refers to all the Ministers and their aides down to the humble Parliamentary Private Secretaries. . . . The 'Cabinet' technically consists of all those politicians invited by the Prime Minister to give collective advice to the Monarch. In reality this means 21–24 ministers chosen by the Prime Minister (Cocker, 1993).

■ THE FUNCTIONS OF THE CABINET

In the political circle, the Cabinet represents an arena where intense debates may take place on a variety of social issues: social policies, energy policy, defence policy, technology, and education, for example. The Cabinet is a vital component in the co-ordination of policy and administration. The determination of policies and the review of existing policies take place within the Cabinet. This does not mean, however, that all policies are discussed and agreed within the Cabinet, but that part of the whole process of policy-making may be located in this particular structure of government. Since there may be only 20–24 members of the Cabinet, it is an impossible task for such a small group to reach a decision on some policies. Consequently, according to Cocker (1993), 'bodies like Cabinet Committees, specialised departments and advisory groups have become so significant in formulating policy, with the Cabinet acting perhaps as the final arbiter in differences not already settled, or as a rubber stamp for decisions already arrived at elsewhere'.

Some functions of Cabinet Committees can be summarised as debating on home affairs and social policy, education and energy policy, economic strategy, the social services, and law and order policy, to name but a few.

■ THE CIVIL SERVICE

The role of the Civil Service in the process of policy-making is a force that should be recognised. Civil servants (scientists, technologists, lawyers, and customs and excise officers, for example) work closely with the ministers who are heads of their departments. Civil servants are known as the 'mandarins' of the Civil Service. They have high-grade administrative posts in government; they have knowledge and power. Although they work to uphold their ministers' interests in the democratic process of policy-making, they have been known to cause deliberate obstruction and to support the departmental—rather than the ministerial—view. Sometimes, civil servants may prevent a particular policy from being developed, if they feel that it is not going to be a popular one.

■ THE FUNCTIONS OF LOCAL GOVERNMENT

Any assessment of governmental social policy processes is incomplete without reference to the important role of local government (local authorities). Central government (Prime minister and cabinet, minister, their departments, the Civil Service), as we have seen, does not operate independently. There is a partnership—based on co-operation and conflict—between these two important statutory structures of society. The conflict is the result of central government policy to restrict expenditure of local authorities and to exercise some form of control over their activities.

In England, the main link between local authorities and central government is the Department of Environment. There are other departments, however, such as the Department for Education and Employment and the Home Office, which are also concerned with various local government functions.

Central government has links with local authorities through contact with regional authorities. These systems of 'regional offices' do not have a significant role in policy-making, with one exception: the regional health authorities, whose function it is to administer health and welfare provisions. These authorities therefore exercise their functions according to directives from central government.

Local authorities are not autonomous; they are dependent to a large extent upon directives from central government. Nevertheless, they are important bodies in making or developing policies. Some Acts of Parliament may provide them with the benefits of implementing some welfare measures. Policy-making in local government is the responsibility of elected members. Councillors often represent the same political parties as at Westminster. Since local authorities act as agencies or enablers of welfare implementation, their contact with the local population gives them a good understanding of people's responses to the services provided, and how effective they are. Any strong resentment, ill-feelings, or discontent from the localities can be transmitted to the appropriate councillors and/or MPs, who will thereafter represent their views in the Commons. Local policies will be assessed, evaluated, and altered after a lengthy process of communication and debates within the local councils, and between the latter and central government as appropriate.

Many local authorities have a network system of 'policy committees', whose aim is to co-ordinate the activities of the authority as a whole.

■ PRESSURE GROUPS

Pressure groups are very simply groups of people who have united their efforts in an informal way to represent their shared views, values, and beliefs regarding specific social issues. Their main aim is to influence Parliament and Government in the way decisions are made and carried out, to the benefit of their members and the causes they support. In attempting to cause social change through changes in social policies, they benefit not only their members, but also other individuals in society who, although not belonging to the group, share similar beliefs about the issues in question. The Greenpeace movement, for example, is a pressure group concerned about the environment and the maintenance of its integrity. Their activities are frequently aimed at raising public and government awareness about the implications of practices (technological or scientific, for example)—the consequences of policies from the government—likely to damage the environment, such as the disposal of nuclear waste.

The activities of pressure groups are wide ranging: they may focus on areas such as politics, finance, employment, ethnic minorities, social welfare, animal welfare, transport, sport, defence, or, as mentioned already, the environment.

Pressure groups are agents of social change. They have a recognised role in the way the country is governed. It is believed that their role is to influence those in power. The Prime Minister, ministers in the House of Commons, and MPs in the constituencies, for example, become the targets of pressure groups.

Pressure groups have become integral in the democratic political structures:

> Hence the growth of pressure, sectional or interest groups was an almost inevitable development accompanying an increasingly democratic system. Political parties may have satisfied a number of aspirations but despite their 'broad church' features could not hope to fulfil the wishes of all citizens. The formation and development of group interests was a partial answer to this problem. It is open to all individuals to exercise their right to influence the ideas and actions of MPs and Ministers by methods that are not illegal. Groups can be much more effective in this direction than individuals (Cocker, 1993).

Pressure groups are sometimes called 'lobbyists': a group of persons who aim at influencing legislators in order to cause changes in social policies on behalf of a particular interest. Norton (1991), for example, made a series of statements concerning pressure groups which demonstrate the nature of their roles: 'Lobbying

of Parliament is thus extensive. Professional lobbying is now, relative to the position before the 1970s, big business. Lobbying firms regularly advertise their services. "Amateur" lobbying by groups—and by constituents—takes place on an even greater scale.'

The growth of pressure groups is a response to the socio-economic problems and policies that affect the welfare of citizens, causing resentment and friction in the community and social unrest. Pressure groups arise to represent the peoples' views, their interests, and their aspirations for better social conditions.

Pressure groups, Norton (1991) noted, can exert influence by resorting to the availability of the departmentally related Select Committees, which have been set up by the House of Commons since the late 1970s:

> For groups outside Westminster, the Committees have acted as magnets. Groups focus their attention on them, submit evidence to them (be it solicited or unsolicited) and may even be invited to send representatives to appear for questioning before the committee. By approaching a Committee, a group may be persuaded to take up an issue—one that government may have little interest in or time for—and hence get the issue on to the agenda of public debate (Norton, 1991).

These channels allow pressure groups to penetrate into the affairs of governmental social policy-making processes. These are opportunities not to be missed, since they open and pave the way towards exposing crucial social policy issues on the agenda for debate, consideration, and, in the long-term, possible implementation. Their action hence may highlight a particular problem or a set of social issues at ground level—or at an individual level. Thus, their influence and actions can sway government. When groups tend to manifest a fairly broad representation of a particular community (e.g. the Confederation of British Industries, CBI), they are consulted by the government and are invited to participate in debates in Whitehall working groups or advisory councils. If legislation is agreed to be essential, proposals are drafted and then distributed to interested groups for analysis, discussions, and comments.

To some extent, the relationship between the government and pressure groups is one of dependency; there is a consultative process whereby the government will attempt to gain the consent and co-operation of as wide a range of organisations as possible, to make sure that the implementation of policies is met in a positive manner by the groups concerned.

Pressure groups are not ignored by the government, because their contribution from grass-roots' level can be invaluable. It is said, for example, that sometimes a department of government is legally obliged to consult with interested groups: 'The government has a duty to consult organised interests, providing the pressure groups involved have a broad enough membership for them to represent a majority view, and that they observe confidentiality about their discussions with the department' (HMSO, 1995).

The expertise of pressure groups is also used by civil service officers. These officers may have either direct or indirect contact with the groups. The advice of these groups is important in the preparation of policy or legislation; the groups may also express their concerns about certain social matters. For example, the Law Society, which is involved in the administration of policy, acts a pressure group: its opinions are important in keeping the government *au fait* with legal matters and developments as they affect the public.

The aims of pressure groups are to utilise as many avenues as possible to influence government, and consequently policy-making.

They approach MPs to express opinions and to ask them to present their views in Parliament or the House of Commons; they gather petitions from the public to protest against government policy and to stimulate action and new initiatives.

▼ Models of Social Welfare Provision

Welfare provision is the result of decisions from social policy making bodies of government. The aim of welfare provision is to ensure the delivery of services to citizens of society. The Welfare State's role is to provide basic security 'from the cradle to the grave'. The provision of services must meet the demand, across as wide a spectrum of social living as possible.

However, it is a fact that although social provision is provided by the State, there are individual actions that contribute towards the alleviation of social problems, and helping those in need. Thus, in Britain one finds philanthropic organisations or individuals who donate to charities, with the objective of helping to reduce social problems and to support those in needs—the poor, the homeless, the unemployed, the disabled, those with mental illhealth, and so on. It is a theme that has been operating for a number of years, as Ware and Goodin (1990) explained: 'At the individual level in 19th century Britain, for instance, we find people making donations to charities (to assist those already in need) and also insuring, through contributions to a friendly society, against certain risks that might place their own family in need.'

Some policies of social-welfare provision, Ware and Goodin (1990) argued, are formulated to meet 'actual needs', whereas others are designed to meet needs from an 'insurance principle'. They identified some models of welfare provision to be:

- the residualist (or needs-based) model;
- the insurance (or contributions-based) model;
- the social citizenship (or rights-based) model.

■ THE RESIDUALIST OR NEEDS-BASED MODEL

This model is founded on the principle that citizens have needs: health needs, employment needs, the need to live in accommodation of an adequate standard, the need to cope with changes in socio-environmental conditions (e.g. relocation, demolition of an estate or slum areas, or the building of a motorway across an area where there is population nearby). A person's need is based on being able to acquire the basic resources to survive: money to buy food and clothing and to obtain some shelter. The state should make provision to attend to such needs, and to prevent deterioration of living standards; hence, individuals who are unable to attain the minimum standard of basic needs should receive support from the state accordingly.

However, it is not so straightforward. Ware and Goodin (1990) explained: 'In so far as the need is for financial assistance, some form of test has to be applied to discover whether a person is in need or not, and this usually involves them having to divulge all the assets available to them ("means testing").' The authors argued that programmes of welfare assistance are not made easily available to individuals, who may be unaware of their entitlement to welfare provision. Furthermore, many people who do apply for benefits refer to the complexities created by jargons within the documen-tation they have to fill in. There is also the factual evidence, at an individual level, of the stigma attached to 'claiming benefits', and reports about the negative attitudes of some staff towards claimants.

In this model, individuals can claim according to a failure to meet basic personal needs. 'State expenditures are simply determined by how far those in need fall below that standard' (Ware and Goodwin, 1990). Benefits are distributed according to present need. Groups in need in society are identified; the poor, the aged, and the sick, for example. Resources will subsequently be allocated to reach such target groups. The policies are expected to consider equal distribution of social welfare facilities to the needy: the 'to-each-according-to-his-needs' philosophy.

■ THE INSURANCE OR CONTRIBUTIONS-BASED MODEL

The difference between this model and the one above is found in the principle that a person who has contributed a set amount of finance in the past is entitled to certain benefits. The contributions, for example as in the National Insurance scheme, do not necessarily have to have been made by the individuals themselves, but could have been made for them by their employers or relatives. In this model, the contributions become the important factors in the delivery of appropriate provision. Ware and Goodin (1990) argued that the 'level of coverage is not related to need, because payments may be made to those who are not in need, while those who are may have no entitlements whatsoever'. For example, an ex-British Steel worker who has £50,000 in the bank and is now unemployed, is entitled to claim unemployment benefits if there is evidence of past contributions to the scheme.

■ SOCIAL CITIZENSHIP OR RIGHTS-BASED MODEL

This model—as the name implies—is related to the belief that a citizen of any community has a right to receive welfare benefits. It is based on the rights of an individual who is a member of any society and can show evidence of permanent residence. There is no means testing, unlike the residualist model.

Although these models provide us with a framework that can be used to assess the validity and effectiveness of welfare provisions, there are limitations to their distinctive features. The needs-based model is fairly similar to the social citizenship model. For example, a social citizen in *need* of healthcare has a *right* to obtain the necessary provision, assuming permanence of residence is proved. With the insurance model, a person who is a social citizen and in need of social welfare provision has the right to claim services not merely on the grounds of being a citizen of the community, but also because he or she has been a contributor to the insurance scheme.

▼ Summary

In this chapter, we considered the nature of social policy; its definition, its features, and its links with the provision of social welfare. An overview of its interdisciplinary nature is outlined, as well as the role of government in the decision-making processes, prior to the implementation of policies that aim at meeting the needs of citizens. A brief survey of the development of the Welfare State is provided to highlight the main background features of the origins of present-day welfare provision. The Beveridge Report of 1942 was mentioned in this context,

since it has always been interpreted as one of the crucial sociopolitical developments of British welfare history.

The role of government in policy-making is emphasised. In particular, the functions of the House of Commons and the Cabinet, and the roles of pressure groups and the Civil Service described. The relationships between local government and central government is explained. It has been argued that the relationships are based on partnership and conflict; the conflict is generated from endeavours of central government to exercise expenditure control on local authorities. The role of local authorities in policy-making processes should not be underestimated. Their close contact with the local population facilitates their assessment of local needs. In this process they are supported by the appropriate councillors, representing the relevant political parties, who have a supportive network of MPs to express their views in the Commons.

The role of the Civil Service in policy-making is as important. Civil servants are high-grade administrative officers employed by government and its ministers. They have crucial roles in policy-making: their experience of political machinery, their regular contact with pressure-group organisations, and their experiences of departmental procedures help them to debate and discuss with relevant ministers the integrity of certain policies and how popular such policies are likely to be.

Pressure groups, too, are influential in policy-making processes. Government departments consult with highly representative pressure-group bodies: one example is the CBI. There is thus a close link between pressure groups and ministers, as well as MPs. Pressure groups regularly contact MPs to discuss issues pertinent to the groups in question and to expose social issues that may affect society as a whole (for example, the effects of nuclear wastes on the environment, awareness of which may be raised by pressure groups such as Greenpeace).

The models of social welfare provision that have been identified are: the residualist (or needs-based) model, the insurance (or contributions-based) model, and the citizenship (or rights-based) model. The needs-based model is concerned with supporting people who are unable to meet a minimum standard of living. The insurance model is founded on financial contributions made by the individual, who is hence guaranteed certain benefits accordingly. The rights-based model is related to being a citizen of a community, who has the rights of welfare, as long as permanence of residence is proved. These models have some overlapping features: every individual of permanent residence has a right to social welfare provision; every individual is likely to experience a certain need for social welfare provision at sometime in life; and most individuals are likely to have contributed to an insurance scheme of some kind.

▼ Application to Clinical Practice

We must not be deflected by the caustic comments of those within the profession who feel that nurse education should encompass purely psychomotor or hands-on skills. Subjects such as social policy, if planned and taught well, are as essential to effective nurse preparation as any traditional subject. To differ on this point merely serves to limit us to being capable assistants to other health care professionals (Gormley, 1995).

Manthorpe (1988) argued the relevance of social policy as applied to district nursing,

too. The social policy knowledge that health-care professionals gain in training gives them insight into the effects of legislative changes on the lives of citizens, increasing their awareness of their own and others' lives and how these are affected by a constantly changing and developing world. Manthorpe (1988) pointed out: 'We are seeing radical social changes that will affect district nurses, their families, their colleagues and above all, their patients and carers.' Gormley (1995) expressed similar beliefs: 'Changes currently taking place in terms of health economics, mixed markets and quality of care packages will be more dramatic than the combined changes of the past half century.'

In what ways can a knowledge of social policy facilitate the delivery of care in any healthcare setting? To what extent can social policy be used to enhance patients' satisfaction, increase the confidence of practitioners, and sharpen their reflective skills?

Gormley (1995) asserted that a sound knowledge of social policy can only help nurses 'to exert the necessary pressure on government to ensure the provision of health education, proper nutrition, safer water, basic sanitation and adequate housing in addition to the preventive, and rehabilitative services that the health service already provides'. In this context, nurses can be seen to act the role of a pressure group.

At the micro-level, nurses' knowledge of social policy can help them to work in closer partnership with other professionals—district nurses, social workers, and mental healthcare workers, for instance—by being able to identify relevant policies to suit the social needs of their clients, to discuss their limitations or effectiveness, and to choose alternative approaches accordingly.

The need to know which benefits are available for specific client groups and the agencies capable of delivering social welfare provision becomes important. Although there are other professionals, such as social workers, whose responsibilities are to support clients with social problems, the nurses' skills and knowledge become complementary. The frequent use of jargon in documentation from benefits agencies should be borne in mind when explaining to patients their entitlement. Spending time with patients who are nearing discharge into the community, to explain the relevant forms to be filled in and what they are used for, would help to reduce the anxieties associated with discharge planning.

Insight into the political framework of government intervention in healthcare delivery could, for example, help the practitioner to anticipate the difficulties patients with particular needs may experience once in the community. This knowledge base can only help in preparing and educating patients who are not familiar with the intricacies of social welfare provision to gain an understanding of what types of services are readily available to them.

On the other hand, there are patients in healthcare settings who possess political awareness. A nurse who is acutely aware of current social issues and government policies, who has some knowledge of legislative processes, can discuss and debate these topics with such patients during therapeutic interactions. Patients have a variety of interests: policy issues may be some of them.

The practitioner's repertoire of reflective skills can also be enhanced. Reflecting on one's psychomotor skills is good and essential; but reflecting by interweaving into one's repertoire the broader sociopolitical framework within which one practices is an essential objective to achieve.

▼ Review Questions

1 Discuss the context within which the making of policy takes place.

2 Discuss the relationships between social policy-making and welfare provision.

▼ References

Abel-Smith B. Assessing the balance sheet. In: Glennerster H, ed. *The future of the Welfare State.* Aldershot: Gower Publishing; 1983:10–23

Brown M, Payne S. *Introduction to social administration in Britain, 7th ed.* London: Unwin Hyman; 1990.

Bulmer M, Lewis J, Piachaud D. *The goals of social policy.* London: Unwin Hyman; 1989.

Butcher T. *Delivering welfare. The governance of the Social Services in the 1990s.* Buckingham: Open University Press; 1995.

Cocker P. *Contemporary British Politics and Government.* London: Tudor; 1993.

Fraser D. *The evolution of the British Welfare State, 2nd ed.* London: Macmillan; 1984.

Gormley K. Social graces. *Nursing Times* 1995, **91**:55–57.

Hill M. *The Welfare State in Britain. A political history since 1945.* Aldershot: Edward Elgar; 1993a.

Hill M. *Understanding social policy, 4th ed.* Oxford: Blackwell; 1993b.

HMSO. *Britain 1995. An official handbook.* London: HMSO; 1994.

Mackintosh M. Introduction. In: Wuyts M, Mackintosh M, Hewitt T, eds. *Development policy and public action.* Milton Keynes: Open University Press; 1992.

Manthorpe J. The social context. *Journal of District Nursing* 1988, **7**(3):18–20.

Midwinter E. *The development of social welfare in Britain.* Buckingham: Open University Press; 1994.

Norton P. *New directions in British politics? Essays on the evolving constitution.* Aldershot: Edward Elgar; 1991.

Pampel F, Williamson J. *Age, class, politics and the Welfare State.* Cambridge: Cambridge University Press; 1989.

Pascall G. *Social policy. A feminist analysis.* London: Routledge; 1986.

Pope R, Pratt A, Hoyle B. *Social welfare in Britain 1885–1985.* Dover, New Hampshire: Croom Helm; 1986.

Rimmer L. Did poverty die when the Welfare State was born? In: Gaffin J, ed. *The nurse and the Welfare State.* Aylesbury: HM+M Publishers; 1981.

Sullivan M. *Modern social policy.* Hemel Hempstead: Harvester Wheatsheaf; 1994.

Ware A, Goodin R. *Needs and welfare.* London: Sage; 1990.

▼ Further Reading

Bennett F. Social policy digest. *Soc Pol* 1996, **25**:105–125.

Huby M, Whyley C. Take-up and the social fund. *Soc Pol* 1996, **25**:1–18.

Jones K. *The making of social policy in Britain 1830–1990.* London: Athlone; 1991.

Page R. The attack on the British Welfare State—more real than imagined? A leveller's tale. *Critical Soc Policy* 1995, issue 44/45:220-228.

15

Health Policy:
Health Needs and Resources

▼ What is Health Policy?

Chapter 14 dealt with social policy or, as it is sometimes called, social administration. As discussed, it has a broad interdisciplinary framework; it embraces policies executed at various levels of social life, by agencies and public organisations, with central government playing a major role in the equation of control, policy-making, and implementation. Health policy is one of the distinct policies circumscribed under the very broad configuration of social policy.

Health is paramount for the survival of the human species; consequently, society finds it imperative to take sufficient measures to secure its continuity. Continuity of health can be assured by the performance of policies from government organisations. The main objectives are to prevent illhealth; to treat illhealth when it occurs; and to take further preventive measures, through health education and health promotion programmes, to reduce the possibilities of its recurrence.

To study health policy, therefore, is to study the ramifications of the development of health services and policies for health: for example, public health services, services for the care of mothers and children, the health insurance and hospital services, the structure of the NHS–their functions, their effectiveness, and the types of expenditures incurred. Other issues associated with this concept are health needs and resources, as well as the methods of allocation and the degree of equality of distribution observed. Primary care and community care are other pertinent issues. Associated with the many areas described so far are topics concerning health reforms and their implications in care distribution.

The aim of this chapter is to present a synopsis of the main features of health policy as applied to the NHS and community care. We first set the scene by briefly surveying the NHS from the time of its inception to 1996. This outlines its background, its progress, its limitations, the types of images it has created, and what is happening now, peoples' perception of its development, and the effectiveness of recommended reforms.

▼ The NHS: Original Structure and Administration

The NHS was created in Britain in 1948 and was a major landmark in British welfare history. It was inspired by the Beveridge Report of 1942. This report was influential in leading a consensus on the view that needs and resources should be mobilised to tackle social problems such as 'want, ignorance and disease'. As a result of the Beveridge report, 'all political parties subscribed to the view that universal access to a comprehensive health care service should form part of the post war settlement' (Laing, 1994).

At the initial evolutionary stage, the hospitals were organised separately to the primary care, and community services fell within the responsibility of local government rather than the Health Service (Paton, 1992).

Laing described it as a 'tripartite' system, with three separate administrative structures:

- Hospital management committees and boards of governors of teaching hospitals, run by the hospitals.
- Community health services operated by local authorities.
- General practitioners (GPs), pharmacists, dentists, and opticians, all of whom worked as independent contractors to executive councils.

The British Medical Association (BMA), exercising its power as one of the major pressure groups in the healthcare system, influenced government at an early stage of the NHS inception to accept their proposals for 'retention of the independent contractor system for GPs: the option of private practice and access to pay beds in NHS hospitals for hospital consultants; a system of distinction awards; a major role in the administration of the service at all levels; and success in resisting local government control' (Ham, 1992). Laing (1994) pointed out that it was hospital doctors' fear of the NHS being under local government control—which could have caused disruption of their clinical autonomy—that led to pressure being applied from that group. This pressure, together with 'the unsuitability of local government areas for administration of hospital service' (Ham, 1992), led to the separation of hospitals from community services, and local authorities losing their administrative control of hospitals.

The belief of the political parties at the time was founded on the original philosophy of Beveridge to create a decentralised, publicly funded healthcare system: to secure equality of healthcare throughout the country. Allsop (1984) summarised the ethos of the NHS philosophy as being based on the State's collective responsibility for comprehensive health services to be provided, with equal access for all its citizens. The National Health Service Act of 1946, Allsop (1984) argued, paved the way towards an increasing commitment from central government to fund a health service that rested on the principles of collectivism, comprehensiveness, equality, and universality. Although these major objectives have not been realised satisfactorily, the foundation of the principles, however, remains 'intrinsic to the idea of a nationalised health care' (Allsop, 1984).

The popularity of this nationalised healthcare system is nationally and internationally recognised. The value placed on its recognised philosophy of 'healthcare for all' has become an important feature—in spite of arguments about its flaws and its increasing proportion of national expenditure. Johnson (1990) pointed out:

> The NHS has a place in our national life. It has always had a particular significance in Fabian and Labour Party circles as is indicated by Titmuss' description of it as 'the most unsordid act of British Social Policy in the 20th century which has allowed and encouraged sentiments of altruism, reciprocity and social duty, to express themselves; to be made explicit and identifiable in measurable patterns of behaviour by all social groups and classes.

The NHS, Klein (1989) reiterated, is internationally unique; it is the 'only national health care system centrally financed and directed, operating in a pluralistic political environment'.

Despite its popularity, the NHS was giving cause for concern from birth; it was not a flawless system. The tripartite system, identified above, was seen as non-integrative, prone to fragmentation and the distancing of healthcare planning and implementation of services. For the next 25 years, Laing (1994) asserted, the

agenda for reform of the NHS was dominated by the perceived need to achieve more effective unification of the three parts. Health policymakers believed that a more integrated healthcare system was a precondition for improving treatment, particularly for patients with chronic conditions whose needs required a coordinated response. Various arguments against the tripartite system were given:

- The lack of integration between hospital and community services interfered or restrained planning and development services.
- Professional isolation: GPs were perceived to maintain distance from 'mainstream hospital practices'.
- Failure to establish a proper management structure and 'an integrated corporate culture' (Strong & Robinson, 1990).
- Although, as Strong and Robinson explained, important advances were made to ensure coordination and distribution of healthcare, the complexity of the system did not give scope for equal distribution of modern facilities across the country: 'Some areas were richly resourced, others poorly provided for.'

However, as Strong and Robinson (1990) pointed out, measures were taken to combat the problems of distribution from the early 1960s to the 1970s. For example, to meet the needs of the local population there were major schemes to build hospitals equipped with modern medical specialties; attempts were made to refocus care planning from a 'vertical' direction to a 'more systematic approach', establishing links among its constituent parts. The authors described how regions were divided into districts, each based around a District General Hospital, but also running other local medical services such as psychiatric hospitals and community nursing; systematic efforts were made to shift resources to the community and to long-term care.

▼ NHS Reforms

■ THE 1974 REORGANISATION

At a very early stage of NHS organisation, in the early 1950s, it became clear to health policy-makers, the media, and the public that the 'days of financial innocence' for the NHS were over. As Klein (1989) put it: 'The realisation that the contrast between infinite opportunities for spending money and all too finite availability of resources had been revealed.' A lack of consideration had been given to the financial implications of setting up the system; the NHS had developed into a bureaucratic organisation.

The 1974 reorganisation became known as the first of a series of major reforms. It must be remembered, however, that in 1966. The Salman report made some changes to the nursing management structure: the institution of a 'Director of Nursing Service' replaced the old 'hospital matron'; and line management sturctures were created.

The 1974 reforms introduced a new corporate structure, 'devised in key part by management consultants and modelled on modern business lines' (Klein, 1989). These reforms took place during a Labour government. According to Le Grand et al. (1991), the reforms did not exploit the opportunity to make radical changes, but included some modifications that showed a 'reversal of policy':

● Decisions were made to phase out private beds in NHS hospitals.

● Medical insurance paid for by the employer was to be taxed as an employee benefit at all levels of remuneration.

The principal concern of policy during the 70s was the re-allocation of resources to the relatively deprived regions and to priority services for the elderly, the mentally ill, and the mentally disabled (Le Grand et al., 1991). Strategic restructuring and the unification of services were other priorities.

The corporate structure was headed by the Department of Health, followed by 14 regional health authorities (RHAs). The RHAs were given finance and hospital-building functions, and their role was to manage 90 area health authorities (AHAs). The AHAs had responsibility for providing community health services—district nursing, health visiting, etc.—and for overseeing the work of the family practice committee. The district management team was the lowest tier in the structure, with a representative function and responsibility to assure a full range of general health and social services. Community health councils (CHCs) were introduced to provide an element of consumer participation. These councils were purely consultative in nature.

Although unification of the tripartite system was largely achieved (Laing, 1994), there was still a separation of community health services from personal services. Jones (1991) argued that the 1974 reorganisation was cumbersome because of the four-tier structure. Although it was considered a major move towards producing efficient and coordinated care, problems and issues still remained (Butler, 1993; Laing, 1994). Concerns were expressed about availability of resources for the long-term funding of the service, to meet local health needs of the population and to ensure medical and nursing treatment to suit needs as required. Furthermore, although the reorganisation included measures to achieve equality of resource distribution to RHAs and AHAs, by the introduction of resource-allocation working parties, according to Laing this did not guarantee an effective method for calculating the relative need of the population for healthcare resources.

■ THE 1982 RESTRUCTURING

When the Conservative government came into office in 1979, they published a consultative document, *Patients First* (DHSS 1979) and incorportated some of the recommendations of the Royal Commission on the NHSS (1979). The AHA tier was removed and the health district became the key accountable body for providing and planning services for their population.

The service, however was being criticised for its inadequacy, the increasing expenditure it was generating, its 'dominance by authoritarian professions, its lack of clear lines of accountability and its sharply demarcated separation from the private sector, and its overwhelming reliance on Treasury funding' (Butler, 1993).

These negative features provided the impetus for the Conservative government, under the administration of Margaret Thatcher, to instigate a thorough scrutiny of the NHS.

In October 1983, there appeared a 25-page report of the NHS Management Inquiry led by Sir Roy Griffiths (Klein, 1989). The report concluded that the service was stagnant and bureaucratic; that consensus decision-making led to long delays in the management process. The prescription (Perrin, 1988) that Griffiths advocated was:

- The fostering of a leadership style of management at all levels down to units.
- A business-style management budget to be developed down to the level of individual clinicians, the natural managers of the hospital services.
- The application of clinical management budgeting, which would lead to a positive impact on improving resource utilisation.

A business style of management—introduced at regional, district, and unit levels—made general managers accountable for their performances; management-budgeting and resource-management programmes were begun (Ham, 1991).

The Griffiths report set the scene for more strategic and decisive NHS reforms in the future. The employment of managers from the top of the corporate structure aimed at increasing the efficiency of the services to suit local demands—a rippling effect, so it was expected, from the top to the bottom of the hierarchy, where care and services are delivered. The foundation for the future of an 'internal market' was laid. As Butler (1993) asserted:

> It laid down the foundations of a management culture of command and obedience that increased the responsiveness of the NHS to political direction. And it created a climate of opinion and practice that finally enabled the government to implement its plan for the internal markets in the NHS in the face of unremitting opposition from all professional groups in the service.

▼ Reforms in the 1990s (the internal market model)

Three White Papers were influential in paving the way towards further draconian reforms of the NHS:

- *Promoting better Health* (1987).
- *Working for Patients* (1989).

- *Caring for People* (1989).

The government maintained that the basic principles of the NHS would remain the same: the availability of health services to all, irrespective of means, and most services free at the point of use (Ham, 1991).

The philosophy of government to increase consumer choice was embodied in the 1987 White Paper *Promoting better Health*: patients would have the freedom to choose and change their GPs. GPs were expected to advertise their services to the consumers. The capitation fee for GPs was increased, from 46% to 60%, in order to increase their incentive to attract patients (Laing, 1994). To maintain their credibility, GPs were also expected to demonstrate health-promoting activities within their departments, as well as to set up preventive programmes to minimise, for example, heart disease and complications of diabetes.

The 1989 White Paper *Working for Patients*—the result of a government review of the NHS—added another impact to the NHS reforms. As Laing (1994) explained, there was widespread criticism of underfunding in those years, particularly from the healthcare professions.

The ethos of this document is embodied in the principles described below:

- To increase competitiveness between purchasers of healthcare services (health authorities, services departments in local authorities, and GPs) and providers of healthcare services [primary healthcare services, directly managed units (non-NHS trusts), NHS trusts, independent hospitals, nursing and residential homes, council-run social services, and large GP practices].
- To instill market principles to make services more responsive to patients.
- To create drive in order to promote greater efficiency and equality in the use of resources.
- To strengthen management arrangements by reviewing health authorities along business lines.
- To make doctors more accountable for their performance.
- To emphasise the implementation of extending resource-management initiatives to involve doctors and nurses in management.
- To introduce medical audit to monitor efficiency of care delivery and resources.

The 1989 White Paper *Caring for people* was a response to the Griffiths report *Community Care: Agenda for Action* published in 1988. It (1989 White paper) aimed at promoting a more efficient service by giving local authorities the lead in the planning of community care (Ham, 1991):

- Local authorities would become enablers and purchasers of care.
- They would be helped in their tasks by the allocation of financial resources.
- They would devise plans for community care.
- They would participate in the assessment and management of care.
- They would work collaboratively with NHS authorities.

The 1991 reorganisation was the culmination of previous reviews and recommendations of White Papers, which created the foundations for using internal market principles.

NHS provision for community care followed the recommendations of the NHS and Community Care Act of 1990. Since the implementation of the act in 1993, services for community care have undergone major changes.

▼ Community Care

In healthcare debates, the term 'community' has been used to demarcate the differentiation between hospital care and primary care (i.e. that delivered by district and community nursing, and by midwifery personnel).

Community care is about providing health and social care services to the population in need. Its goal is to make the best use of available scarce resources to implement methods of intervention aimed at empowering the individual in his or her community setting. To achieve this goal, a multidisciplinary team approach is crucial; the holistic needs of people can only be met when there is collaboration between health and social care agencies (Nocon, 1994).

The aim of the NHS and Community Care Act of 1990 was to stimulate the provision of, and produce better integration among, health services, in particular between hospitals and community services. However, Lawson (1993) argued that the impact by the end of the community care reforms generally was significantly less than originally intended. He went on to outline the possible causes:

- Inadequate financial resources and a lack of prioritisation concerning community care needs.
- Delays in implementation.
- Uncertainty about future financing of community care, caused by a non-confident attitude regarding the adequacy of resources to be transferred from the Department of Social Security (DSS).

Lart and Means (1993) pointed out that charging for services, like home care, day care, meals-on-wheels, and aids and adaptations, became a crucial issue for local authorities in planning and implementing community care. It contradicted the theoretical underpinnings of the philosophy of free welfare provision.

It must be appreciated, however, that community care is not solely a concept of statutory care provision, developed and facilitated by local authorities and other agencies: community care also includes aspects of care delivered by the 'informal sector'. Johnson (1990) stated:

> More often than not community care means care by families especially nuclear families. Within the informal sector, bonds of kinship support the strongest reciprocal obligations . . . To deny the importance of the family as a source of care would be to ignore the accumulated evidence of several decades. Nevertheless, informal care by families faces considerable pressure at present and this is likely to intensify during the 1990s.

A distinction is also made regarding what community care is: care *in* the community or care *by* the community. Very often it means the care given *in* the community by kin and networks of friends and neighbours. On the other hand, care delivered by statutory agencies—primary healthcare and hospital trusts—can be considered as given *by* the community, since the term 'community' could easily encompass all groups of individuals in a social setting (community hospitals, residential homes, nursing homes, etc.), as well as local authorities, and other agencies. However, whatever approaches are used, care requires the urgent and imperative collaboration between statutory staff who are immediately involved in the provision of services.

Hence, a multidisciplinary team approach should be considered, in any healthcare delivery, to include the contribution of both formal and informal carers. As Nocon (1994) pointed out:

> The contribution of informal carers has itself been frequently taken for granted, and their participation in service planning has been minimal. The voice of users, similarly has seldom been heard, yet if services are to be appropriate and effective, it is essential

that users are fully involved in decisions about both service planning and delivery.

The concept of collaboration and partnership in care should also be reflected in the ways health and social care are made accessible to users. Northway (1996) argued that the effects of the reforms advocated by the White Paper *Caring for People* are now being felt. She made particular reference to the division that has been created between health and social care. The divide has obvious implications for the adequacy of health and social care delivery, as well as causing tension between the agencies involved regarding where responsibilities lie.

The principles of the reform advocated by the NHs and Community Care Act of 1990 are based on the belief that individuals should be provided with access to facilities to satisfy their health and social needs. Northway (1996) explained that this was to be accomplished through the introduction of care management, under which needs would be identified and an individual package of care devised. It was emphasised that a written plan should be produced, detailing the services to be provided, and that the views and preferences of clients should be considered.

These clinical objectives can only be met when care organisations in the community— health professionals, social services, and voluntary agencies—maintain effective and collaborative discussion concerning the best approaches to be used in the assessment and planning of care. At present there is a fragmentation of service due to a lack of differentiation between healthcare and social care. A broad interpretation of healthcare would comprise the physical, psychological, spiritual, and social aspects. However, as Northway (1996) explained, the term is often interpreted to mean measures aimed at curing sickness and the management of symptoms of illhealth and

disability based purely on a medical model. Social care, on the other hand, is seen to be 'non-medical', concerned with the maintenance of an individual's social-life activities.

It is difficult for healthcare professionals easily to accept this demarcation. Their training and clinical professionalism have instilled and developed in them beliefs and values associated with holistic care intervention—the belief that the 'whole' person's needs must be accepted, assessed, and identified.

Close collaboration between services, to ensure that the complex health and social needs of people are met, is not presently happening for the following reasons:

- There is a shortfall in understanding regarding the effects of a lack of social care on the health of the person, and vice versa.
- There are resource implications (funding): strain caused by financial considerations limits agencies' involvement in care. Economic constraints are thus implicated.
- Social care may be charged for: healthcare is still mainly free at the point of delivery.
- District nurses are undertaking non-nursing work because of the lack of services offered by other agencies, in an attempt to 'cover gaps' in social-care provision.
- Charging for social care will affect the uptake of provision by specific client groups who are unable to pay. A financial assessment to identify affordability will further discourage uptake.
- The lack of coordination between care agencies causes fragmentation and loss of care continuity. Northway (1996) explained how some patients being discharged into community settings from 'acute hospitals' do not have appropriate community care being arranged.

Northway (1996) distinguished some positive innovations to alleviate the dilemmas faced by local authorities and health organisations in relation to the health and social care divide:

- Joint commissioning: aimed at creating joint agreements between agencies for commissioning services for a client group.
- Locality purchasing: aimed at purchasing healthcare services tailored to personal needs.
- Cash payments: a proposal by government to allow social services departments to make cash payments to disabled people instead of providing community care services. This would give clients more autonomy in purchasing services specific to their health and social needs.

The reforms are attracting dissatisfaction, not only among healthcare professionals in the community and in local authorities, but among GPs as well (Leese & Bosanquet, 1996). These authors conducted a study to investigate the views of group practice GPs regarding the effects of the 1990 contract and fundholding on general practice organisation. They concluded that GPs were generally unhappy with the NHS reforms, as evidenced by their continued opposition, their concerns about levels of workload and administration, and their desire to retire early. On the other hand, there were some positive outcomes from the reforms: 'A sizeable minority of group practice respondents (38%) agreed that the quality of services provided in general practices had improved considerably since the introduction of the 1990 contract.'

▼ The Future of Health Policy

There is no doubt that health policies of the future will undergo further major changes; it would be unrealistic to argue otherwise. The identified changes that have occurred in the distant past show us that health services are not fixed entities; that health administrative structures are not permanent features; that health policies should not be interpreted solely along traditional methods, but should be reassessed, redefined, re-evaluated, adapted, and transformed, to reflect present and future needs.

The Welfare State is a well-established system in British society, but there is some doubt—in political circles, in the media, and among academics—whether it will continue to survive in the 1990s and beyond. Le Grand (1991), commenting on the integrity of the Welfare State, wrote: 'It seems reasonable to describe the Welfare State over the period 1973–1987 as a success. It survived: key parts even thrived. Welfare outcomes rose: some inequalities diminished and others were far less than they would have been had there been no Welfare State.'

I would point out that from the late 1980s to present time—in spite of the vast amount of literature on recent reforms, and the exposure of dissatisfaction among users and providers of health services—there have been some positive outcomes from the changes. These include increased managerial responsibilities; tighter budgetary control; opportunities to apply business methods in health practices; increased accountability; opportunities to develop professional collaboration and partnership with other agencies; opportunities for consumers to exercise choice to suit their needs. Furthermore, as Laing (1994) pointed out, funding was given to agents acting on behalf of consumers (as with GP fundholders buying services on behalf of their patients).

These are some of the positive developments. For further developments to be pursued along the lines of efficiency and equity at the point of delivery, health policy of the future should consider methods aimed at increasing the credibility of the 'internal market' model of health services; for example, 'access to accurate information on costs and quality, appropriate motivation on the part of both purchasers and providers' (Laing, 1994).

This 'quasi market' (another term used to mean the 'internal market' mechanism) will in the future—if developed as anticipated—increase competitiveness for provision from independent agencies. Le Grand (1991) opined:

> If these reforms are carried through to their logical conclusion, the Welfare State in the 1990s will be one where local authorities will not own and operate schools, houses and residential homes, and where health authorities will not own and operate hospitals ...

Instead:

> Private and voluntary institutions will be financed by local and Central government, as they compete for custom. There will be a shift from the State as funder, perhaps only as a residual role as provider, which will have an impact on the way services are delivered and employees treated.

Socio-economic factors will have an impact on care services and resources. Poverty, unemployment, homelessness, road-traffic accidents, and disabilities of various kinds—psychological and physical—are perennial problems. The increase in the elderly population, particularly those aged 80 years and over, will impinge on the availability of scarce health resources: 'Even if some improvement in the overall health of 80 year olds is allowed for, there is likely to be a substantial rise in the demands for health and social care from this group and hence from the third age overall, (Le Grand, 1991).

There are other social factors that health policy-makers must anticipate and prepare for. For example, the increase in air travel has facilitated population mobility from one corner of the world to another. The implications for health are wide ranging. We have already experienced, and still are experiencing, the impact of AIDS on humans, and the drain that this has on financial resources. The possibility of humankind's exposure to other—yet unknown—diseases, as well as unknown bacteria and viruses, must be recognised and acted upon if preventive health is to be exercised.

Although modern medical technology can cope with many pathological and environmental conditions that affect humankind, the refinement of equipment to increase its sensitivity and effectiveness in combating diseases is imperative. The use of computerisation in healthcare services, for example, has helped to accelerate the identification of diseases by using methods of imagery and ultrasound scan. Technological innovation, although initially extremely expensive, produces major resources used by many healthcare organisations to meet needs. For example, Ham (1992) described how lasers have been applied most effectively in eye surgery, in the removal of skin blemishes, and by chest surgeons to clear airways that have become blocked because of lung cancer.

These changes in the healthcare system demand a high level of specialisation and training for clinicians. For professionals to specialise in specific fields of scientific innovation and advances, resources must be mobilised accordingly. Health policies must therefore be designed with a futuristic outlook, in readiness for other highly technological innovations. The allocation of resources has to respond to future demands.

Modernisation in healthcare systems is sometimes viewed with incredulity by users of health services, who have been accustomed to traditional methods of healthcare: the 'as-in-the-old-days' attitude. Health policies of the future should be reliant on as broad a set of perspectives as possible, obtained from users of health and social services. This may be achieved by tapping into the benefits of systematic research findings.

It is the responsibility of healthcare providers to want to obtain the views of service users (Mc Iver, 1991). This ambition becomes even more imperative in view of recent NHS reforms. Draconian changes, as we have experienced in the Health Services, should be encountered with robust systems of evaluation: the application of systematic research programmes to analyse the views of users, as well as providers, and the findings to be collated and subsequently utilised for future health policies.

A basic initial approach towards this major undertaking of obtaining accurate information from users and providers would consist of, using McIver's terms, an identification of 'conceptual and methodological issues' to be resolved:

- Obtaining a representative sample of users.
- Asking the right questions.
- Asking questions in an appropriate manner.
- Understanding and interpreting the data correctly.

The recruitment of highly experienced researchers from not only the healthcare systems, but also from the business world, will strengthen the process. If a business type of management is to be developed in healthcare, such an eclectic approach would give opportunities to combine ideas from other professions in problem-solving research, with the ultimate aim of developing a better, more efficient, and equitable healthcare service.

The content of medical and nursing literature exposes clear concerns about the effects of reforms on the patients. However, it is equally important that the impact of reforms on the personnel in the Health Services is assessed. Social change is stressful. Personnel have to alter their 'traditional' methods of tackling professional problems. A business style of management— tight budgetary control, constraints on resources, a consumer charter, constraints on staffing level, the tension and conflict caused by regrading—become stressors for professionals in Health Services.

Health policies of the future should contain a clause specific to the possible needs of healthcare professionals for counselling and specialised training free at the point of delivery and for support in undertaking new and challenging tasks. Research in this area is therefore essential.

The opinions of professionals and users of the service are integral to the process of health policy. For example, Ong (1993) commented:

> An important example of research which starts by asking local people and workers what they think, need and want in relation to health policy and provision is the West Lambeth study on Clapham, London . . . The study intended to enable people to redefine health and health needs, in order that the results would influence planners and policy makers. It used a 'bottom up' approach and emphasised the necessity of including lay perspectives in formulating a complete picture of health inequities.

Consideration of the lay definition of health is necessary as this will give an insight into the public's perception of the services offered by health and social care agencies. These findings are invaluable for future health planning.

Similarly, the professionals' health views, and their personal experiences of healthcare and social care at the point of delivery, are important. They are the managers of healthcare; they are the key agents of change in the NHS (Spurgeon & Barwell, 1991); their contribution will help to enhance future policies.

We have seen how medical advances and technology are influencing the Health Services, with new innovative ideas in care provision and facilities. At an even more futuristic level, as we enter the twenty-first century, the wind of social change will gather more pace. In the field of space sciences, experts are studying and analysing the possibilities of establishing people (other scientists, technologists, biochemists, etc.) in space laboratories. Astronauts and cosmonauts are expected to survive in an alien environment, surrounded by technological gadgetry. The impact of weightlessness on health, the stress factors linked with the isolation of space travels, and the sociopsychological environment of working in satellite laboratories, are some of the issues health policy-makers of the future will need to anticipate. Thus, as extraterrestrial human activities accelerate and expand to encounter new frontiers, health services of the future should develop and expand accordingly, to accommodate future needs.

It is possible that the NHS of the future will have extraterrestrial units in space to cater for the healthcare needs of a minority group—the scientists doing research in their space laboratories. Medical and nursing personnel will undoubtedly need specialised training to match developments such as these. Human needs for health and safety will remain the same. The causes of illhealth will become more extensive, as humankind faces new and challenging territories. The perennial problems of shortfalls in resources and funding, and their uneven distribution, will continue to make headlines in medical and nursing literature.

▼ Summary

The aim of health policy is to ensure that an integrated system of health services is in operation; a system that will meet the healthcare and social needs of a given population. To study health policy means gaining an insight and understanding of the ways and methods used to deliver welfare provision. The dimensions of health policy are varied, and include facets such as public health services, maternal and child care services, the health insurance and hospital services, the NHS and its administrative structures and reforms, as well as community care. The emphasis of health policy also includes an assessment of the needs and resources, and how the latter are distributed to meet target groups in society, for example, the elderly, the disabled, and the mentally ill.

It has been pointed out that the NHS of the 1940s, 1970s, and 1980s was not effectively administered. The first reforms started with the 1974 reorganisation under a Labour government. Some changes were made in the structure of the NHS. There were 14 regional health authorities, 90 area health authorities (AHAs), and then district management teams, with the Department of Health representing control from central government. In addition, community health councils were instituted to represent consumers' views.

Although the 1974 reorganisation was considered a major reform, it had its weaknesses. The concerns about resource allocation were not solved. There was still inequality of distribution. The introduction of resource-allocation working parties, to ensure an effective method for calculating the relative need of populations for healthcare resources, was deemed to be inadequate.

The 1982 reorganisation was an attempt to solve the problems of the 1974 reforms. The 1982 changes took place under a Conservative government led by Mrs Thatcher. In the 1982 reforms, the AHAs were abolished. The government wanted to bring an element of business-type management into the NHS. The Griffiths report of 1983 confirmed that the time was ripe to implement changes along business lines. The report concluded that the health services were stagnant, and that consensus decision-making was causing delays in the management process. The Griffiths report prescribed a leadership style of management.

It is argued that the initial changes encouraged by the report paved the way for more strategic and decisive reforms of the NHS. Three White Papers influenced this process: *Promoting better Health* (1987), *Working for Patients* (1989), and *Caring for People* (1989). These papers, and the NHS and Community Care Act of 1990, led to the 1991 reforms. An internal market model of management was introduced into the NHS. Providers of care were identified as Trust hospitals, primary healthcare services, independent hospitals, nursing and residential homes, and large GP practices, for example. Purchasers of services were the health authorities, services departments in local authorities, and GPs.

Other changes included the creation of a drive to promote more efficient use of resources, the strengthening of management arrangements by regular reviews, the introduction of medical audits, and an increase in professional accountability.

The impact of the new reforms, as reflected in the literature, has been to cause discontent and dissatisfaction about the services provided.

Financial constraints, lack of prioritisation concerning community care needs, and fragmentation of activities between healthcare and social care are some of the reasons given. Healthcare is free at the point of delivery, whereas some types of social care are not free. Some professionals in the community are trying to bridge the gaps between services by undertaking tasks that other agencies should be doing. It is argued that a system of collaboration and partnership would go a long way to improving the services.

In spite of negative responses from some quarters, the new reforms do have some positive features: increased responsibilities and opportunities to develop a business style of management, via internal market principles, to improve efficiency in patient care. Some endeavours to improve the services are evident in schemes such as joint commissioning, cash payments, and locality purchasing.

The future of health policy lies in keeping pace with the latest developments in health and social care services. It is necessary for health policy-makers to seek the views of users and providers. Therefore, systematic research must be undertaken before the implementation of other reforms.

Medical and scientific advances, demographic changes, and increases in the elderly population are some issues to be assessed when designing future health policies.

▼ Application to Clinical Practice

Changes on a massive scale, as the ones we are experiencing in the NHS, are bound to affect patients and professionals alike. In spite of changes, patient care remains first and foremost in the minds of providers of service. To provide an efficient service, healthcare professionals must first examine their own beliefs about the recent NHS changes. They should identify and assess (self-assessment) factors they feel could undermine their confidence in delivering care; for example, anxieties regarding resource management, lack of knowledge on the complexities of the internal market mechanism, or their roles in the new structures. Another issue that may impinge on practice is reliance on traditional methods of care not founded on research findings. The reforms advocate an efficient and cost-effective service, with the client in the centre of the internal market model. Professionals who are unsure about their roles will need to organise support-group sessions to discuss their needs for a supportive network and to debate the recent health-service changes and how these changes can improve their own efficiency at a clinical level. If training and further professional developments are required, it is the duty of unit managers to ascertain the provision of regular updating through workshops, study days, and appropriate courses.

The dominant theme in health care is 'empowerment of patients and clients, backed by the belief that professionals should be working in partnership with those they seek to serve' (Wright, 1995). This philosophy integrates well with the previously mentioned philosophy of collaboration and partnership in relation to health and social care services. Since the patient is the main focus of care, it is advisable to use this orientation for several reasons:

- Involving patients in nursing practice gives professionals opportunities to discover issues from the patient's perspectives. The information obtained could be vital for either present or future care intervention.

- The planning of changes to be implemented can be discussed and analysed, and constraints (e.g. resource availability) identified.
- It enhances patients' knowledge and skills to participate collaboratively in their care, empowering them in the process.

The involvement of patients in nursing practice can potentially minimise the boundaries between professionals and users of the service (Wright, 1995). The achievement of this aim can occur only in the process of renegotiation, re-identification, and re-evaluation of changing beliefs regarding health and social care. Patients nowadays are more acutely aware of health practices, due to media coverage. Their understanding of current issues should not be underestimated.

To cross boundaries, Wright (1995) commented:

> It is critical to include those who have influence over the service and its resources such as politicians, commissioning health authorities, fundholding general practitioners and family health service authorities. Local volunteer groups and patients' representatives should also be included, and links should be forged with other agencies such as social services.

It is evident that a multidisciplinary team approach is essential. Effective communication networks become priorities. The relaying of vital information from one agency to another will prevent duplication and uncertainty in relation to proposed plans of action or changes likely to affect patient care. It may be necessary for professionals 'to reach out', to work and mediate with other members of the multidisciplinary team, senior managers, and personnel from other specialties (Wright, 1995).

Other measures that may facilitate accessibility to health services, and increase the credibility of both health and social services, consist of professionals travelling to localities and meeting users in their neighbourhood, to assess health and social needs. In this way, workers in health and social care will be in a better position to assess and understand the 'racial, environmental, social, economic and political issues affecting health' (Wright, 1995).

Since users and providers of services are living in times of change, implementation rests on sensitive management at all levels. Spurgeon and Barwell (1991), writing on the role of general managers in the management of change, stated:

> To manage change the use of open meetings is essential, in the communication process of explaining the new systems; to develop relations with others including District General Manager, Unit General Managers and authority members; and building a network of contacts through which the organisation might be influenced.

A similar model of management can be used at hospital ward and community centre levels. Managers directly involved in care delivery, and their staff, have a need to express their views about change implementation; the constraints they experience in their day-to-day nursing and medical activities; their possible needs for explanation and support when they encounter clinical situations that may cause negative impact on patient care; for example, problems with discharge planning, such as a failure to identify appropriate agencies that will take responsibilities for undertaking either the health or social care of patients. Situations like these need to be exposed in debates among staff in clinical practice. A 'bottom-up' approach is necessary. The transmission of concerns from the 'shop floor' through appro-

priate channels of the management hierarchy should be done. Spoken communication, although important and speedy, has been known to become distorted by the time the message finally reaches the desired destination. Written communication should follow any spoken transmission of information to prevent fragmentation, distortion, and misinformation.

In the past, management courses have tended to be offered to clinical managers (ward sisters, charge nurses, unit managers). In view of the reforms in the NHS, every practitioner of nursing and medicine needs training in basic management principles. These principles can be applied at the most basic level of the organisation—the bedside—and will contribute to the management of care delivery, with the client and significant others as participating agents.

▼ Review Questions

1 Explore the reasons for the NHS reforms from 1974 to the present time.

2 'The views of users and providers of health services are important.' Discuss this statement in relation to recent NHS reforms.

3 Examine the importance of future health policies in the context of medical and scientific advances.

▼ References

Allsop J. *Health policy and the National Health Service.* London: Longman; 1984.

Butler J. A case study in the NHS: working for patients. In: Taylor-Gooby P, Lawson R, eds. *Markets and managers. New issues in the delivery of welfare.* Buckingham: Open University Press; 1993.

DHSS (1979) *Patients First.* A consultative document, London: HMSO.

DHSS (1987) *Promoting better Health Care.* London: HMSO.

DHSS (1989) *Caring for People.* London: HMSO.

DHSS (1989) *Working for Patients.* London: HMSO.

Griffiths R. *NHS Management Enquiry Report.* London: HMSO; 1987

Ham C. *The new National Health Service organisation and management.* Oxford: Readcliffe; 1991.

Ham C. *Health policy in Britain. The politics and organisation of the NHS, 3rd ed.* Basingstoke: Macmillan; 1992.

Johnson N. *Reconstructing the Welfare State. A decade of change 1980–1990.* Hemel Hempstead: Harvester-Wheatsheaf: 1990.

Klein R. *The politics of the NHS, 2nd ed.* London: Longman Group; 1989.

Laing W. *Managing the NHS. Past, present and agenda for the future.* London: OHE; 1994.

Lart R, Means R. User empowerment and buying community care; reflections on the emerging debate about charging policies. In: Page R, Deakin N, eds. *The costs of welfare.* Aldershot: Avebury; 1993.

Lawson R. The new technology of management in the personal social services. In: Taylor-Gooby P, Lawson R, eds. *Markets and managers. New issues in the delivery of welfare.* Buckingham: Open University Press; 1993.

Leese B, Bosanquet N. Changes in general practice organisation: a survey of general practitioners' view on the 1990 contract and fundholding. *Br J Gen Pract* 1996, **46**:95–99.

Le Grand J. The State of Welfare In: Barr N, Evandrou M, *et al. The State of Welfare. The Welfare State in Britain since 1974.* Oxford University Press: New York; 1991;338–360.

McIver S. *An introduction to obtaining the views of users of health services.* London: Kings' Fund Centre; 1991.

Nocon A. *Collaboration in community care in the 1990s.* Sunderland: BEP; 1994.

Northway R. The health and social care divide: bridging the gap. *Nurs Stand* 1996, **10,21**:43–47.

Ong B. *The practice of health services research.* London: Chapman & Hall; 1993.

Paton C. *Competition and planning in the NHS. The danger of unplanned markets.* London: Chapman & Hall; 1992.

Perrin J. *Resource management in the NHS.* London: Chapman & Hall; 1988.

Spurgeon P, *Implementing change in the NHS.* A guide for general mangagers: London: Chapman & Hall; 1991.

Strong P, Robinson J. *The NHS under new management.* Buckingham: Open University Press; 1990.

Wright S. *'We thought we knew. . . Involving patients in nursing practice.* London: King's Fund Centre; 1995.

▼ Further Reading

Le Grand J, Winter D, Woolley F. The NHS: safe in whose hands? In: Barr N, Coulter F, Evandrou M. *The state of welfare, the Welfare State in Britain since 1974.* New York: Oxford University Press; 1991:88–134.

Patrick D, Erikson P. *Health status and health policy. Allocating resources to health care.* Oxford: Oxford University Press; 1993.

Peck E, Spurgeon P. *NHS trusts in practice.* Essex: Longman; 1993.

Robinson R, Le Grand J. *Evaluating the NHS reforms.* Berkshire: King's Fund Institute/ Policy Journals; 1993.

Taylor D. *Understanding the NHS* in the 1980s. London: OHE; 1984.

Index